Ocular examination

BASIS AND TECHNIQUE

Ocular examination

BASIS AND TECHNIQUE

Arthur H. Keeney, M.D., D.Sc.

Professor of Ophthalmology, University
of Louisville, School of Medicine,
Louisville, Kentucky

Second edition

WITH 200 ILLUSTRATIONS

The C. V. Mosby Company

Saint Louis   1976

Second edition

Copyright © 1976 by The C. V. Mosby Company

Previous edition copyrighted 1970

Printed in the United States of America

Distributed in Great Britain by Henry Kimpton, London

Library of Congress Cataloging in Publication Data

Keeney, Arthur Hail, 1920-
    Ocular examination: basis and technique.

    Bibliography: p.
    Includes index.
    1. Eye—Examination. I. Title. [DNLM: 1. Eye diseases—Diagnosis. 2. Ophthalmology—Instrumentation. WW141 K260]
RE75.K44 1976   617.7'1   76-7518
ISBN 0-8016-2632-3

GW/CB/B 9 8 7 6 5 4 3 2 1

Contributors

BEN P. HOUSER, Jr., M.D.

Wills Eye Hospital and Research Institute, Philadelphia, Pennsylvania

THEODORE LAWWILL, M.D.

Chief, Electrophysiology Laboratory, University of Louisville, School of Medicine, Louisville, Kentucky

PATRICK R. O'CONNOR, M.D.

Chief, Retina Service, University of Louisville, School of Medicine, Louisville, Kentucky

JOSEPH U. TOGLIA, M.D.

Associate Professor of Neurology and Otorhinology, Temple University School of Medicine, Philadelphia, Pennsylvania

WAYNE W. WONG, M.D.

Staff Ophthalmologist, Queen's Medical Center, Honolulu, Hawaii

Preface

The second edition of this book, like its predecessor, is addressed to two major levels of ophthalmic examination. The first level is the initial examination by the primary eye examiner—the front-line practitioner and his assistants or the resident physician in training who must master and learn to perform each technique efficiently. The second level is the subspecialty or consultation examination by an ophthalmologist who makes a "pet" of a particular disease group or whose work is limited entirely to one subject area.

In every case, the philosophy of approach is to achieve the optimal number of examining procedures in the minimum number of patient visits and with the least movement of the patient within the examining offices. Professional workers can move more rapidly and without issuance of instructions than can perplexed and uncertain patients. Chapter 1 is therefore devoted to the layout, organization, and equipment of the examining office.

The present rate of advance in optic, mechanical, electronic, and physiologic knowledge of the visual system renders necessary the updating of this volume. This 5-year cycle happily corresponds with William Osler's "quinquennial braindusting" for all scholar-practitioners, as well as workaday cycles of our American National Standards Institute, and its Z80 Ophthalmic Standards, which require revision at least every 5 years.

A significant number of diagnostic instruments have disappeared and others have been superseded since publication of the first edition. Fiber optics, though inefficient in light conduction, have removed heat from many critical areas and thus have earned their expensive incorporation into such instruments as indirect ophthalmoscopes, goniolenses, and contact transilluminators. The search for automation and objectivity has progressed, though not yet with complete satisfaction in perimeters, refractometers, and devices to measure visual acuity. Practical uses of evoked cortical responses for refraction, visual field studies, or the detection of malingerers are still a bit beyond the capability of usual office equipment. Ultrasound via the compact Bronson-Turner unit has gained acceptance in the office but is now challenged for morphologic detail and enormous range of gray scale by the Roentgen EMI scan—particularly in its current third generation refinements. Halogen and other high-intensity lights for ophthalmoscopes and slit lamps reveal defects earlier but may be painfully bright or raise questions of photic damage.

Current systems of medical and visual services have increased interest in the roles of ophthalmic aides, assistants, or technologists. Traditionally the American ophthalmologist has relied on four basic sources of help in his profession:

1. An intelligent and efficient Girl Friday, who most commonly is not a registered nurse but who meets a wide spectrum of needs in assisting patients.
2. An operating room scrub assistant, who now more commonly is a scrub technologist or occasionally is a practical nurse rather than the previous registered nurse.
3. The optician, as the skilled professional in spectacles, contact lenses, low-vision aids, and prosthetic designs; and, more recently, the ocul(arist, who has

evolved from this group as a unique artist-craftsman devoting all of his energies to design and fabrication of artificial eyes, orbital replacements, and special ocular prostheses. Since 1947 a significant number of these individuals have been certified by their own American Board of Opticianry at the primary level of Ophthalmic Optician, or the advanced level of Master of Ophthalmic Optics.

4. Least commonly, the orthoptist, who may be a former nurse or individual with college background who has pursued an academic year of instruction usually given in a department of ophthalmology at a school of medicine. This individual then gains required clinical experience during a 1-year traineeship in an orthoptic department. The training programs and the candidates are examined on a national basis by the American Orthoptic Council.

Since a difficult birth in 1970, the Joint Commission on Allied Health Personnel in Ophthalmology has been struggling to reach some homeostasis through endocrine changes of prepuberty. Over an initial 5 years, however, several hundred skilled ophthalmic assistants and a few hundred ophthalmic technicians are now certified by JCAHPO on the basis of national written and practical examinations. These data gatherers, similar to x-ray and laboratory technicians, valuably assist in visual care.

Examinations covered in this book represent practical working techniques. The book does not purport to be encyclopedic in listing every eponymic variation of instrument or technique, nor historically replete in prototypes. My personal preferences and biases —for example, my own Near Vision Test Card—reflect more than 25 years of active practice and are by design part of this volume. Hopefully these are leavened, here and there, in sections authored by associates who have plowed their single furrows to exquisite excellence.

The eye is a unique and matchless organ of inquiry. In its naked and unaided outward range, it is able to resolve the craters of the recently perambulated moon and the minimal separable intervals between stars that are millions of light years away. To the unaided examiner inquiring inwardly, ocular motility, pupillary action, even the color and composition of the ocular coast display the story of half the cranial nerves, index the occurrence of jaundice, anemia, or polycythemia, and differentiate many variations in disturbances of the pituitary and thyroid systems. Relatively simple optic tools of the past century enormously multiply the fruits of these inquiries. More sophisticated instruments of the moment uncover many more subtleties and commensurately extend the examiner's responsibilities for early detection of disorder and avoidance of visual catastrophe.

This book is primarily centered upon instrumental techniques that increase the examiner's clinical penetration of the visual system. In most sections, some outline of normalcy and normal variation in structure and function is included as a baseline from which pathologic deviations are measured. To the reader with some familiarity in this area, terseness of presentation is offered to make the value of orderly review more palatable.

Retinoscopy and refraction, though inherent components of ocular examination, are treated extensively in other separate publications and are therefore not detailed here. The same is true of bacteriology, virology, and radiology, which must frequently be brought into full-scale study of the visual system. The initial steps and the detailed extensions that the examiner must accomplish in his clinical setting are the core of this volume.

Continually I am indebted to trustees, senior university officers, and, increasingly of late, the taxpayers who directly and indirectly nurture our educational institutions. From gestation of the first edition I continue my appreciation of the Board of Directors and the professional family of the Wills Eye Hospital and Research Institute of Philadelphia. Particularly I acknowledge the labors of Mr. Donald C. Rubel, President of the Board, and Mr. William P. Cairo, Vice President, who directly facilitated the productivity of those years, with no tangible compensation other than personal satisfaction. Very visible appreciation accrues to Mrs. Anthony Kidawa, Mrs. Patricia Upham, and Mrs. Richard Haberkost, who appear most frequently in these pages as model patients photographed during examination.

My closest companion both in creativity and confinement through these volumes has, of course, been Dr. Virginia Keeney, whose decades of alternations between wife, mother, and civic worker on one hand and physician, counselor, and critic on the other have been of enormous value.

Initial assistance of staff members of the Wills Eye Hospital from Dr. Lov K. Sarin of the Retina Service, Mr. Terrance L. Tomer, Retinal Photographer, Dr. Joseph U. Toglia, Neurootologist, Dr. Arnold B. Popkin of the Electrophysiology Service, and Dr. Ben P. Houser, Jr., former Chief Resident at Wills, have been extended by Dr. Wayne W. Wong of Honolulu and new colleagues at the University of Louisville. I particularly thank Dr. Patrick R. O'Connor, Chief of the Retina Service, and Dr. Theodore Lawwill, Chief of the Electrophysiology laboratory in the Department of Ophthalmology at the University of Louisville, School of Medicine. For three decades, those closest to me and most responsible for stimulating the quest for better understanding have been thousands of wonderful patients and dozens of catalytic residents. To both I am perpetually indebted. Also, individual manufacturers and distributors of equipment have been generous and cooperative in supplying materials on request. Their technical and engineering contributions to ocular diagnosis are essential.

In the final responsibilities and labors of preparing the manuscript I am deeply indebted to my Office Administrator, Mrs. Nancy Westmoreland, and to the secretarial staff, particularly represented by Mrs. Ann Worley. I appreciate their patience and good spirits through countless revisions, changes, and deadlines. Hopefully the elaborations and increased details of this edition will prove useful to the tyro and also to the alert and seasoned clinician whose usually inundated life calls for a tight synthesis of good and efficient practice. In such hope we may garner in the years ahead more effective knowledge for that date rather than be confined to old saws of previous years.

Arthur H. Keeney

Contents

Ocular examination

BASIS AND TECHNIQUE

Basic principles

Basic preparation for the examination

THE EXAMINER

"A misleading symptom is misleading only to one able to be misled."

SIR HENEAGE OGILVIE

The most important basic preparation to examination is thorough understanding of normal variations and disease processes. Well-organized knowledge, analytic curiosity, probing skills, consideration, and ingenuity can circumvent a lack of equipment and devices. Instruments are merely extensions of the neurosensory capability of the examiner and, like the finest electron microscope, are worthless without the interpretations of a perceptive eye and intelligent brain. The optimal formal education of the examiner is not an end in itself but merely a base line of provisional data on which must be built a lifetime of further refinement, increasing knowledge, and seasoned judgment. No instrument or group of instruments can exceed the inherent abilities of the examiner. *

SPACE FOR THE EXAMINING AREA
General examining room

Ophthalmic examining space should be inviting and gracious to help make the patient feel at ease. Tiny rooms cluttered with equipment and optic mirrors are dehumanizing and mechanical; narrow pie-shaped

*More personal guidelines for dress, deportment, responsibility, and general activity of the examiner can be obtained from the instruction of Lord Chamberlain Polonius to his son, Laertes, in Shakespeare's *Hamlet* Act I, Scene iii.

rooms compressing to projection chart widths at the far end are oppressive.

The examining room should ideally be 24 ft. long. This distance may be measured diagonally within shorter walls or lengthwise in a room no narrower than 9 ft. This allows the examiner to move behind the examining chair or to lower the chair back for recumbent procedures. The available "lane length" of 20 ft. from the patient's eye to the projection screen is minimal for standardization of acuity notations, motility notations, and the practical simulation of ocular resolving power at infinity. This distance is distinctly inadequate for eliciting divergence excess types of intermittent exotropia, and therefore the space must include a window where binocularity under remote fixation (preferably a block or more away and under bright illumination) can be assessed.

Equipment in the examining room must necessarily be extensive to achieve maximum efficiency of one-stop service, in terms of both minimum number of visits to the office and movement within the office. For optic reasons, equipment surfaces should be dull or matte and of black, dark gray, or subdued dark tones. This reduces annoying light reflections and distractions to both patient and examiner. Nothing could be more optically illogical and bedazzling than to attempt intraocular examinations near a large picture window with polished, gay coral instruments, as shown in some manufacturer's catalogs. Also, for patient reassurance and relaxation, cold chrome and hospital pastels should be avoided.

Small instruments, knives, scissors, and

Fig. 1-1. Solid front cabinetry removes knives and offensive instruments from immediate view. A, Jenkel-Davidson cabinet. (Jenkel-Davidson House of Vision, San Francisco, California 94119); B, Da-Laur combination cabinetry. (Needham Heights, Massachusetts 02194.)

syringes should be stored in solid-door cabinets. Neither children nor adults are made happy by the display of punctum dilators or chalazion curettes in military columns (Fig. 1-1). These should be appropriately grouped, wrapped, labeled, sterilized, and then stored in the cabinets.

The use of woods such as walnut, mahogany, ash, or chestnut with upholstering colors such as tan, deep red, gray, umber, or muted greens minimizes the sometimes painful suggestion of shots and sutures. Also, this affords an attractive method of designating examining rooms by woods or colors. (Though an esthete might make faint pause over being sent to the gray or the blue room, no one really wants to be consigned numerically to room two or geographically to the back room; however, almost everyone is satisfied to be escorted to the walnut room.)

Illumination in the examining room should be predominantly artificial, usually subdued, and under intensity control. It is essential, however, that the room be rendered quite dark for procedures such as indirect ophthalmoscopy; therefore, venetian blinds should be of the interlocking and light-proof type, supplemented by full-length lined drapes at each side of the window to eliminate light-streaking at the edges. Subdued light from an indirect source behind a cornice is less desirable than that from a table lamp with an opaque shade, because the latter is generally warmer and allows the patient or relative to read by its localized intensity while awaiting the examiner's entrance or for drops to take effect.

Access for the examiner and the patient is preferably by different doors. The patient should be able to enter and leave from a corridor or alcove off the reception area. This should be arranged so that others in the reception area do not look directly into the examining room when the door is opened. The examiner, on the other hand, should enter and leave by a back corridor or small interchange room where he can receive information about the next patient, calls, or other messages. Some doctors like to keep a dictating system in such inbetween rooms so that notes may be promptly dictated after the patient is seen.

Seating in the examining room must not only provide full access to the patient in either the sitting or recumbent position but should also provide mobility space for the examiner, who generally uses a stool with large casters (small casters catch in rugs) with a back. (The back on the stool becomes increasingly comforting in latter hours of the day and with advancing years of practice.) There should also be pleasant adjacent seating for at least *three* relatives or attendants within each examining room. Here a medium-sized or three-cushion davenport is particularly appropriate because (1) a single patient or family unit is being served and (2) it affords a place for fainting or ill individuals to recline. The common pattern of several members of the family accompanying a youngster or an elderly patient often provides a quick index of hereditary problems in the family and saves repetition of explanation to different generations. Don't be trapped by letting a mate or grown sibling remain out in the reception area when a lengthy explanation must be given. The eye is conspicuously involved or is an index organ in a high percentage of heritable diseases. Adjacent seating for several family members may greatly expedite genetic diagnosis and increase the effectiveness of genetic counseling.

A small washbasin, such as a stainless steel "trailer sink," should be in every examining room so that the doctor may wash his hands in the presence of the patient. Its base can be attractively boxed to the floor, obscuring unsightly plumbing and giving storage space for paper towels, tissues, and so on.* A mirror should also be in every examining room so that ladies may adjust their hair or hats after the doctor leaves.

Special examining room

Each patient care room in an office or clinic should be fitted for the accomplish-

*Benson Optical Co., Minneapolis, Minnesota 55440; Da-Laur, Inc., Needham Heights, Massachusetts 02194.

ment of as many procedures as possible. This also applies to minor surgical undertakings and to those procedures that can well be delegated to a technologist. Thus neither patient nor staff time is lost in moving people from room to room. Exceptions are needed, however, such as in the employment of large or complex equipment (dark adaptometers, Tübinger perimeters, and ultrasound) or of instruments that must be electrically shielded (for electroretinography or electroencephalography); where technologists will spend relatively long periods with patients (orthoptic studies, electronic tonometry, fluorescein angiography, electrooculography, and contact lens fitting), or where patients may merely remain in the office for protracted periods (mydriatic instillations, water provocative tests, and subcutaneous Prostigmin tests).

It is not efficient planning to set aside a separate room for special study of strabismus, retinal detachment, or glaucoma. Even the special consultant in these fields should accomplish his investigations in a flexible and multiple-purpose room. He may consign some procedures, however, to other office areas where the technologist and patient are removed from distractions and disturbances. In large clinics with multiple examiners, it is generally advantageous to equip groups of separate rooms in which associated technologists do their work. This applies most immediately to contact lens fitting, tonography, fluorescein angiography, orthoptics, and electrophysiology.

NONEXAMINING SPACES IN THE SUITE
Reception area

Appurtenances and decor in the reception area should be inviting and domestic or club-like rather than sterile and professional. Reception room furniture should be covered with a good, fabric-backed, flexible plastic such as Naugahyde because it (1) harbors less dust and allergens than wool, (2) adds softness that wooden or molded furniture cannot give, (3) is less expensive than leather or wool upholstery, (4) will

last longer, and (5) cleans easily with only soap and water. Chrome-like furniture should not be used because of its cold and commercial feeling. Cane, though more artistic, is impractical because of frequent breaks and chronic need for recaning.

Seating is most commonly needed for singles or doubles, and the two-cushion settee or loveseat will reassuringly accommodate two adults plus an apprehensive child patient. There is little invitation to the larger davenport, particularly the three-seater, when strangers occupying each end block all access to side tables and the last man in is faced with elbow-rubbing center isolation.

A children's table, round (to reduce corner injuries and proprietary sides) and of solid hard wood, with four to six solid children's chairs should be placed in one corner of the reception area, perhaps semipartitioned off by a sturdy wrought-iron trellis or half-height book shelves. Several good youth magazines will earn you gratitude from the children and also younger mothers who want to get with it and sit on the children's chairs. (More mature parents or grandparents will appreciate a few adult-size chairs overlooking the children's unit.)

The number of reception spaces should be in a ratio of approximately seven to each examining chair. Thus the minimum should be about seven; with two examiners using four units, there should be nearly twenty-eight reception spaces, including the children's unit. Three to ten of the total should be in a separate "mydriatic room" if possible. This reduces any shock of a jammed waiting room for entering patients and gains semiprivacy for the occasional scene of a child resisting drops. In this mydriatic room where many patients are precluded from reading, a truly high-fidelity sound system may be an appreciated comfort and divertissement to the captives.

The reception desk should be in direct view from the patient's entrance door and afford surveillance of the entire reception area. It needs a slightly elevated, protective front "barrier" to keep small hands or the idly curious adult from delving into work materials. If the receptionist must also answer the telephone, as is often done, she should have a "hush booth" or recessed alcove so that every incoming call is not a matter for public display or reception room entertainment. The receptionist's telephone should be impossible to reach from the waiting area, to avoid preemption by patients.

The reception area is the nerve center of a busy office; here a gracious nonprofessional must make semiprofessional decisions regarding the urgency of calls that would interrupt work in progress, problems that must be meshed into crowded schedules, and complaints that can safely be postponed for decision. She must be schooled in the separation of *true emergencies* (chemical burns, acute glaucoma, lacerated eyes, vascular occlusions), *urgencies*, both medical and social (retinal detachments, uveitis, lacrimal infections, departures for Africa, out-of-state grandmothers of patient families who will only be in town for 10 days but who have chronic glaucoma plus cataracts), and *elective problems* (periodic change in spectacles, blepharochalasis, cataract rechecks, involution of the macula, old ptosis).

The appointment book should be large and open and lie completely flat on the secretary's desk. It should show at least a whole day on one page or at most the entire week on the total open pages in direct view. Time intervals are preferably printed in units of 15 minutes. Minimal information listed should be the patient's full name, the nature of the visit (new examination, follow-up visit, glasses recheck, postoperative sutures), and the telephone number where the patient could be reached in case it is necessary to cancel or to reschedule appointments. Entries should always be made with a pencil, which is preferably tied or chained to the book. Though the receptionist should not be trapped with a small or crowded appointment book page, she should keep for the doctor's reference a vest-pocket counterpart of this book indicating surgical schedules, hospital admissions, luncheon commitments, and out-of-town schedules. She should steal this from his pocket at least twice a week to be sure it is up-to-date.

Though good commercial reception and appointment books may be purchased from many suppliers, after a few years in practice it will be preferable for the physician to design, with his receptionists, an appointment book geared to his particular demands.

Lighting in the reception area should be slightly subdued because many patients may have irritable eyes or dilated pupils. This also affords a gentle transition into the further subdued light of the examining room. Windows with glass curtains or partially turned (not light-tight) venetian blinds preserve some relief from claustrophobia and yet reduce brightness. A few table lamps with opaque shades facilitate reading for those who want to browse through the fresh and unusual magazines.

Piped-in music of low fidelity is often resented by intelligent persons rendered captive to another individual's preselection. Such obligate aural salads are less appropriate to the professional office than to the commercial world, and the expense might more productively be directed to interesting and current literature.

All hats, overcoats, and extra garments that the patient may wish to remove should be handled *before* the patient is seated in the examining chair and *before* the physician enters the room. The most practical place is an alcove with hat shelves between the reception room and the corridor entrance to the examining area. Coats and raingear should never be permitted to take up reception seats for both esthetic and economic reasons. Women must always be reminded to keep their purses with them, and patients insisting on taking outer gear back into the examining areas should be accommodated rather than debated. There should be a closet for the doctor and the staff away from the reception area.

Bookkeeping

Though an accounting firm, office management service, or, in recent years, some banks should ultimately, properly, and with conservation of the doctor's time supervise all fiscal procedures, it is essential to have some bookkeeping resource immediately available. Here routine charges can be posted and explained, cash payments can be received and receipted, status of accounts can be updated and revised, minor problems can be answered and corrected. This area should be available along the path of the departing patient, but not in the open reception area where frank and clear discussion of finances, essential to the well-being of most patients, might be embarrassing. Courtesy here is essential, and, in the event of questioning, the accounting aide should immediately express the possibility of an office error that she will be pleased to check. Though a small chair may be moved from nearby, no chairs should be placed at this desk, as they encourage lingering and unneeded conversation both by the staff and patients.

Lavatories

Facilities for patients should be available within the building, preferably on the same floor, but *not* within the suite. An office lavatory is essential to conserve the time of the office staff, for the occasionally ill patient with nausea and vomiting of angle-closure glaucoma, or following Prostigmin testing. The lavatory should be small, contain an adequate wall mirror, and preferably be painted throughout in a uniform and unattractive shade of red or purple. This has remarkable value in discouraging staff members from lingering.

Typing and correspondence

The doctor should never economize on professional height and properly designed desks and seating for secretarial help. Whether time-efficiency is best served by dictating notes after seeing a patient or by writing notes with many abbreviations during the examination, there will continue to be increasing numbers of forms, letters, and patient reports to prepare. Every referring practitioner, resident, intern, or other professional colleague deserves a brief (pref-

erably one page, single-spaced) understandable report of the findings, recommendations, and reasons therefore. A few excellent secretaries can be taught to formulate such letters from examination notes—this has danger, however, of uncomplimentary routinism being detected by those who refer patients repeatedly. In most cases these letters should be dictated personally, and thus a progressive load of typing evolves. Efficiency is best served not by direct dictation to a secretary but by the use of identical dictating equipment on the examiner's desk, between examining rooms, in his car, and at home. Both written materials and instructions thus accumulated on a catch-as-catch-can basis wherever the doctor is, reach the typist without interrupting either person.

The typing space should be isolated from phone calls but accessible by intercom. Often the best location for this space is off the corridor between examining rooms or adjacent to the mydriatic room. The typist may double to attend the mydriatic room and relieve others in the office. It is valuable to have some flexible person such as this to fill in when other members of the staff are absent.

Intercommunications

Each inner room—excluding the lavatory and mydriatic room—should be equipped with a station of a separate intercom system. Squawk boxes and loud-speaker systems, no matter how subdued, are not appropriate to the private and confidential nature of activities in the office. The instrument should be of one-piece or French phone design to be completely controlled with one hand or caught easily between the ear and shoulder.

The use of telephone circuitry for intercom purposes seems simple and frugal. Actually, it is complicated and perpetually expensive. Whenever telephone circuits are used for intercommunications, this precludes use of the telephones for their outside purposes and prevents office staff members from delivering confidential spoken messages simultaneously while the doctor is talking on an outside line. With separate intercom instruments, it is possible to hold one to each ear in order to receive comments or information from the aide while handling a problem via the telephone. Of course, with either separate intercoms or intercom circuits on the telephone, it is possible to get the often-needed assistance of the appointment secretary or office aide on the same line with a major call. Remember also, the monthly charge for each button and each light goes on forever, whereas I have had the satisfaction of using substantial office intercom phones without a penny of maintenance for more than a decade.

The telephone extension in each office where patients are received should be without a dial. The doctor's own calls will be dialed by his secretary, and the available

dial in a room where a patient is waiting his arrival is often an inducement to initiate a nonoffice call that ties up the office line and often has to be terminated with loss of the examiner's time on entering the room or with some embarrassment on the part of the patient.

Both the telephone and the separate intercommunication phone should be located where they can be reached from the examining chair without rising or moving.

BASIC EXAMINING EQUIPMENT

Certain basic examining equipment needs to be present in any examining room for either initial ophthalmic examination or subspecialty and consultation examination. Selecting, modifying, or designing equipment is part of the fun and a manifestation

Fig. 1-2. Example of custom-fitted, hard plastic case containing basic portable diagnostic instruments, transformer, and small assortment of drugs. At left from bottom upward are: retinoscope, ophthalmodynamometer, transilluminator, direct ophthalmoscope, +30-diopter lens, and three-mirror contact lens. At right are power handle for retinoscope, sphygmomanometer, percussion hammer, binocular indirect ophthalmoscope, and loupe. (Designed by John H. Weaver, M.D.)

of the individual's penetration. As early as possible in training years, the young practitioner should initiate appraisal of portable instruments and begin their purchase. He thus becomes familiar with performance and design limitations of major hand equipment. He works more readily and easily with his own instruments and learns their care and repair. These common items essential for every resident include (1) a giant (hand) ophthalmoscope, (2) an indirect binocular ophthalmoscope, (3) a multiple-mirrored contact lens for examining the angle and fundus, (4) a Schiøtz tonometer, (5) a surgical loupe, (6) a good retinoscope, (7) a simple exophthalmometer, and (8), as the British say, a splendid inspection torch. Before completion of training he should add (1) his first, simple external camera, (2) an ophthalmodynamometer, (3) an electric keratoscope or Placido's disc, (4) a hand rotary prism or prism bars, and (5) a MIRA fiber optics transilluminator.* He should also be using and evaluating major examining units such as slit lamps, refractors, and lensometers from various manufacturers so that well-reasoned orders can be placed several months before intended use. Thus the basic hand tools to equip the first of minimally two or ultimately three or more complete examining units in an office are familiar acquisitions or the components of a portable case (Fig. 1-2) early in professional life.

The initial as well as each subsequently fitted examining room should have not only as full equipment as possible for "one-stop service" but should also have compact grouping of the maximum amount of equipment to minimize movement by the examiner and to avoid movement by the patient. This generally necessitates stand-mounted (Figs. 1-3 and 1-4) (hydraulic or electric) instruments, with the second choice being wall-mounted (spring-counterbalanced) instruments. Wall-mounted projectors and cabinetry are desirable to conserve valuable floor space and to reduce floor clutter; however,

*This supersedes the painfully warm Lancaster incandescent bulb transilluminator.

Fig. 1-3. Reliance spring-mounted refractor and slit lamp floor stand, which must be bolted to floor. (Model No. 7700-IC, Reliance Koenigkramer Co., Cincinnati, Ohio 45216.)

wall-mounted refractors and slit lamps tie the examining chair and the patient so close to the wall that the chair rotation (90 degrees) for 1-meter tangent screen examination is not practical. Similarly, these restrict the desirable arc of access when the chair back is dropped to place the patient horizontal for indirect ophthalmoscopy.

A sturdy compromise is the Benson Refraction Pole, which conserves space and money by eliminating the bulky base of conventional instrument stands. This will

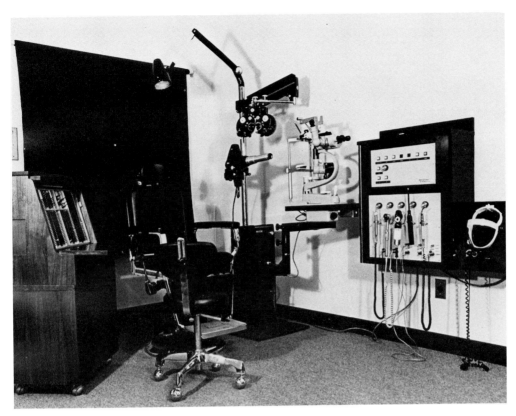

Fig. 1-4. Major examining equipment grouped close to patient and within arm's reach of the seated examiner. Large casters on doctor's stool aid quick positioning. Stein-Keeler Auto Switch unit is shown mounted on wall at right. (Wills Eye Hospital, Philadelphia, Pennsylvania 19130.)

easily accommodate three counter-balanced arms for refractor, slit lamp, and other instruments. Its secure anchorage to ceiling and floor reduces the mechanical problems of oscillation or vibration at the free, upper end of a floor-based stand.

The automation conscious examiner will like a built-in Stein Autoswitch unit, which, in production form, carries receptacles for six hand examining units. Each holder is so wired that simply lifting the instrument will (1) turn it on, (2) darken the room to an appropriately preselected level, (3) turn on a suitably located fixation light with distinctive color, and (4) actuate a reminder light on the control panel indicating that both the instrument and the fixation light are on. All of these actions are reversed instantly when the instrument is returned to its hanger. The row of buttons at the top are wired for actions such as turning on a flashing fixation light for children or lighting the slit lamp and at the same time appropriately dimming the room (Fig. 1-5).*

The examining chair should be relatively narrow, with only short, elbowrest type armpieces. This allows the doctor to roll quite near, as is necessary for direct ophthalmoscopy, lacrimal irrigations, and similar close control maneuvers. Since the chair is narrow, the elbowrests or any sidepieces must be hinged to turn away from the occasional broad beam of alimentary overindulgence. The chair should be comfortably padded and without an extending footrest, or at most with an inconspicuous folded

*Manufactured by Diversatronics, Inc., Wynnewood, Pennsylvania 19096 and distributed by Keeler Optical Products, Broomall, Pennsylvania 19008.

Fig. 1-5. Guyton-Carlson electrically controlled diagnostic unit with 33-cm. arc perimeter swung upward from patient. (Carlson Manufacturing Co., Royal Oaks, Michigan 48067.)

rest to be turned out only when obligatory. Furniture projections such as footrests may easily trip the unwary patient, just as comfortably long armrests traumatize the examiner's abdomen. A headrest, usually adjustable, is indispensable for indentation tonometry, orbital tonometry, esthesiometry, and even the occasional psychologic retreater apprehensive about fingers or instruments approaching his eyes. Both the chair and the space must allow full reclining range of the back. The chair's height also

must be adjustable, preferably by a foot-pump hydraulic system rather than electrically. This is not only healthy for the sedentary examiner but also reduces service costs and interruptions as well as capital outlay.

Except for the built-in electro-mechanical elevations system (20 to 29 in.), the American Optical Corporation's Compact Chair generally meets these requirements and offers a full 360° rotation, whereas the more expensive Custom Motorized Chair will rotate

Fig. 1-6. Reliance Koenigkramer Chair, No. 665, combines comfort with dimensions small enough to permit close access of examiner. Further conservation of floor space is achieved by mounting chair on floor stand (Reliance Combo 2000; 45″ base size) and eliminating a separate base for the chair. (FF Koenigkramer, Cincinnati, Ohio 45216.)

Fig. 1-7. Compact examining chair (SMR Maxi Chair introduced in 1969; currently modified model is G-II) may be adjusted from lowest seat position 18 in. above floor to a maximum elevation of 38 in. Chair is fully reclining to the semi-Fowler position. Footrest is retracted in low position as illustrated but extends outward when chair is elevated or reclined. Loose upholstery cushioning slides over structural elements of the chair during adjustment to avoid disturbing patient's clothing. Chair rotates 360 degrees. Headrest is adjusted forward and backward. (Surgical, Mechanical, Research Inc., Newport Beach, California 92663.)

only 210°. The Compact Chair is well counter-balanced, and distractingly reflective bright enamels and fabrics can be avoided with effort. Similar substantial chairs are also available as Koenigkramer Reliance 665 (Fig. 1-6). The Bausch and Lomb Libra Chair is more suitably accessible than its telebrachial and overweight relative, Orion.

Closely grouped to the examining chair are the obligate, heavy items: refractor, trial case, lensometer, slit lamp, and tangent screen. In spite of the obvious efficiency and facility of modern refractors, the trial case—and less often the trial frame—continues to be indispensable for retinoscopy of small children, handling the patient with spinal deformity, and refining high dioptric corrections (such as in the aphakic patient) over his spectacles. The trial case should not be a compromise economy kit but should provide a full range of lenses with compensated base curves, to simulate as closely as possible what the patient will finally wear.

Small items for the examining desk such as punctum dilators, lacrimal cannulas, sterile fluorescein paper strips, individually packaged sterile cotton-tipped applicators, a nasal speculum, and opaque and red clip-on lenses are built up in keeping with the examiner's preference and practice. Similarly, a selection of minor surgical instruments for chalazia, suture removal, and

biopsy must be accumulated in accordance with individual needs.

The age of a practitioner's patient population tends to increase with his own years in practice. Thus in early years, strabismic children of young parents are seen frequently, and later one sees more problems of senile cataracts, glaucoma, and involutional retinal problems. Concomitantly the myopic problems of school children give way to needs for high dioptric magnifying adds and low vision aids. In these advancing years, presbycusis often follows presbyopia and many patients present with spectacle-mounted hearing aids. When these are removed for eye examination, a substitution aid is handy to have. A small stethoscope-type unit (Loud and Clear) is distributed by Titmus Optical Company.* Its insertion in the patient's ear does not interfere with the eye examination, avoids shouting matches, and restores comforting contact.

A small kit of emergency drugs stored with a tourniquet and alcohol sponges may some day be lifesaving. The kit should include atropine, morphine, epinephrine, Na Amytal, and nitroglycerin. Similarly, an emergency portable oxygen tank fitted with a disposable face mask and nonrebreathing valves should be available in the office.

*Petersburg, Virginia 23807.

Indications for diagnostic examination steps

THE PATIENT'S HISTORY

Proper examination requires the systematic application of successive diagnostic maneuvers or steps. From the hundreds of possible and variously productive tests that can be catalogued, it is essential to select efficiently the germane and needed procedures. Two things enable the clinician to do this appropriately and with significant security. The first is the patient's *history*, properly evoked and verified, if necessary, internally, by cross questions to elicit corroborating details, or externally, by obtaining old records, hospital summaries, or slides of previous tissue specimens. (Copies of pathology reports should be received with suspicion as secondary evidence because they (1) may come from nonrepresentative sections of a lesion, (2) are subject to differences in interpretation by various pathologists, (3) sometimes are precast by interpretations no longer consonant with better understanding of the process, and (4) may be plagued by even more clerical errors than appear between lensometer readings from a pair of spectacles and a crumpled old copy of a prescription that the patient carries.) The second is that sense of correlation known as *clinical judgment*, which grows in proportion to a practitioner's years of self-critical diagnostics, periodically refined by review of his data and accomplishments.

"A clinician is complex. He is part craftsman, part practical scientist, and part historian."

THOMAS ADDIS (1881-1949)

Obtaining the history

Chief complaints are the first subjective leads obtained in the diagnostic examination. The clinician should note several items of objective information as he crosses the examining room to the patient—or, with less conservation of his time, as the patient comes to the examining position. For example, searching movements of the patient's eye and head in scrutinizing the doctor immediately suggest impairment of central vision, whereas failure of the patient to recognize the examiner's out-streched hand in greeting is a tip-off to major field loss. Both for mental analysis and for commitment to record, complaints should be reduced to succinct and compressed expressions, refined in specific details such as severity, intermittency, or character and dated as to onset. Thus no patient may state his complaints as "painless progressive impairment of vision for 4 years, more marked o.d. than o.s." but this capsules the salient features for differential diagnosis of senile nuclear cataracts; "intermittent painful blurring of vision o.d. with redness and watery discharge for 4 years" aims the studies toward recurrent uveitis.

To weigh both accuracy and significance, it is often best if the patient—whether young child or aged grandparent—describes his own symptoms rather than having them interpreted and edited by a hopefully helpful adult. Similarly, undue influence on the independence of the diagnosis is often avoided by tactfully turning the patient's narrative away from recounts of previous professional advice. Where the name of an earlier examiner is volunteered, it may expedite obtaining desired details later and should therefore be quietly recorded. If the name is not volunteered, do not probe, because the patient may consider this a violation of confidence or prejudicial to the examiner's own thinking. Innocuously noting where previous care was rendered may serve fully to obtain old records with less suggestion of prying.

History of the present illness should add specific details in relation to each chief complaint. If the chief complaint is "dull, bioccipital, and bifrontal headaches intermittently for 2 years," the further details should specify the severity in some degree, the presence or absence of aura, the duration of episodes and periods of relief, any association with use of the eyes either for near or far, complications such as nausea and vomiting, and concomitants such as nasal stuffiness or allergy. Lack of clear characterization of the complaint or lack of interference with usual activities is important in indicating less significance or a more functional than organic base.

Previous operations, surgical complications, and specific drugs with dosage and frequency should be noted in sufficient detail and date to evaluate past efficiency and to relate to future therapy.

Past history should outline any other or unrelated eye injuries or disturbances. The age and circumstances of wearing glasses should be recorded. Recently worn and unwearable spectacles should be verified on the lensometer with particular attention to prismatic elements (prescribed or inadvertent). They should also be checked on the face, particularly for fit on the bridge, centration of the visual axis with the optic center, and characteristics of any segments.

Medical history should particularly annotate systemic disease relating to vision, such as diabetes, thyroid disturbances, tumors, or vascular alterations. Medications being taken and any drug idiosyncrasy should always be noted. A special area on the record cover or card, such as vertically on the right hand edge, should bear notation in bold letters of drug allergy or sensitivity.

Family history should stress heritable ocular diseases (such as macular disturbances, color blindness, congenital defects, retinal detachments, cataract, or strabismus) and familial systemic diseases (such as diabetes,

hypertension, and the like). Where serious visual defects are incompletely understood in remotely located siblings or cousins, it is helpful family counseling as well as assistance in diagnosis to request follow-through correspondence.

METHODOLOGY OF HISTORY INTERVIEW

Most productive clinicians prefer to have an intelligent and courteous aide record not only identifying vital statistics (never asking a lady's age in earshot of a public area) or fixed-field information, but also the previously discussed details of complaints, present illness, and past, medical, and family histories. The aide may check any medications with the patient and phone R_{χ} numbers to druggists for verification of unlabeled prescriptions. Any alert high school student can be trained to neutralize spectacles or, if they should be lost or broken, to phone for recent prescriptions. She may also check visual acuity with and without glasses if so trained and instructed.

By virtue of intimate knowledge of disease, the skilled examiner can elicit most pertinent details of disease quite directly. He may prefer to invest additional time this way rather than to delegate the preliminary chores. Even with delegation, he must verify and amplify some details of the history as developed.

Short and complex ophthalmic record forms requiring more than seven pages may be found in other eye texts or obtained from commercial record companies. Printers and business form manufacturers are eager to sell forms printed to individual preference. In many cases, allocated record spaces will be insufficient for complex aspects or unneeded by the astute clinician. For initial and less complicated ophthalmic examination, plain white record forms, preferably 5 × 8 in. or 8½ × 11 in. (standard correspondence paper size), give the best flexibility of space and conservation of storage needs. Specific components of the examination may be conspicuously identified, where indicated, by a series of rubber stamps (refraction, fundus outline, lid sketch, muscle diagram, and so on) available commercially or on individual design (Fig. 2-1). Preprinted record forms, preferably in identifying colors, are desirable for the more structured subspecialty or consultation examinations such as strabismus, retinal detachment, glaucoma, uveitis, corneal disease, and plastic work. Records lightly shaded in various colors are also expeditious in identifying different members in a group practice.

The technique of having an accompanying secretary make shorthand notes from observations during the examination is recommended for cold efficiency. The secretary and her note pad conspicuously disrupt the confidentiality of patient relations though safeguarding the male examiner who is otherwise often alone with patients. Where anterooms or alcoves are available just outside of examination areas, it is preferable that the doctor use a dictating unit there between patients. A few hand-recorded notes, dates, and numbers such as tension, refraction, or exophthalmometry tend to ensure better accuracy of the ultimate record.

A valuable safeguard against confusion of right and left is the well-established convention of examining and recording details of the *right* eye first. Even if this eye is gone, the first notation should be a description of the socket or postsurgical site.

Study should be given by the individual starting practice to the use of computer-compatible information forms. Several types have had considerable trial, as the old Hollerith IBM cards, which can accommodate up to 250 bits of information per card and which have been used by the Lovelace Foundation* with twelve separate cards for history, external examination, fundus, glaucoma, refraction, and so forth. Other mark-sense devices may represent even more voluminous check lists. Large information

*Albuquerque, New Mexico 87108.

Fig. 2-1. Examples of rubber stamp devices useful on plain record forms for refraction and posterior pole fundus findings. Other types are available commercially and on individual design.

scoring sheets inevitably present a forbidding specter of boxes to be checked, but they can be completed in a few minutes by one who has gained familiarity with the alternatives, and they commit diagnostic efforts and data to the ultimate potential of machine reading efficiency. Color coding of individual forms again aids identification in preparation and in manual handling of small numbers of forms. System developments are available to reduce or to eliminate the time-consuming and expensive handling of laborious checklists and key punch recording of data (fixed field length methods). Special typewriters (costing $2,000 to $3,000) based on standard keyboards have been available for several years to type out hard copy on usual paper for routine use and at the same time prepare punch paper tape in machine language. This variable field length technique imposes essentially no restrictions on the amount or type of verbal or numerical data that may be included. The paper tape, after necessary editing or correcting from the hard copy, is then used to place the information on magnetic tape for computer storage, analysis, and retrieval. Several thousand reports or about 4,000 pages of narrative can be placed on a single reel of magnetic tape ($35) and retained indefinitely.

Increasing requests for detailed reports by insurance companies, intermediary agencies, pre-employment programs, driver licensing authorities, workman's compensation, the Social Security Administration, and the courts seek a pseudo-uniformity in all diagnostic and treatment services. In truth, physiologic and pathologic processes in patients are nonuniform, and at best, Gaussian. Similarly, neurosensory attributes and interpretive processes of examiners differ significantly. This leads to variations, both in type and sequence, of procedures followed in patient care. Nonetheless, doctors who are today athwart the increasing demands for systematic reports must use some standardization and coding in procedural terminology. Current Procedural Terminology published now in its third (1973) edition by the American Medical Association Committee on Computer Systems in Medicine and the Division of Medical Practice is a fundamental document for such coding. The 109 page Terminology for Reporting Indexing, Retrieval of Services and Procedures in Ophthalmology, published by the American Academy of Ophthalmology and Otolaryngology* in 1975, is the most detailed guidebook for diagnostic and surgical procedures in the ophthalmic field. Though this is not a nomenclature of disease, it does provide cross references to the two diagnostic codes most commonly used by hospitals and health agencies in the United States:

International Classification of Disease Adapted, (ICDA), 8th Revision, for use in the United States, Dept. H.E.W., U.S. Public Health Service, Pub. No. 1693, 1968 (available from U.S. Government Printing Office, Washington, D.C. 20402).

Hospital Adaptation of ICDA, (H-ICDA), ed. 2, Commission on Professional and Hospital Activities 1974 (available from CPHA, 1968 Green Road, Ann Arbor, Michigan 48105).

Appropriate five-digit code numbers, usually with the several potential and alphabetically indicated modifiers, are used for many diagnostic procedures in nearly all of the states, superseding four-digit coding of the older California Relative Value Studies.

SEMANTIC AWARENESS IN VISUAL EXAMINATIONS

WAYNE W. WONG, M.D.

"I know that you believe you understand what you think I said, but I'm not sure you realize that what you heard is not what I meant."
ANONYMOUS, 1969

Ocular examination provides rich opportunity for both objective determinations and subjective verifications. Frequently in visual components of examination, the subjective elements are vitally important to ultimate patient comfort and tolerance. Assessing

*15 Second St., N.W., Rochester, Minnesota 55901.

subjective complaints and subjective responses requires acute penetration and deciphering of the semantics involved. Both objective analysis (such as external inspection, ophthalmoscopy, and retinoscopy) and subjective responses (such as optotypes, Maddox rod, stereoacuity, "better or worse" comparison of two lenses, duochrome, cross cylinder, and Simultantest) should be related. They are pivotal to medical records, proceeding to additionally indicated steps and securing ultimate visual comfort. The vital help and inherent hindrance of language during subjective procedures are replete with frustrating and even humorous reactions. These have provided an experiential lore for most mature examiners. The beginner must be aware of psycholinguistic factors, their potential for misleading, and the most efficient phrases to minimize semantic obstacles.

OBTAINING A HISTORY

Before any words are spoken, an interaction between patient and examiner—a nonverbal phase of communication—occurs that plays an important part in decisions to be made about the patient and his problems. The manner of the patient's entrance, his facial expression, and even his mode of attire initiate both an informative and a reactive process. A counterpart reaction occurs in the patient, but at this time his reaction is of secondary importance since he is seeking help and has placed himself in a submissive role.

The history-taking begins as the patient starts verbalizing the reasons for his visit. It expands, for better or for worse, as the patient searches for words to express his feelings or adds small stories or phrases that enter his mind. The examiner should be attuned to both appropriateness and relevancy of such extensions or else he may abruptly frustrate the patient's attempted delineations by impatience or by an omnipotent attitude (Lee, 1941). He further must remember that any word may have a list of uses and meanings, and he must be aware that what is being said may not

represent what he assumes it does. Transmitting an "all-knowing" attitude makes the patient either disdain or feel no need to elaborate further details such as the relative degree of pain or discomfort he has experienced. Patient No. 1 is not the same as patient No. 2 nor patient No. 3, either medically or according to indexing principles of general semantics (Johnson, 1946; Korzybski, 1950).

Many patients who come for visual examination do not identify visual deficiency as the reason for their visit; rather they relate their visit to a list of symptoms of discomfort about the eyes or head that they think to be of ocular origin. The examiner, therefore, must *scan* the patient's problems as the patient believes he sees them. The real reason for the visit may be consciously or inadvertently submerged in a host of less relevant descriptions. The manner, more than the order, in which the patient's complaints are enumerated often gives the direction in which diagnostic steps must proceed, if one but takes time to listen actively and applies the effort to listen analytically.

Korzybski (1950) coined a term to characterize communications as "time-binders" in which the understanding of words bridges the gap of time. Through long training we enter an environment of words used so often that we fail to realize how a simple isolated word from a particular patient refers to a moving complex of events involving people and things. "Whiplash" is an illustration. Reference literature here is both vague and studded with small specifics such as impaired accommodation or unequal pupils. These patients have a similarity of history. They are involved in a rear-end automobile crash, often of a relatively minor nature. Symptoms may not be noted on the day of the crash, but over the following days there is a complaint of neck pain and then vague visual symptoms frequently indicated by the word "dizzy," which may mean a multitude of sensations such as disequilibrium, vertigo, diplopia, a fainting feeling, a pulling feeling about the eyes, etc. Such cases often involve liability and the examiner must try to sift the real from the imaginary. He must search and prod the language to find words that both the examiner and the patient agree nearly fit the symptoms.

When a patient says "pain," he is thinking of a specific kind of pain in his experience; we cannot feel the identical "pain." Too often we become bracketed by linguistic conditioning and listen to a patient in terms of premature generalizations, such as "a poor historian," "a perfectionist," "a chronic complainer," "a low I.Q.," or "a nut." Once a patient's complaint is classified so subjectively, listening is impaired and induced deafness becomes a barrier to better understanding. Labels for human beings should be avoided.

Obtaining a visual record

The primary function in ophthalmic care is the preservation of vision. While a patient is under professional care, it is obligatory to have a record of visual function on the first examination, for whatever reason, and also after treatment, especially after surgery. We will ultimately ask, "What can you see?" The word *see*, however, is basically ambiguous. In accepted usage, the term implies recognition of graded characters of the smallest size from a standard distance of 20 feet or 6 meters. In the United States and Canada this is usually recorded in a Snellen fraction; in Europe a decimal notation is common. Another meaning of *see* is the recognition of the immediate environment, perhaps not in minute detail, but enough to determine if the surrounding objects are of concern for that individual at that moment. An example of this is an individual who has 20/100 uncorrected vision yet prefers to drive a car without correction and does so well enough to enjoy a crash-free record earned with his parafoveal and peripheral vision.

Determining uncorrected vision on the Snellen chart requires a subjective response, which must receive critical analysis. The mere request to read the letters evokes a host of semantic reactions that vary with each individual. The poor question, "Can

you see the letters in the bottom line?" often results in a mere affirmative answer. Similarly, when asked to read the letters on the bottom line, many patients will answer that they "can see the letters but can't read them." A perfectionist whose life and interest require attention to small details tends to concentrate and linger silently on a particular letter until positive that he is absolutely correct before verbalizing the letter. Others decline to guess or hazard a "mistake" in reading the letters, and if there is the slightest question that they might be "wrong," they will remain silent while mentally trying to identify the letters correctly. Such patients, when asked "What do you *think* the letters look like?" or "Let's see how well you can *guess*," will often read the entire row correctly.

This response occurs because anything we see is in part independent of what is being seen and in part determined by the characteristics of stored past experiences. For example, the rows of letters in some projector slides end with a code number. Many patients cannot conceive of a row of letters that may have a numeral for the last symbol; consequently, they try to make the terminal numeral into a letter, such as calling "2" a "backward s" or "z." If several rows of letters or an entire chart must be presented, it is often most efficient to say "Please read aloud the smallest letters you *can* see." It is better to expose only one line of letters at a time, beginning if possible with sufficiently large stimuli to afford the encouragement of success before proceeding rapidly to letters approaching the limits of resolution.

Some fatiguing patients fail to grasp that the purpose of the Snellen chart is to determine the smallest symbols that *can* be read. Such patients often wish to waste effort in reading entire lines or, under test of the second eye, may insist on reading the entire chart again, beginning with the largest letter. These mental attitudes and rigidities reveal not only personality patterns but barriers that must be overcome in order to record visual acuity.

To encourage and elicit maximal acuity

in an elderly individual or the new aphakic patient or following ocular disease, we should patiently prod the patient onto "the next line" or through isolated rather than crowded lines of letters. For Federal Aviation Administration examination of flyers or even for driver licensing, however, we should identify the level of immediate or definitive and prompt response. If a patient must be cajoled, pushed, and laboriously brought to read a smaller line to qualify for transport vision, both he and the examiner are failing to recognize the responsibility of *prompt* visual decision.

Determination of central acuity is so subject to variables that it is helpful to seek specificity not only in the fractions recorded but in the type of symbols used, that is, serif or nonserif letters, equal difficulty letters developed by Louise Sloan in 1959, numbers, letters in isolation or row, and so on. This is particularly important in industrial injuries where vision as recorded before and after an accident plays a major role in the settlement. One must detect the low-grade myopic patient whose usual habit is to squint or frown ever so slightly to read the 20/70 line and then, with momentary glimpses of the smaller letters or figures through his temporary stenopeic eyelid–pupillary slit, quickly scan and read the 20/40 line. A similar situation occurs with a young hyperopic patient whose accommodative effort momentarily brings better reading. Such subtle maneuvers often are not involved following an eye injury because the patient is inescapably aware of possible compensatory settlement. Recorded vision should be so noted that another examiner on another date may repeat the testing under essentially similar conditions.

Too many workman's compensation cases have been brought to court because a doctor treating the initial injury did not record vision. When the injury is of such severity as to require emergency hospitalization or when Snellen charts are not immediately available, then some form of near vision record as "able to read headlines or newsprint" is better than no record.

Snellen's* real contribution was to standardize the size and form of test letters with relation to the distance from the observer. When this standardization was accepted, examiners could communicate with colleagues in other parts of the world and know they were approaching comparable measures. This reduced confusion concerning acuity and its notation. However, all 20/20 visions are not equal. A person who correctly reads the 20/20 line letters with a normal rate and cadence distinctly exceeds a patient who also reads correctly the same line while laboriously picking out each letter with much ocular and cerebral effort.

Visual acuity notations often should be amplified by adjectives describing the manner in which "best" visual acuity is achieved. When the patient is unable to "read" an entire row of letters, the number read correctly out of the total on that row may be recorded. For instance, if there are ten letters on the 20/20 line and the patient with effort reads correctly only four, his acuity is more meaningfully recorded as "20/20, four out of ten with effort," rather than merely "20/20−." Since all charts do not have the same number of letters on each row, recording the total number of letters on the row adds exactness. Reading a Snellen line fully and in usual cadence and rhythm should be designated without modification as "20/20," "20/15," and so on; descriptions such as "slow," "hesitantly," "with great effort," or "poorly" will reveal for subsequent examination the functional level in which the patient responded on that day.

There is a distinctly different effect of "pleasing" or "praising" words in contrast to "disgruntled" or "angry" words in encouraging a patient to read another line. Verbalized concurrence or encouragement as "That is very good; now try the next line," yields better results than such statements as "Is that all you can see?" expressed in a derogatory or impatient tone. If we use the

*Snellen, H., Test-types for the determination of acuteness of vision, 1st ed., 1862.

same patience and effort in coaxing the best visual response out of less complicated office patients as we use in postsurgical patients, we can elicit better Snellen and other visual responses.

Ideally, a different set of letters or numbers should be used for each eye, and traditionally the right is examined first. If different letters cannot be used for each eye, the poorer eye should be tested first so that the second eye will not have the benefit of visual recall from the first. Once the visual stimuli of a row of letters are consciously or subliminally recognized in the cerebral cortex, their influence cannot be removed.

The examiner must be alert for subtle changes in the visual efficiency in the presence of 20/20 acuity. A patient may use terms like "a web before my eye," "it seems funny," "there is a haze or smoke before my eye," "it looks faint," or "washed out." If such descriptions persist in the light of seemingly normal morphology (fundus, vitreous, lens, and cornea), one must then pursue possibly incipient neuro-ophthalmic problems. Particularly when these visual symptoms are new and the patient can't describe them other than in vague terms, they must be heard with empathy and not cast aside as neurotic.

The "dominance" of one eye in relation to the other is a confusing area because instrumental techniques for identifying the dominant or the controlling eye are numerous, and determination may be *subjective* or *objective*. In a binocular individual, there is commonly a favored or preferred eye, only crudely or roughly analogous to the preferred or stronger extremities. One sees this when recording uncorrected vision, for one eye may be able to read two or three lines or more on the Snellen chart than does the other, and yet both eyes end up with the identical prescription lenses. There may be *central* or *peripheral* suppression of vision in the nonpreferred eye or local pathology (either current or antecedent) responsible for reduced acuity of one eye.

When a diagnosis is made and explanation undertaken, the examiner must consider the impact of particular words on the patient. The word *cataract* is used too frequently in routine clinical activity and to some patients implies blindness with all its unpleasantness and hardships. There is often little realization that the term *cataract* as commonly used specifies an opacity of the usually clear lens that may vary from a few peripheral dots not affecting vision, to a dense white intumescent lens requiring semi-emergency surgery. Likewise, the term *glaucoma* indicates an increase in intraocular pressure that may vary from borderline tension easily controlled with medications and without loss of vision, to absolute glaucoma and blindness that may be inherited. By describing an early cataract as a "slight clouding or haziness of the lens," the presence of "small white spokes or spots in the lens," the lens is "a bit milky or opalescent," one is less likely to precipitate fear or an anxiety crisis. Other words should be scrupulously avoided altogether. Thus the words *senile* and *degenerative* are unacceptable; conditions relating to all such changes are far better referred to as "the inroads of distinguishing maturity."

Subjective phase of refraction

Objective refractometers* have not become popular because subjective response plays a more important part than do instrumental findings. For the final prescription, most examiners rely increasingly on subjective responses in proportion to the patient's maturity, intelligence, and analytic capacity. By careful questioning while test-

*Refractometers or optometers such as the Hartinger Coincidence Refractionometer (Carl Zeiss) or the Eye Refractometer (Rodenstock) are still subjective to the extent of dependence upon personal interpretations by the examiner. The new (1972) infrared Ophthalmetron of Safir (Bausch and Lomb) is objective both from the point of view of the patient and the examiner. During the course of a 3-second reading of retinal image clarity as seen in modified ophthalmoscopy, it automatically prints out a continuous curve of refractive power through a rotation of 180 degrees. Dioptric values above and below zero are recorded on the abscissa, and axis notations are indicated on the ordinate.

ing visual responses in the subjective phase, one can often elicit the metamorphopsia of early macular changes. With proper questions, differences in intensity of color or hue between the two eyes (which may be more pronounced than the "brighter eye phenomenon") can be elicited from the patient with early optic nerve damage (toxic, ischemic, or compressive) before field loss or structural changes in the optic nerve head are visible. Neuro-ophthalmic disorders frequently pose a communicative obstacle between examiner and patient, particularly in the sensory as contrasted with the more objective motor aspects. Early diagnoses are missed because the examiner fails to recognize that the patient's words do not fit into his academic pigeonholes.

This phase of ocular examination is also steeped in neurolinguistic reactions. If the examiner anticipates the alternative reactions, both accuracy and speed are gained while adverse reactions and fatigue are reduced. In a myopic patient at his final lens or end point of refraction, adding a $-.25$ sphere will often evoke the remark, "That is better." However, if the examiner specifically asks if the test letters appear "smaller and darker" or "more sharply outlined and farther away" (rather than bigger and easier to see), an affirmative answer is evidence of overcorrection.

Often a patient will find it seemingly impossible to determine which is the better lens when adding or subtracting as little as a .25 sphere, but he will respond definitively when questioned in the negative—"Does this make it worse?" Also, more accurate differential plus increased patient relaxation and confidence are obtained if the examiner states that the lenses are very close and briefly compliments the patient on making a differential. Empathy with the task must be shown promptly, and there is never reason to berate or chastise the patient for not reaching a decision. In the hyperopic adult, the final prescription should be the lens that is "comfortable" when reading the 20/20 or best line. The accommodative power of each hyperopic patient varies with age,

energy, and previous lens wearing. The end point must be verified subjectively. This is best done quickly and by asking, after increasing the power by a .25 sphere, whether this makes the letters "more comfortable or bigger and easier to see." If it does, then he is a candidate for the greater strength.

Often in refinement of an "end point," when the patient is asked which of two lenses is "better," there is confusion, particularly if a long line of letters is exposed. The examiner should verbally direct the patient's attention to a particular *pair* of letters or narrow the projected test line, thus concentrating the area of resolution and yet providing a necessary shift in fixation to avoid retinal fatigue. If there is still some hesitation, attention may be briefly channeled to the vertical bars and the horizontal bar of the letter "H" so that comparison is reduced to horizontal and vertical components. This affords opportunity to compare this image of "H" with one stored in his brain. In such decisions it is best not to push to a line beyond practical resolution but to use a slightly larger letter that affords resolution with less effort.

New and subjective optometers with continuously variable sphere (as developed by Louis Alvarez) and cylinder (as developed by William Humphry) power are introducing a do-it-yourself system in which the patient focuses or aligns simple targets. The use of visible light, rather than infrared as in the automated objective refractors, reduces the error introduced by specific refraction of the long wave length infrared light. These instruments necessitate considerable patient cooperation. The elegant and manually operated Vision Analyzer of Humphry Instruments, Inc., Berkeley, California, uses a concave mirror at an 8-ft. test distance. This analyzer eliminates real lenses or lens holders near the patient's face. From the table-size console, a dual projection optical system presents virtual (phantom) lenses either at a suitable distance for glasses or directly on the cornea for fitting contact lenses. The projection may be superimposed on the patient's own spectacles as desirable in high ametropia. Fogging may be incorporated. One eye may be examined at a time, or both eyes simultaneously. A table-top model is under development by the American Optical Corporation.

Brighter eye phenomenon

After each eye has been corrected optimally to 20/20 or better, there normally is further improvement in acuity when the eyes are tested binocularly. The patient may be able to read an additional line or read with greater facility and cadence. Such performance automatically screens out significant heterophoria at that test distance. The patient may remark, however, that one eye "sees better" than the other. Time and fatigue are reduced if the examiner elicits the patient's meaning of "better." Difference of resolving power is not involved, because the patient has demonstrated ability to read 20/20 or better with each eye. However, if one eye is covered while the patient is reading the test chart and then the cover quickly changed to the opposite eye, the patient may be made aware that blackness of letters, brightness of the background, or overall field differs between the two eyes. He may even report a faint difference in color value between the two eyes so that the image from one seems slightly browner or muted. The "brighter eye" is usually the eye the patient calls the "better eye."

The patient, if need be, can be reassured then that the "brighter eye" phenomenon is a normal or physiologic variation and has nothing to do with visual acuity. This "brighter eye" phenomenon is a quantitative variable of the image that does not lend itself to clinical measurement but that can be studied under laboratory conditions. It is related to the variables called hue, saturation, and brightness (in terminology endorsed by the Optical Society of America) (Evans, 1948). It is a peripheral or "sensory dominance" (input) in contrast to "motor dominance" of an eye that is used for sighting a gun or similar aligning. This phenomenon is related to that which occurs when a person is suddenly exposed to bright lights and shows a preference for "seeing" with one eye by closing the other, such as when walking from a dark room into bright sunlight or being suddenly roused out of a sound sleep with the room lights turned on. The child with divergence excess exotropia classically shows this by closing one eye in bright light.

Semantic reaction to the word "see"

The ability to "see" is both a peripheral optic accomplishment and a cerebral process of registration, classification, and association in Brodmann's areas 17, 18, and 19. We only "see" or perceive what we have learned to interpret. This requires functions of the angular gyrus and the surrounding temporoparietal lobe. Clinical refractive examination embraces many of these central nervous system elements, but refraction per se measures only the optic components on the visual or fixation axis of foveal vision.

Parafoveal, paramacular, perimacular, and peripheral vision, however, are more important end-organ and optic components for spatial orientation, travel, and nonreading activities. Some patients having "old shoe" familiarity with 20/200 uncorrected binocular vision prefer to go about their daily duties and even driving without refractive correction, because they "need glasses only for reading." The word "see" has different meanings to different people. It is important that the patient be enabled to convey, and the examiner be alert to appreciate, the range of visual task relations for that specific patient to his "seeing." Though the 20/200 uncorrected patient may be safe and comfortable at a party, he certainly cannot resolve freeway control signs quickly enough or at sufficient distance to avoid initiating a chain of rear-end crashes.

Contact lens patients with only 20/30 or even 20/40 vision resulting from residual posterior corneal or lenticular astigmatism often feel they "see better" with their contact lenses than when enjoying 20/20+ vision with spectacles. This may be related in part to the wider field, size difference, or relief from spectacle frame scotomas afforded by contact lenses. It may also result from motivation and the fact that 20/20 by itself is far from the only criterion for routine or casual "seeing." Twenty/twenty aphakic vision may be crippling or very restrictive and disturbing to the spatial relations of an elderly person who was mobile and well-adjusted to his broader and less magnified visual world with 20/70 phakic vision. Or it may be no problem to the well-adjusted hyperope who has endured +6 to +8 lenses since childhood.

An individual's total "seeing" relates to several components of optic and also cerebral patterns to which he has adapted and familiarized himself. Though words will always be inadequate, one must earnestly seek to explain and interpret aphakic vision to a patient before cataract surgery. Based specifically on his previous refractive status,

this must be in terms of differences in size, brightness, nearness, color, and prism displacement. Even brief forewarning prior to surgery will help to reduce postoperative disturbances but can never replace the actual experience of being aphakic.

Responsibility of the examiner

The examiner's responsibility extends until the patient has stabilized and optimized himself in a visual world and is adapted to a set of glasses that he uses with real functional advantage, with protection to his eyes, and without discomfort. The patient also tends to hold him responsible for any error induced by the optician. Any discomfiture related to new spectacles must be heard with an unprejudiced mind and without fear of bruising one's ego. It is necessary to be

Fig. 2-2. Lens measure shown in use with its three points applied to concave surface of a lens measuring nearly −3 diopters in its horizontal axis. With contact established in this fashion, lens measure is rotated through 180 degrees to check for consistency of spherical surface or to measure variations in diopterage that would indicate cylindric component.

sure that the prescription was (1) correctly derived, (2) properly related to previously correct or incorrect spectacles, (3) accurately written, and (4) precisely rendered into spectacles. The examiner must verify power, interpupillary distance, base curve (Fig. 2-2), and prescribed or induced imbalance. The visual distress created by a new set of spectacles on a base curve different from that to which he has been adapted, may be difficult to verbalize with other than simple words such as "these glasses feel funny, strange, or different." If asked whether or not objects tend to slant, curve, or float, positive answers may indicate altered base curves or lens warpage without change in dioptric power. The patient's description of the circumstances under which his symptoms occur often will pinpoint the causes of discomfort—if the physician listens with discriminatory discernment.

Importance of listening to patients' complaints

Bifocals must never be insisted upon by the examiner, but the reasons for considering them should be explained. The patient should be given a choice of buying such pairs of glasses as he wants, but the advantages and disadvantages must be *understood* by him. The word "bifocals" often causes a strong psycholinguistic reaction; some patients will even refuse to try to understand their described benefits. Such patients, often women who associate bifocals with aging, may pleasantly accept a separate pair of "reading glasses" or demiglasses and less easily adapt to "invisible bifocals" such as the "Younger," "Varilux," "Progressor," and "Omnifocal" lenses.

On the other hand, when intermediate viewing becomes a problem, the word "trifocals" may bring a reaction of utter despair to such patients. If "bifocals" sound troublesome, "trifocals" must be three times worse. Complaints associated with multifocals may be lessened by proper instruction when the patient is handed his first prescription. Often a patient has difficulty in verbalizing his problems of intermediate distance viewing

but can readily demonstrate this when asked to recount his visual demands when this discomfort occurs. It is often informative if he will dramatize what he does in his office with letters, adding machine tape, people in the room, at the piano, and so on.

When a patient complains of reading discomfort with bifocals, it is important to inspect the glasses as the patient wears them. Top edges of the bifocals must be horizontal and a pantoscopic tilt of at least 15 degrees should be present to bring the lower edges of the eyepieces close to the zygomatic eminences. The presbyopic patient often cannot see that he is looking through the bifocals for distance viewing or through only one segment if the frames are not seated correctly on the face. Vague complaints that are difficult to verbalize may be caused by a change in either base curve or the shape of the bifocals. If a patient has been using a Ful-vue, flat-top bifocal for years and his new lenses are Kryptok, he will have complaints because of the "image jump" from distance to near viewing. The use of minus cylinders in one pair of spectacles and plus cylinders in another will often cause symptoms that are difficult for the patient to describe, as it is a novel experience for which he has neither linguistic equipment nor standard of comparison to describe the "different" visual sensation. The lensometer is of no help here, but a lens measure (Fig. 2-2) applied to the old lens and the new lens may clearly reveal different base curves as the cause of distress.

In myopia, a change of lens to a higher power may create sensations of smallness or the floors appearing to "float" and objects appearing to "move" quickly with each head movement. These sensations usually disappear in a few days as the brain becomes adapted to the altered image schemes created by the new lenses. If these symptoms persist, then we should compare the base curves of the old lens with the new one; if there is a significant difference, the new lens should be reground as closely to the old base curve as possible. Such a difference may be encountered when plastic lenses are used because the various manufacturers of plastic lenses each have varying base curves for different power ranges. For example, if a patient has become accustomed to the Armolite plastic lens and his new pair is American Optical Company's AOlite plastic lens, even though he is able to read the 20/20 line without difficulty he may complain of discomfort because of the difference in base curves used in molding. The brain, being accustomed to the perceived image through one set of base curves or plus cylinder lenses, finds it difficult to adapt to another set of base curves or minus cylinders. If the examiner is unaware of this and the patient is unable to describe this sensation with other than vague or everyday words, a label of psychoneurosis is easily and erroneously attached to the patient. This produces dissatisfaction for patient, examiner, and optician.

Another situation difficult for the patient to describe is the vague discomfort, particularly noted by a hyperopic patient, when reading or looking at near objects. In such cases the eyepieces may be fitted perpendicular to the ground; and as the eyes rotate downward to read, there is an induced oblique astigmatism. This will disappear immediately if the bottom of the lenses is tilted (pantoscoped) closer to the cheeks so that the visual axis strikes the glasses near the theoretically desirable perpendicular for all lines of gaze.

After one has eliminated each mechanical and optic source of discomfort, it is still necessary to listen to the patient to rule out psychologic factors. It is not uncommon for a patient, particularly a woman, to be dissatisfied with the type, style, or color of frame she has selected. The patient may be reluctant or unable to verbalize this directly and hence may be unhappy with her "glasses." Occasionally a patient may have a deeply rooted or near pathologic fixation in search of "one pair of glasses" that will resolve all problems. Such a patient may refuse to accept the reality of other ocular or central nervous system disease to the degree that she has seen half a dozen eye examiners and with fanatic zeal is continuing her search for the elusive "one pair of glasses." Such a patient requires a psychiatrist.

Summary

Those of us entrusted with the eyesight of fellow humans must be constantly aware that each patient differs in his past experiences and will respond in a different manner. In our world of words, meanings are constantly shaded or altered by individual backgrounds and experiences. Because of such different personal make-up, each will react differently to a given situation. We must also become aware of our own reactions to the patient, the significance of the manner in which the patient presents his problems, and the variables in his verbalization. Visual acuity notations should use short descriptive terms in addition to the usual Snellen fraction for a more exacting appraisal. When both examiner and examinee have an approximately common image of the problem, both the establishment of visual acuity and identification of correction can be interesting, pleasant, efficient, and rewarding.

REFERENCES

Cullmann, B., Benes, F., et al.: Rational documentation of ophthalmologic examination (optical mark's reader forms) Klin. Mbl. Angenheilk. **164:**829-837, 1974.

Johnson, W.: People in quandries, New York, 1946, Harper & Row, Publishers.

Knight, C. L., Hoyt, W. F., and Wilson, C. B.: Syndrome of incipient prechiasmal optic nerve compression, Arch. Ophthalmol. **87:**1-11, 1972.

Korzybski, A.: Manhood of humanity, ed. 2, Garden City, New York, 1950, Country Life Press.

Korzybski, A.: Science and sanity, ed. 4, Garden City, New York, 1958, Country Life Press.

Lee, I. J.: Language habits in human affairs, New York, 1941, Harper & Row, Publishers.

The initial examination

Much is learned in the immediate confrontation with the patient, in far less time than it can be described, simply by the Sherlock Holmes technique of critical observation plus clinical judgment. The ocular apparatus, being located accessibly on a surface area of the body and being transparent in much of its structure, lends itself to accurate verification or cross-checking of diagnostic findings by subjective and objective techniques. The fact that the eyes and orbits are also in a frontal area in the upper portion of the body makes for easy examining access in a conventional chair and with minimum social concerns of disrobing. By the same token, this may lull the examiner into omitting necessary physical steps such as looking at the axillary skin folds in the presence of angioid streaks, holding a youngster upside down when evaluating a deep hemangioma, or having the patient recumbent with at least 270 degrees of access about the head for indirect ophthalmoscopy.

A general impression of the patient's development, health, and mental ability is attained both by observation and by his manner and accuracy in responding to examining procedures. Often a fairly good estimate of the intelligence quotient and even occupation is derived in the course of ocular examination. General body posture and particular head position (such as face turning, elevation, or depression of the chin) give clues to neuromuscular disturbances and to imbalances of the extraocular muscles. Noting scars of previous injuries or surgery will tell more about what can be improved in the future than will most patients' prolonged narrative of what happened in the past. Similarly, skin disturbances, enlargement of glands, and even subtle disturbances in form or functions of facial components serve as guideposts to increase the directness of historic questions and diagnostic steps.

PRELIMINARY INSPECTION

After reading the notes previously recorded by the aide, brief introductory exchanges, and verification of seemingly salient points, directness is served by a preliminary but systematic examination of the adnexa and anterior segments with the aid of a bright focal penlight or "inspection torch." Whether this takes place in the office with available high-intensity bracket magnifiers (Luxo, Dazor, Fresnel-Burton) or in an emergency room with small surgical lights (Rene, Castle, American Sterilizer), these diffuse sources should be avoided because they produce photophobic responses, lid closure, avoidance movements of the head, and temporary dazzling impairment of retinal sensitivity.

Small professional pocketlights (Welch-Allyn or Oculus, Standard Pocketlight [AA batteries], Focusing Pocketlight [AA batteries], Mite-T-Lite [AAA alkaline batteries], Keeler Pen Torch [nylon body with screw-on focalizer], Ultralite Deluxe Pocketlight by Concept [AAA alkaline batteries; Fig. 3-1]) or the more cumbersome (and expensive) transformer-based units such as the Barkan hammer light, Ortho-Lite, Mayou focal illuminator, and Rayner Premier Hand Lamp have the important advantage of providing narrowly concentrated light beams with almost no dazzling effect except when particularly directed into the pupil to test pupillary reactions. (The thick-handled rechargeable pocketlights generally take up too much desk space and are awkward pocket stretchers.) Small diameter tips such as the

Fig. 3-1. Ultra-lite with slip on cobalt filter and 1 mm. pin hole attachments. Weight 1 oz.; lifetime guarantee. (Concept, Clearwater, Florida 33516.)

Fig. 3-2. Example of spectacle-mounted loupe with adjustable interpupillary distance. (Neitz Instruments Co., Ltd., Tokyo, Japan.)

Finnoff nosepiece, National curved, straight, and angulated metal extensions, or Mayou curved and straight tips have usefulness for transilluminating possible cystoid masses on the lid or iris and even for checking an occasional paranasal sinus for cloudiness that may be causing orbital symptoms. As an alternative, a hand ophthalmoscope may be used for this inspection. By rotating the +20-diopter lens into position, localized magnification of 5× is obtained when the instrument and the examiner's eye are brought to 1 in. from the ocular surface. Magnification of 2× to 3× with a clip-on loupe (Telesight, Keeler), a headband, or spectacle-mounted aid (May, Oculus, Beebe Binocular loupe, Bausch and Lomb DuaLoupe, Dana) helps this survey but should not be used under 2× because of limited value nor much over 3× because of limited range (Fig. 3-2).

An ingenious and lightweight spectacle mounting was introduced by Keeler in 1970 to accommodate an interchangeable loupe magnifier, or a small indirect ophthalmoscope similar to the Schultz-Crock (p. 191).

Stereo vision and coordinated illumination are afforded compactly with either of the two "plug-in" units. The Sola Surgical Loupe (2× magnification at 33 cm.) is available without illumination and with standard tungsten lamp or high intensity quartz-halogen lamp (Fig. 3-3). The latter provides essentially double illumination at a higher filament temperature and "whiter" light. This, however, requires double power supply and reduces usual life time of the rechargeable pack from 2 to 1 hour of continuous use.

Fig. 3-3. Sola Commido Interchangeable Unit. 2× Galilean telescopic loupes are centered over each eye of the observer, when the slides are pushed in from either side of the carriage. First surface mirrors for indirect ophthalmoscopy are positioned by pulling both slides laterally. This physically moves the telescopes outward. Interpupillary distances are adjustable from 58 to 74 mm. Available with quartz halogen or standard lamp.

The lightweight, flat, foldable, metalframe Zeiss or Cameron 2× loupe with an 8-in. working distance may be slipped on with or without conventional spectacles. It has a real working asset of pocket portability in most hard spectacle cases. The physician's habit of keeping one of these and a penlight in his suit jacket is an advantage for neighborhood foreign body problems, anterior segment problems on rounds, and even splinter assistance for the children.

The heavy but inexpensive hair crumplers with padded headbands and side shields (Berger Magni-Focuser, B & L Magna-Visor, Donegan OptiVisor, Donegan Optiloupe) are better suited to industrial inspection lines than intermittent office use. A heavier (13.5 oz.) and expensive exception to the head-mounted units is the 8× "Beckerscope" with 8-in. working distance, as designed by Stanley C. Becker in 1969; this is suitable as a mobile, miniature surgical microscope and is available with dual fiber optic illumination. It can be worn over spectacles or correction may be corporated in the unit. The slightly more recent Xonix head-mounted microscope with fiber optic illumination affords zoom magnification of 6× to 12× with field diameter of 28 mm. to 18 mm. Working distance is 10 in. from the objective lenses or 13 in. from the eye. Both of these prismatic binocular systems tax the upper limits of magnification that are practical without the stabilization or movement control obtained in a floor- or ceiling-mounted system.

The old technique of a condensing lens for illumination in one hand and a magnifying glass (Ukaim, Hastings, Coddington) in the other precludes most opportunities for manipulations and is not recommended. Similarly most of the old, hand, monocular slit lamps (Bausch and Lomb 7.5×, Bishop-Harman 12×, Krimsky 10× "feather weight," Bettman and McNair 8-25×, Zeiss Jena 6×) afford neither good slit characteristics nor use flexibility. (One recent exception for mobile clinic work is the Kowa portable slit lamp with power supply and carrying case, which is a $700 to $1,000 investment; see p. 85.)

The preliminary inspection—which can be accomplished while talking to the patient—should grossly survey:

1. Symmetry and mobility of the face, especially about the orbits
2. Condition of the skin, particularly the lids
3. Condition of the brows and lashes (for movement, loss, scaling, color, malposition)
4. Position and action of the lids (without touching them)
5. Position of the lacrimal puncta and evidence of lacrimal disturbances
6. Condition of the conjunctiva (for congestion, edema, masses)
7. Preauricular nodes (if the face must be steadied or elevated, the examiner can do this with the fingers of each hand palpating these nodes for enlargement and tenderness at the same time)
8. Position and movement of the globes (for exophthalmos and muscle action)
9. Condition of the cornea (for brightness, irregularity, scars)
10. Gross characteristics of the anterior chamber (for obliteration, hemorrhage, masses)
11. Condition of the lens (for dislocation, opacity, and partial or complete absence)

The alterations of pathologic disturbances in the eye, as elsewhere in the body, present almost limitless variations, degrees of severity, and stages of activity. For basic simplification, however, all biologic disorders can be reduced to nine types. The examiner must always be ready to recount these groups when faced with a lesion of unidentified cause. The nine basic disorders include:

1. Congenital defects
2. Infections
3. Allergies
4. Injuries
5. Vascular defects
6. Neoplasms
7. Degenerations
8. Endocrine disturbances
9. Vitamin deficiencies

The ocular examiner has one additional aspect of physiology beyond the preceding nine classifications; this is the special area of optic or visual disturbance. Each of the above mechanisms can affect optic and visual function of the eyes. Therefore the examiner must recognize their roles as well as the unique optical elements of the visual system.

Negative findings should not be recorded. Positive findings, which may be noted tersely if desired, bracket subsequent questions to significant areas and indicate the examining procedures apt to be productive. Thus noting active tearing or epiphora eliminates a rose bengal test for lacrimal deficiency, noting acute allergic lid edema contraindicates refractive procedures, or noting a dark limbal mass obligates transillumination.

INFANTS, NEWBORNS, AND PREMATURE BABIES

The timing of initial eye examination has been directed to the newborn nursery and particularly the premature nursery by retrolental fibroplasia in the late 1940s and early 1950s. Though ophthalmia neonatorum should be essentially eliminated by silver nitrate or other prophylactic installations in the delivery room, an optimal safeguard against unsuspected congenital defects would be careful eye examinations of all infants at birth. The high requirements for ophthalmic manpower and the low percentage yield of pathology, however, make it appropriate for alert obstetricians, pediatricians, and nursery personnel to accomplish preliminary eye screening. The ophthalmologist examining infants of 1 lb. to 9 lbs. must accomplish both external and fundus survey. Good pupillary dilatation is needed for the latter. Even though the anterior chambers appear shallow, angle closure is rare in infants. Systemic tolerance to conjunctival installations is also good. My preference is a drop of topical anesthetic (Ophthaine or Ophthetic) in each eye followed by two installations of 1% Mydriacyl and two installations of 4% Homatropine or 2.5% Neosynephrine. These should be administered at intervals of 5 minutes. The Sauer infant's speculum held open by spring tension frees the hand and is much easier to use than separate lid retractors. If tempted by frugality to substitute paper clips for lid retractors, try instead the safer, spring tension wire speculum of Alfonso. Though its tips resemble paper clips, there is much less danger of mechanical injuries.

The indirect binocular ophthalmoscope greatly reduces difficulties of restive eye movements or nystagmus, but Lawton Smith's "patience technique" for direct ophthalmoscopy should be used for posterior pole detail. Slightly prolonged observation allows fundus features to go by often enough until they are well understood or the activity subsides. Repeated, quiet reassurances might lull the infant, but will certainly reassure a helping mother.

Positioning of the infants either in the office or in the nursery is remarkably convenient using the lap technique with the infant on its back. The head is toward the examiner and resting on his knees. The mother holds both hands of the infant, and with her arms and elbows restrains the wiggling body. When slightly larger, the youngster's legs may be spread around the mother's waist and retained by her elbows. Patients in this position may avoid the greater hazards of examination under general anesthesia.

VISUAL ACUITY
Basic concepts

Immediately following amplification of notes in the history and the simultaneous completion of preliminary inspection, visual acuity should be checked (if this was not previously done by the aide). This should precede any manipulation of the globe (which the patient might later claim as related to his visual loss) or intraocular examination (where the dazzle of lights might affect attempts to establish visual acuity shortly thereafter).

On a parity with though usually less urgent than pain, loss of vision is the demanding concern of the patient. Therefore it is essential to record acuity in detail on the initial examination and as part of every general physical examination. This should be done first without the spectacle correction (sc) and then with correction (cc), always approaching the right eye first. On each follow-up examination acuity is usually checked, but it is done primarily for distance and with the appropriate distance spectacle correction in place. Distance acuity is more significant and reproducible than near acuity and is less subject to the variables that alter near acuity (illumination, pupillary size, refraction, accommodation).

Basis of measuring acuity

Clinical measurements of visual acuity are based on historic convention and utility, recognizing from astronomic observations that the minimum separable capability of a healthy human eye is approximately 1 minute of arc. Robert Hooke (1635-1703, distinguished "Experimenter" of the Royal Society of England) made the first measurements of the "minimum visual angle" based on the ability of an emmetropic eye to achieve resolution of binary stars. Under exquisite laboratory conditions this capability may range downward to 15 or 30 seconds of arc; study of interconal distance at the fovea generally would support such a functional ability. The aligning power or ability of the eye to detect a break in a contour, however, is about five times finer or accurate within 3 seconds of arc. This aligning power is used to make readings on vernier scales.

Utilizing the average and commonplace minimum separable distance of 1 minute of arc, test letters such as Es are constructed in which each of the total five horizontal strokes and spaces subtend 1 minute, and the overall letter subtends 5 minutes. Commonly the largest letters used in office testing are sized to subtend 5 minutes at a distance of 200 ft., and the smallest subtend 5 minutes at 10 ft. To test the eye in a position of focal rest or without accommodative muscle effort, the test distance should simulate infinity. For practicality and again by historic convention, this is commonly taken to be a test distance of 20 ft.

Using the Snellen notation, acuity is expressed by first recording the test distance (commonly 20 ft.) and then recording the distance at which the smallest letter seen should be read by an average normal eye. Thus at a test distance of 20 ft., if the patient can see only the letter that should be seen at 200 ft., his Snellen notation is 20/200. (In the metric system this would be 6/60.) If he reads at 20 ft. the size letters that the average person can see, the Snellen notation is 20/20 (or 6/6). If he sees considerably better than average and can recognize letters that the average person must approach within 10 ft. to recognize, his Snellen notation is 20/10 (6/3).

Pin Hole Acuity (Scheiner's Test, 1619)

As a single method of minimizing refractive abberation and even many irregularities in the media, an opaque disc with a 1 mm. central pin hole opening will often reveal the maximum resolving power of the retina. The pin hole disc, placed in a lens position before the eye, may also be used to determine if a refractive correction as developed in a trial frame or refractor is yielding best corrected acuity. If vision through the pin hole aperture is improved, then further refinement in the lens combination is probably needed. This test becomes less reliable in persons of advanced age because it reduces needed increasing light levels for vision. Pausing a few moments for the older patient to adapt, however, will reduce some of this disadvantage.

Notation of visual levels below 20/200

If the patient cannot recognize the largest letter available (commonly the 20/200 letter), it is helpful to walk the patient slowly toward the chart, noting the distance at which he first recognizes the letter. If this is at 8 ft., the Snellen notation is 8/200. When the patient cannot see the largest letter at any distance, the examiner may spread his fingers in good light and estimate the most remote distance at which the patient counts fingers (such as, C.F. at 3 ft.). Failing this, the patient is asked to detect hand movements, usually horizontal or vertical,

and note is made of the maximum distance at which this is possible (for instance, H.M. at 2 ft.).

The next lowest quality of vision is the preservation of *light projection* or localization of light in space. This may be noted as "accurate light projection" or "temporal light projection only." The final and minimal visual response is *light perception* only and may be expressed as "L.P. only" or its absence as "no L.P." If a patient with markedly limited acuity can localize doorways, tell where windows and bright lights are located, doesn't stumble over major objects of furniture, and by aligning power can tell curbs and sidewalks, it is a significant functional guide to note "travel vision." This is far more valuable than retention of mere light perception and projection.

Illiterate and preschool techniques

For a patient who is illiterate or competent only in another language, a size series of so-called "illiterate Es" may be used, asking the patient to indicate in which direction the fingers or openings point. This can also be done with children down to the age of 3 or 3½ if they are bright and cooperative, or by the age of 4 if somewhat dull or reluctant. Charts and individual cards with schematized pictures such as those developed by Henry Allen in 1961 are advantageously designed for the 2½- to 3½-year-old at the attention range of 30 to 200 in. but are influenced by family cultural patterns and are slightly less accurate than illiterate Es. Sets of 12 durable single character cards 4 × 5 in. in size presenting an umbrella, an apple, and a house each on four cards give steps of Snellen approximation (20/200, 20/100, 20/50, 20/40, 20/30, 20/20, 20/15, and 20/10). At 5 ft. these serve well for low vision diagnosis (20/40 to 20/400) or at 1 ft. will simulate 20/200 to 20/2000 (New York Association of the Blind, New York, New York 10022). Sjögren's hand test (1939) made of simplified block prints of the hand with fingers outstretched on each of six cards are graduated in levels from 20/120 to 20/20 for use at 20 ft., but patients tend to lose attention at this more remote range and the cards again are slightly less accurate than the Es. Since horizontal direction sense develops later than vertical orientation in children, the use of illiterate Es incorporates a source of error eliminated by O. Ffooks in his matching three symbol cubes. These present a circle, a square, and a triangle, which are accurately related to Snellen standard, nonserif illiterate Es from 20/20 to 20/200. They are also available in an 8-page booklet extending their capacity to 20/15.

Aphakic vision or visual performance after cataract extraction

Patients who are to undergo lens extraction should be forewarned of resultant alteration in visual function either with aphakic spectacles or contact lenses. The examiner must be attuned to the optical bases for these noticeable postsurgical changes. Because the lenticular component of refraction is effectively moved a few mm. forward with a contact lens and even farther forward with aphakic spectacle lens, there will be size increments of several percent, particularly with the spectacle correction. The visual world thus will seem larger or closer. Visual field studies show distinct constriction in the high-plus, spectacle corrected aphake who had no or only a modest refractive error before operation. With a contact lens, visual field restrictions are distinctly less. A hyperoptic patient of 6 to 9 diopters who has adapted throughout life to lens and frame constriction of fields, may find relatively little difficulty in utilizing the increased plus of his aphakic spectacles.

Loss of central vision following optimal refractive correction for aphakia is due almost entirely to one of five factors: (1) cystoid macular edema, which is the most common cause and appears several months after extraction—the loss may be as much as 50% but the prognosis is for significant recovery over 12 mos. to 18 mos. (2) ischemic optic neuropathy that has a fixed and unencouraging prognosis, (3) chorioretinal wrinkling caused by hypotonia, (4) macular pucker caused by contraction of a thin preretinal membrane, or (5) senile involution of the macula (degeneration of Haab) that may exacerbate after surgery.

Equipment for distance visual acuity measurements

Countless distance test devices (Ives, Wall and Ochs, Cardsell), wall charts (Dennett, Cowan, Sloan, Ewing, A.M.A., Landolt, Berens, and Beach), and illuminated cabinets (Green, Black, Rogers, DaLaur Good-Lite, Graham Field) are still cataloged for measuring distance acuity. All, however, were superseded by a first generation of complex projection devices (Clason, Ferree-Rand). Now a second generation of Project-O-Charts (American Optical), Compact Acuity Projectors (Bausch and Lomb), Rodavist (Rodenstock), Biotronics 100 slide random access projector, Kodak-Eljtanar 80 slide unit, or T/O-Matic (Titmus) make the previous devices truly obsolete. The Remote Control American Optical Custom Project-O-Chart (1971) offers two dials, each with 15 square apertures that can be sequenced by the examiner. A choice of about 60 slides can be inserted in the two discs and then modified for single horizontal lines, astigmatic rotation, polarization, or axis contrast. A new fingertip control panel (1975) gives rapid random access to 28 different character slides by clear and illuminated touch buttons.

Easily washable metal projection screens no longer carry exploring children's fingerprints. Projection slides are available in any combination of letters, numbers, illiterate Es, Allen figures, Landolt Cs, Sjögren's hands, duochrome, astigmatic tests, and astigmatic dials. Lens quality and projection clarity exceed the definition previously attained in variously smudged, yellowed, or dirty test cards. It would no longer be possible for the late Walter Lancaster to write that projectors "will please those who are satisfied with mediocrity, and place convenience first." Indeed remarkable convenience and reduction in time-fatigue for the patient are served by availability of projector mountings for wall, desk, and floor or incorporation in major diagnostic ensembles. Where these still may not be in easy reach of the examiner, electric remote controls are available. Commonly these motor-driven changes are made more slowly than can be done by the dexterous hand of the alert examiner who quickly perceives the approximate test level to which the projector should be changed.

Inherent advantages of the projector over the wall chart include (1) avoidance of the chart being exposed for inadvertent memorization; (2) complete control of the optotypes without leaving the examining position; (3) essentially limitless combinations of optotypes, polarized stereopsis tests, polarized phoria tests, color tests, fixation or attention devices, and other tests; (4) display of single test figures, which often aid the senescent and hesitant; or (5) display of full lines for the vigorous performer or to bring out the "crowding phenomenon" (von Noorden), which may reveal subtle amblyopia in children who perform better or even normally with isolated symbols.

Louise Sloan has shown that nonserif or Gothic letters, particularly when arranged in groups of similar complexity, give more consistent and accurate results, though they are 5% to 10% easier to recognize than the original serif capitals used by Snellen. Letters and numbers in the patient's own language most closely relate to his daily seeing requirements and therefore are the most practical optotypes. Clearly some letters such as I, L, and T are much easier to recognize, whereas W, M, and X are much more difficult. The Sloan recommendation to use only the ten letters—D, K, R, H, V, C, N, Z, S, O—makes for better uniformity of difficulty in successive test lines or type sizes.

Because visual resolving power increases with light intensity (within limits), some effort should be made to standardize the level of test screen illumination between 20 and 80 footcandles. The importance of precision in such illumination is largely outweighed by (1) the enormous light adaptation capacity of the healthy human retina, which under laboratory conditions may reach 100,000-fold, and (2) age-linked changes in retinal sensitivity, which essentially require doubled intensity for visual recognition under dim illumination for each 13 years of adult life. Any planned changes in screen illumination, however, should be accomplished with an iris diaphragm in the projector and not by rheostat. Reducing current to the bulb changes its temperature and color emission characteristics, thus introducing a chromatic variable. Because it is both impractical and unrepresentative of usual conditions, refraction should not be done in the dark. Contrast, however, is one of the basic variables in measuring acuity. Higher contrast is needed with advancing age or lower levels of luminance. Surrounding light should be less than 30% of chart illumination. Glare and stray incident light should be eliminated from the test area. Contrast of letters to background should be held at a good .85 to .95. Remember also the spectacle correction giving best contrast sensitivity may not give the best Snellen acuity. When stray light cannot be consistently blocked out, an opaque box—open end toward the patient—should be built about the projection screen and extend forward about 1 ft. This acts as a light shield.

Several screening charts such as the line of transilluminated charts by Good-Lite Company* or their more recent Insta-Line Chart with remote control linear illumination, similar to the old Green's Illuminated Vision charts, are suitable for presenting any one of several preset lines at a time.

Zoom lens projections systems (Auto Nikon 50-300 mm. Zoom) offer continuous rather than stepwise numbering for central visual acuity. This, however, exceeds clinical significance and clinical reliability in the generation of small test divisions. This also presents a major variable in different levels of brightness.

For efficient checking of either near or distance acuity with spectacle correction in place, an inexpensive clip-on occluder should

*Forest Park, Illinois 60130.

NEAR VISION TEST CARD

UNIVERSITY OF LOUISVILLE

12

WHEN IN THE COURSE OF HUMAN EVENTS, IT BECOMES NECESSARY FOR

11

ONE PEOPLE TO DISSOLVE THE POLITICAL BANDS WHICH HAVE CONNECTED THEM

9

WITH ANOTHER, AND TO ASSUME AMONG THE POWERS OF THE EARTH, THE SEPARATE AND EQUAL STATION TO

7

WHICH THE LAWS OF NATURE AND OF NATURE'S GOD ENTITLE THEM, A DECENT RESPECT TO THE OPINIONS OF MANKIND REQUIRES THAT THEY SHOULD DECLARE THE

6

CAUSES WHICH IMPEL THEM TO THE SEPARATION   WE HOLD THESE TRUTHS TO BE SELF-EVIDENT, THAT ALL MEN ARE CREATED EQUAL, THAT THEY ARE ENDOWED BY THEIR CREATOR WITH CERTAIN UNALIENABLE

5

RIGHTS, THAT AMONG THESE ARE LIFE, LIBERTY, AND THE PURSUIT OF HAPPINESS   THAT TO SECURE THESE RIGHTS, GOVERNMENTS ARE INSTITUTED AMONG MEN, DERIVING THEIR JUST POWERS FROM THE CONSENT OF THE GOVERNED,

3

THAT, WHENEVER ANY FORM OF GOVERNMENT BECOMES DESTRUCTIVE OF THESE ENDS, IT IS THE RIGHT OF THE PEOPLE TO ALTER OR TO ABOLISH IT, AND TO INSTITUTE NEW GOVERNMENT, LAYING ITS FOUNDATION ON SUCH PRINCIPLES AND ORGANIZING ITS POWERS IN SUCH FORM, AS TO THEM SHALL SEEM MOST LIKELY TO

CHART TO BE HELD
14 INCHES FROM EYE

COPYRIGHT   1958
GUILD OF PRESCRIPTION
OPTICIANS OF AMERICA INC.

Fig. 3-4. Front side of author's disposable near vision test card with matte finish (reduced one-fifth). (Distributed by Opticians Association of America, Washington, D.C. 20036.)

NEAR VISION TEST CARD

UNIVERSITY OF LOUISVILLE

REVISED JAEGER STANDARD	NEAR SNELLEN NOTATION	METRIC DISTANCE	DISTANCE SNELLEN APPROXIMATION	DECIMAL NOTATION	A. M. A. 1955 NEAR VISUAL EFFICIENCY
12	14/89 (in.)	2.25 M.	20/130 (ft.)	0.15	10%

WHEN IN THE COURSE OF HUMAN EVENTS, IT BECOMES NECESSARY FOR

11	14/79	2.0	20/120	0.2	13%

ONE PEOPLE TO DISSOLVE THE POLITICAL BANDS WHICH HAVE CONNECTED THEM

9	14/60	1.5	20/85	0.22	20%

WITH ANOTHER, AND TO ASSUME AMONG THE POWERS OF THE EARTH, THE SEPARATE AND EQUAL STATION TO

7	14/42	1.05	20/60	0.35	40%

WHICH THE LAWS OF NATURE AND OF NATURE'S GOD ENTITLE THEM. A DECENT RESPECT TO THE OPINIONS OF MANKIND REQUIRES THAT THEY SHOULD DECLARE THE

6	14/35	.82	20/50	0.4	50%

CAUSES WHICH IMPEL THEM TO THE SEPARATION. WE HOLD THESE TRUTHS TO BE SELF-EVIDENT, THAT ALL MEN ARE CREATED EQUAL, THAT THEY ARE ENDOWED BY THEIR CREATOR WITH CERTAIN UNALIENABLE

5	14/28	.75	20/40	0.5	90%

RIGHTS, THAT AMONG THESE ARE LIFE, LIBERTY, AND THE PURSUIT OF HAPPINESS. THAT TO SECURE THESE RIGHTS, GOVERNMENTS ARE INSTITUTED AMONG MEN, DERIVING THEIR JUST POWERS FROM THE CONSENT OF THE GOVERNED,

3	14/21	.53	20/30	0.6	95%

THAT, WHENEVER ANY FORM OF GOVERNMENT BECOMES DESTRUCTIVE OF THESE ENDS, IT IS THE RIGHT OF THE PEOPLE TO ALTER OR TO ABOLISH IT, AND TO INSTITUTE NEW GOVERNMENT, LAYING ITS FOUNDATION ON SUCH PRINCIPLES AND ORGANIZING ITS POWERS IN SUCH FORM, AS TO THEM SHALL SEEM MOST LIKELY TO

1	14/14	.37	20/20	1.0	100%

EFFECT THEIR SAFETY AND HAPPINESS. PRUDENCE, INDEED, WILL DICTATE THAT GOVERNMENTS LONG ESTABLISHED SHOULD NOT BE CHANGED FOR LIGHT AND TRANSIENT CAUSES AND ACCORDINGLY ALL EXPERIENCE HATH SHOWN, THAT MANKIND ARE MORE DISPOSED TO SUFFER, WHILE EVILS ARE SUFFERABLE, THAN TO RIGHT THEMSELVES BY ABOLISHING THE FORMS TO WHICH THEY ARE ACCUSTOMED. BUT WHEN A LONG TRAIN OF ABUSES AND USURPATIONS

CHART TO BE HELD
14 INCHES FROM EYE

ENGINEERED AND PRODUCED BY
COURIER-JOURNAL LITHO CO., LOUISVILLE 16, KY.

Fig. 3-4, cont'd. Back side of author's disposable near vision test card.

be used to block out the eye not being tested. This leaves the examiner's hands free for projector and notes. Of further value in refining a high dioptric lens is the Halberg (3 cell) trial clip attachable to the spectacle eyepiece for the eye under examination. This increases refractive precision and is especially convenient in determining presbyopic adds over distance corrections or modifying aphakic lenses as worn.

Near visual acuity

Critically derived measurements of near acuity are functionally important not only for quantitation of bifocal strength but also because many occupational and educational demands are primarily for near, because low vision aids are more frequently needed for near than for distance, and because calculations of visual impairment for compensation and insurance purposes weigh both distance and near acuity. Measurements of near acuity are less reproducible (coefficient of reliability, 0.75 to 0.78) and are affected more than measurements simulating infinity (coefficient of reliability, 0.95 to 0.97) by pupillary size, illumination levels, accommodative requirements, refractive errors and type of distance correction, and the impairments of presbyopia. These variables negate somewhat even the most precise size reduction of the 5-minute distance optotype to correspond with the same visual angle at a near reading distance. Dozens of proper names* obfuscate both literature and cataloges to such a degree that the proper numbering of type sizes from *one* as the smallest appears on some cards completely reversed and on others supplanted by metric distances or Snellen-like designation in inches such as 14/14. Near test confusion was particularly eponymized by the 1854 "Schriftscalen" of Eduard Jaeger, which was merely a series of variously sized type selected from

*Landolt, Reid, E. Fuchs, Kuchler, Smee, Striedingen, Birkhauser, Golvin, Miller, Friedman, Evans, Schweigger, Benjamin Franklin, Boettcher, Berens, Hutchinson, Fink, Lebensohn, Guibor, Sloan, Studt-Abel, Good-Lite, Keeler, Stimson, and so on.

materials on hand at the convenience of Jaeger's printer.

Near acuity notations should be based on the Snellen principle of a 1-minute arc of minimal resolution and, for practical comparison to reading needs, should present sentence structure and word arrangements simulating conventional near tasks. The examiner should also be freed from need to look with the patient at the card for verification, thus avoiding time loss or awkward repositioning of either patient or examiner. The card should have a matte finish or minimal glare surface (though dull surfaces commonly predispose to ink spreading, which is intolerable in the small type sizes). My inexpensive card (Fig. 3-4) meets these essentials, provides a Revised Jaeger Standard of notation, gives physiologic approximations for near or distance notations, and includes a rounded-off version of Visual Efficiency (A.M.A.).

Near testing should be done immediately after recording uncorrected distance acuity and before creating the near point disturbances that accompany dilation of the pupils. Excellent near acuity with poor distance acuity at any age suggests myopia and very little astigmatism. Contrariwise, good distance acuity and poor near acuity suggests moderate hyperopia (with little or no astigmatism), presbyopia (usually beginning in the forties), or accommodative (nerve III) impairment. Comparably poor acuity at both near and distance suggests significant astigmatism or significant pathology. Thus the near determination may verify the distance acuity or immediately yield further diagnostic leads.

In near examinations, care must be taken to provide comfortable reading light on the test material, usually in a ratio about threefold greater than the room light. Within moderate limits, resolving power or clinical manifestation of acuity is proportional to increasing illumination. Added light often helps the maturing patient with early involutional disease of the macula but may distinctly handicap the more mature patient with nuclear (axial) lens opacities.

The most definitive examination of near acuity comes after optimal distance correction has been determined and with such correction in place. Once the patient has been properly rendered emmetropic for distance—and there are no cycloplegic effects—a relatively precise, age-correlated near point (punctum proximum) can be measured and the indicated dioptric power of lens adds determined for near working distances. If the near test card is mounted on an "accommodation arm" or extension of a refractor, it is necessary to check adequate focal light on the test card when it is changed from the right (first) to the left (second) eye or when the card must be brought closer than the usual reading distance of 13 to 15 in. to assist subnormal vision by magnification or added dioptric power.

As a valuable check on the accuracy of distance refraction correction, the monocular near blur point should be at almost identical distances in front of each eye. For the average presbyopic patient on monocular testing, this should be set at 14 in.; when both eyes are uncovered (binocular verification) the patient will usually demonstrate a closer blur point by about an inch. If the monocular near blur points are unequal, this first suggests re-examination of the distance correction and only secondarily suggests unequal accommodative power. The latter should be further evidenced by cataractous changes, unequal pupils, or other findings of third nerve impairment.

The position for measuring near acuity has been overemphasized by traditional examiners who are oriented exclusively to trial frame techniques rather than refractors *and* trial frames. Aside from motility problems, particularly those associated with V, A, or X phenomena, there is neither theoretic nor practical necessity to make near measurements in vertically altered lines of gaze rather than through a properly positioned refractor. It is essential to know the patient's occupational near range requirements; rarely these will be *upward* in certain control engineers or electronic specialists actually working at times inside

equipment with overhead elements. Measurements through a refractor generally give more precise linear control than can be secured with a trial frame. Additionally, the frame with two or three lenses slipped in place and often with insufficient pantoscopic tilt of the eyepiece produces misleading marginal aberrations that underestimate the final near acuity achievable with a single lens having its lower edge properly tilted almost into contact with the malar eminences.

PRELIMINARY EXAMINATION OF BROWS, LIDS, CONJUNCTIVA, AND ADNEXA
Brows

Configuration of the brow is normally symmetric and should be observed for loss of hair, particularly from the temporal ends. Hypothyroidism is often responsible for such loss and is further indicated by roughness or puffiness of the skin. In areas where leprosy is endemic, it is frequent to find loss of the eyebrows as one of the early and classic manifestations of the disease.

Seborrhea of the brows is often a concomitant of similar disturbances producing oily scales throughout the scalp and along the cilia of the lids. This is a frequent cause of chronic marginal blepharitis.

Movement of the brows should be noted for evidence of integrity of the upper divisions of the facial nerve, which also supply the orbicularis oculi muscle, which is responsible for closing the lids. Unilateral impairment of brow movement indicates peripheral rather than central impairment of nerve VII because the brows receive bilateral central innervation.

Lids
Lid structure

The lids participate in essentially all of the dermatologic disturbances that plague the body. The skin of the lids is the thinnest and most delicate of any skin surface and therefore some dermatologic diseases present here with greater functional disturbance than similar processes elsewhere. The chronic dry scaling of atopic dermatitis or neuro-dermatitis produces darkening and inelasticity of the lids, which is also prognostically related to the development of dermatogenic cataracts.

Mechanical disturbances involving relaxation and redundancy must be noted for their weight, unattractive appearance, and, particularly in the upper lids, their awning-like restriction of upward field. When this is a relaxation of the skin alone, it is commonly called *dermatochalasis*. When it relates to recurrent lid edema or is compounded by two or three pockets of fat herniation forward through defects in the septum orbitale (or rarely when it is related to systemic trichinosis), it is referred to as *blepharochalasis*. The weight of these disturbances in the lower lid may pull the lid border from the globe, causing a mechanical ectropion. If the lower tear punctum is also dragged forward, this is marked by epiphora over the lid border onto the cheek. Correct diagnosis of cause may eliminate disturbances producing intermittent edema, but the most frequent varieties are related to maturity. Here, correct diagnosis, followed by appropriate excision and septal repair if needed, usually leads to major cosmetic and significant functional improvement.

Redness and parchment-like consistency of the lid skin with minor swelling and moderate itching suggest an allergic or sensitivity reaction. This may be accompanied by pale edema (chemosis) of the conjunctiva. Such findings call for diagnostic elimination of all possible skin allergens including soaps and cosmetics, search for environmental allergens, and, often, skin testing for hypersensitivity.

Any skin tumor or cancer that develops elsewhere may also appear in the lids, and the lower lid is particularly susceptible to basal cell carcinoma. All painless circumscribed areas of skin thickening without discoloration should be considered to be possible malignancies until proved otherwise. The yellowish infiltration of xanthelasma, particularly radiating from the inner canthal area, may be associated with elevated serum lipid fractions. Any such circumscribed yellowish or lipid-type deposition calls for careful study of serum cholesterol and other lipids in order to decide whether medical therapy or surgical excision is needed.

Edema or painless diffuse swelling of the lids in the absence of trauma or inflammation indicates a check for systemic retention of fluid as in heart or kidney failure. The eye examiner should extend the inspection to the pretibial area in search of pitting edema—always of pathologic importance—as revealed by digital pressure.

Painful, tender, and inflamed masses in the lid suggest infections or possibly occult foreign bodies. Palpation of fluid-filled or fluctuant masses without pulsation suggests incision for drainage and possible culturing of released material if it appears purulent.

Chronic redness and irritation is often overlooked when resulting from low-grade chronic inflammation in the lash follicles or the meibomian (tarsal) glands. All such irritable eyes and lids should have careful inspection of the lashes for scaly or seborrheic debris about their bases. This is related rarely to pediculosis of the lashes or commonly to *Demodex* mites in the follicles, which may be evidenced by excreta on the cilia. In doubtful cases of chronic lid border irritation a few lashes may be pulled individually and their bulbs inspected under the high power of the slit lamp ($30\times$ to $40\times$) to reveal the *Demodex*, which has a body diameter slightly less than the diameter of the cilia.

Lumpiness or thickening in the vertical patterns of the meibomian glands as seen through the tarsal conjunctiva or secretions localized over their orifices on the lid borders suggests chronic inflammation of these glands and indicates a need for mechanical expression. This is easiest done by the examiner's thumbnails bringing the conjunctival surfaces of the upper and lower lids together. Gentle pressure, though somewhat uncomfortable to the patient, will often deliver through the lid border orifices offending and inspissated secretions that must be eliminated before clearing of lowgrade infections can be expected. Bacteriologic culturing and testing of colonies for antibiotic sensitivity is not obligatory in initial therapy. If adequate response is not achieved in a few weeks of treatment, however, then careful bacteriologic and sensitivity studies are indicated.

Lid function

Following evaluation of the appearance, structure, and abnormalities of the lid substance, it is essential to evaluate the closing and opening mechanisms. Impairments of closing predispose the cornea to drying, ulceration, and secondary infection, whereas impairments of opening may render the eye visually useless.

Orbicularis function and lid closure. Facial (nerve VII) paralysis or Bell's palsy is usually a peripheral interruption in the nerve interfering with brow motion as well as orbicularis closure. Physiologically, the lid borders should come into smooth apposition without forceful exertion. When there is poor closure some corneal protection is afforded by the physiologic Bell's phenomenon of upward rotation of the eye on attempted closure.

In questionable or mild orbicularis paresis, closure strength of this muscle should be qualitatively and comparatively assessed. The examiner should separate the patient's lids with the thumb and first finger of each hand, spreading the lids toward the bony orbital rim. The patient is exhorted to close both lids as forcefully as possible. By varying the separation force of the thumb and forefingers, the examiner attains a quantification of innervational force.*

Ectropion and lid relaxation from other than facial nerve impairment should be evaluated for senile (atonic) or other causative mechanisms. Sometimes cicatricial scarring below the lid border actively pulls the lid away from the globe with the similar disruptive effect of causing lacrimal

*Less recommended are a variety of lid border dynamometers, contact shells with rubber balloons, and contact levers as by D. Miller, H. K. Muller, H. Jacobs, and W. Straub and E. W. Burton.

punctal eversion. This leads to epiphora. Cicatricial scarring may follow lacerations, thermal or chemical burns, or postradiation atrophy, which is usually accompanied by epilation and depigmentation.

Exaggerated closure may be unilateral or bilateral and, at times, very incapacitating. Protective *ptosis* or *lid closure* may be initiated by corneal ulceration and chronic or acute injuries to the epithelium. This appears bilateral following epithelium damage from ultraviolet exposure, such as actinic keratoconjunctivitis, welder's flash, or snow blindness. It is diagnosed by fluorescein staining, which shows punctate destruction of the epithelium, particularly in the exposed interpalpebral area. Acute extraocular muscle paralysis often produces voluntary unilateral protective closure. This is diagnosed by the patient's ability to open the eye on request, thus revealing an ocular deviation and a subjective complaint of diplopia.

Severe photophobic disturbances usually relate to active disease involvement of the cornea. Classically, the extreme photophobia of childhood or youth that causes a youngster to crawl under the bed or to bury his face in a pillow relates to bilateral interstitial keratitis of congenital syphilis, phlyctenular keratitis with round cell infiltrations of the limbus or cornea, or congenital glaucoma with stretching of the globe. The diagnosis of one of these three conditions can almost be guaranteed on the basis of history from the parents and the avoidance behavior of the child. In areas where acute trachoma is endemic, this process may also create similar, though slightly less, photophobia in its initial stages.

Blepharospasm may result from acute trigeminal nerve irritation by foreign bodies or abrasions, but under these circumstances it is unilateral and relieved by diagnostic instillation of topical anesthetics. Essential or functional blepharospasm is usually a severe bilateral problem of psychiatric origin causing great withdrawal and distress by the patient and those around him. The patient often affects digital elevation of his lids but, on quiet discussion, may be shown to have voluntary opening power. In more entrenched blepharospasms (sometimes referred to as conversion hysteria) there is total inability to open the lids. A local anesthetic block of the facial nerve or brief general anesthesia is necessary to gain visualization of the globe in order to rule out pathology in it. The individual with advanced parkinsonism may also be plagued by bilateral blepharospasm.

Levator function and lid opening

Ptosis. Elevation of the upper lid is normally carried out by the levator muscle, which has common embryologic origin with the superior rectus muscle and also shares with it common innervation by the superior division of the oculomotor or third cranial nerve. Examination of the ptotic individual requires careful estimation of residual levator function, which must be differentiated from frontalis muscle assistance. It is usually necessary for the examiner to hold the soft tissues in the brow region firmly against the underlying bone of the skull in order to eliminate frontalis muscle activity in a patient who has resorted to this in compensation for a levator impairment. Localized muscular dystrophy is often suggested when the superior rectus muscle is impaired concurrently with the levator and a hypotropia exists.

Evaluation of ptosis also requires careful examination of downward rotations, because localized levator dystrophies and fibrous replacements of the elastic muscle tissue often limit the downward excursion of the lid during depressed gaze. This is called lagophthalmos. Such lid limitation in downward gaze accompanying ptosis will restrict the amount of surgical resection of the levator that can be done in planning for improvement of the primary position.

It is helpful to measure the vertical width of the interpalpebral fissure at its midpoint in the (1) primary position, (2) maximally depressed gaze, and (3) maximally elevated gaze, in order to quantitate in millimeters the amount of ptosis and lid lag in each eye.

Though congenital (bilateral or unilateral) and often hereditary ptosis is the most com-

mon anomaly of the lids, differential consideration must always be given to neurogenic and myasthenic mechanisms. Congenital ptosis remains throughout life, is affected only slightly by fatigue, and may become worse in late adult years. Testing for myasthenia gravis should be done particularly in older males and younger females having a history indicating increasing ptosis with fatigue. Usually the disease is acquired rather than congenital. One of the simplest tests in the partially ptotic individual is to open and close the lids rapidly twenty or thirty times. This usually increases the ptosis in myasthenia gravis. Variable diplopia (caused by involvement of extraocular muscles), jaw weakness, and difficulty in swallowing are further diagnostic signs of myasthenia.

The most specific test is intravenous injection of edrophonium chloride (Tensilon,* 10 mg./ml.) in dosages of 1 to 10 mg. For adults, the entire 1-ml. test dose (10 mg.) is taken into a tuberculin syringe and the needle inserted into an antecubital vein. Two milligrams is given and the needle is left in place. A positive improvement in ptosis should be noted within 45 seconds; if this is not seen, then the remaining 8 mg. is injected. Failure to attain distinct improvement in the ptosis after this second injection is a valid negative test. Dosage should be reduced by weight for children, administering 1 mg. for a weight of 75 pounds. All effects are usually over within a few minutes.

A less pleasant and more time-consuming alternate test, established by M. B. Walker in 1934, involves the use of neostigmine bromide (Prostigmin,* 1-ml. vials of 1:1,000, 1:2,000, and 1:4,000) by subcutaneous or intramuscular injection. One or two milligrams in an adult usually produces improvement in 15 to 30 minutes. Children may at times require the full adult dose, but the amount may be scaled down to 1/50 mg. in the newborn. All effects are usually over in 45 to 60 minutes.

Side effects of nausea, vomiting, intestinal

---

*Roche Laboratories, Nutley, New Jersey 07110.

peristalsis, urinary evacuation, bradycardia, and bronchial secretions are infrequent but more marked with Prostigmin than with Tensilon. A syringe containing 1 mg. atropine sulfate ready for intravenous or subcutaneous injection should be available whenever such cholinergic agents are injected.

Upper lid tucking or lid retraction. As the reverse of blepharoptosis, some patients present with tucking of the upper lids and deepening of the upper lid folds. This is usually bilateral, though frequently asymmetric, and classically is associated with hyperophthalmic Graves' disease (thyrotoxic exophthalmos) and its concomitants of tachycardia, nervousness, heat intolerance, and weight loss. With nystagmus, paralysis of upward gaze, or multiple sclerosis, such lid retraction may be evidence of major pathology in the brainstem.

Conjunctiva

The conjunctiva, normally a smooth, glistening, and essentially transparent mucosal layer, flexibly unites the lids and globes with well-moistened appositional surfaces. It extends from tight attachment on the inner surface of the lids (palpebral portion), through loose folds in the fornices (cul-de-sac portion), to an intermediate degree of attachment to the anterior globe (bulbar portion). In the circumferential area extending 2 or 3 mm. from the limbus, it becomes firmly attached to the globe.

In the bulbar and lower lid portions it is easily accessible to direct inspection by instructed rotation of the globe and gentle downward traction of the lower lid. Inspection of the upper palpebral and cul-de-sac portions is slightly more difficult because of the protective reflexes and the presence of the levator structures blending with the upper tarsal plate. In sensitive individuals, those with some lid spasm, or those harboring acute pathology behind the lid, it is often necessary to instill a topical anesthetic before everting the lid.

Eversion is done while asking the patient to look downward. The examiner grasps the upper cilia between the thumb and forefinger of one hand and "flips" the upper lid with finger pressure directed downward against the upper edge of the tarsal plate. Often this pressure can be directed more precisely or more effectively with the end of a cotton-tipped applicator or match stem (Fig. 3-5, *A*). This eversion still does not expose the upper cul-de-sac, which may harbor foreign bodies as large as a BB. For such exposure a lid everter such as the Walker (Fig. 3-5, *B*, right and left) or a lid retractor such as the Desmarres must be pressed gently above the upper edge of the tarsal plate (Fig. 3-5, *C*) and the lid pulled upward over the instrument. The curved end of the instrument then will press forward the cul-de-sac tissues, permitting identification and removal of foreign debris or study of the characteristics of this area where lymphomatous masses and chronic viral inflammations may be manifest.

The conjunctiva is the portion of the eye most frequently involved in bacterial and viral inflammations. Fortunately, these inflammations tend to be contained and generally accessible to microbiologic diagnosis; they endanger vision only by corneal extension. Unfortunately, most conjunctival infections produce very little immune reaction and tend to involve the similar epithelium of the cornea, but the process here is commonly mild. At times, however, it can be rapidly destructive and resistant to most antibiotic therapy. Practically every pathogen that attacks the body can be harbored in or infect the conjunctiva. In addition a few pathogens, particularly viruses such as the large trachoma virus, seem to appear almost exclusively in the conjunctiva or cornea.*

The spectrum of neoplastic disease in the conjunctiva is also similar to that of tumors affecting epithelial membranes elsewhere. Fortunately, the conjunctiva is easily available for excisional biopsy of suspect lesions. This may be done rather widely because

---

*Epidemiologic studies of the 1970s suggest an identical virus may also cause significant infection of the cervix and vagina.

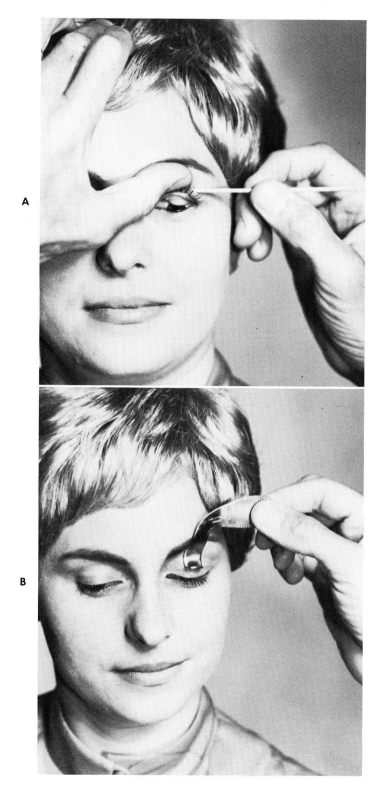

Fig. 3-5. A, Eversion of upper lid with aid of applicator directing pressure at upper edge of tarsal plate. B, Walker lid everter for left upper lid. C, Double eversion of upper lid exposing conjunctiva of the cul-de-sac over curved tip of Walker everter.

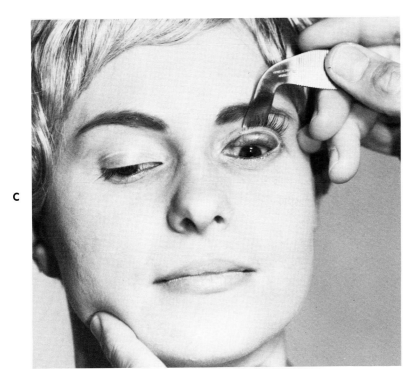

c

Fig. 3-5, cont'd. For legend see opposite page.

of the easy mobility of bulbar and cul-de-sac conjunctiva to cover defects. In melanotic changes possibly indicating malignancy, almost half of the bulbar conjunctiva may be excised and still afford easy repair by sliding to cover the defect.

Adnexa

Lacrimal glands. Normally the lacrimal glands are inconspicuous in their location at the superior temporal portion of the orbital rim. The upper lid configuration, which commonly gives an S-shaped curve to the upper lid with downward depression in the outer third of the border, should be noted for swellings in this area. Ordinarily, on eversion of the upper lids, with the gaze directed straight down, the lacrimal glands do not herniate. If the gaze, however, is directed down and to the opposite side and the upper lid retracted temporally while it is everted, it is usually possible to visualize the palpebral lobe of the gland. In advanced years, there is a physiologic tendency for the gland to drop downward and be visualized more easily. As in many other ocular evaluations, it is most important to compare the appearance of the right and left structures.

In young people, the gland may be involved in congenital, benign tumors. In mid- and later life, the glands may be symmetrically enlarged with blood dyscrasias. The lacrimal glands are histologically almost identical to the salivary glands and generally may show any pathologic process or malignancy that the salivary glands can develop. Such local malignancies are most often unilateral, and the highly lethal mixed cell tumor is one of the more common. Tender, red, and painful swelling of localized infection or abscess occurs but is unusual.

Preauricular gland. The preauricular gland, a lymph node, is generally located anterior to the tragus of the ear or over the condyle of the mandible. It is the first interceptor station of lymphatic drainage from the lids, conjunctiva, and associated superficial adnexal structures. Thus both acute and chronic infections of the lids or conjunctiva may cause enlargement, lowgrade pain, moderate tenderness, and rarely redness at this site. The gland is ordinarily neither tender nor palpable unless involved by inflammatory disease. Its involvement is an index of the severity of the infectious process. It rarely participates in diffuse disturbances of the lymphatic system.

Orbit

The orbit is a complex, rigid, conic receptacle constituted by seven bones and primarily serving as a protective housing for the globe and its appendages. Its major anterior opening or "base" affords access to the globe plus suspension for the lids. Its major posterior opening or optic foramen at the orbital apex affords passageway for the optic nerve and its attendant supporting structures, connecting via the optic chiasm to the brain. Two further major openings, the superior orbital (sphenoidal) fissure and the inferior orbital (sphenomaxillary) fissure, are of diagnostic and x-ray importance. Several medium-sized openings (infraorbital canal, superior orbital foramen or notch, the nasolacrimal canal) may also be identified by special x-ray examinations, but numerous and more variable small openings for arteries, veins, and nerves are generally of obscure diagnostic identification.

Thickness of the orbital bones varies widely from the extremely thin lamina papyracea of the ethmoid bone, which may actually contain bony dehiscences, to the usually strong and massive superior orbital margin. With advancing years, there is thinning of the periosteum and also of the bone, particularly in the roof and lateral wall areas.

Angulations of the orbital bones vary widely from outward angulation in embryologic life and early childhood to various final positions that may be measured on submentovertex x-ray films (p. 240). This varies not only among individuals but also among races. The mechanical position or angulation of the orbits appears to have a positional influence on the globes in about one-fourth of nonparalytic and nonaccommodative horizontal strabismus patients.

Because the orbit has common boundaries with paranasal sinuses above (frontal), medially (ethmoids), and below (maxillary), it is vulnerable to the transmission of infection or neoplasm from these structures.

Diagnostic examination of the orbit (see also pp. 238-243) primarily involves the following:

A. Preliminary inspection for:
   1. Lid swelling and distortion: this may be collateral edema from deep orbital cellulitis, paranasal sinus infection, mechanical stretching of the lids by a tumor mass, or secondary to kidney or heart decompensation.
   2. Secretions and discharge from the conjunctiva or from the homolateral nasal passage: the latter may represent primary nasal disease extending into the orbit or, less commonly, drainage from lacrimal infection into the nose.
   3. Disturbances of the rim contours: these may be from traumatic fracture displacement, neoplastic erosion (better seen on x ray), or, rarely, inflammatory thickening of the periosteum.
   4. Congestion and edema of the conjunctiva: this may be caused by superficial and local infection or by deeper infection that has extended across the conjunctival barrier.
   5. Vascular anomalies evident in the lids or conjunctiva: these may be histologically benign hemangiomas or serious distensions of deep vessels following carotid artery–cavernous sinus fistula.
   6. Exophthalmic displacement of the globe: this may be directly forward, such as from a mass within the muscle cone, or obliquely, in relation to masses localized elsewhere in the orbit.
   7. Impaired rotation of the globe in any direction: orbital tumors and inflammatory disturbances may directly in-

vade and limit these muscles or by their mass may inhibit rotation in their direction. At other times, inflammation, trauma, or neoplasm may interrupt the nerve supply to given extraocular muscles without mechanical restrictions; in these cases, passive or forced ductions by the examiner are usually free.

B. Palpation of the orbit for:
1. Any masses accessible to the exploring fingertip applied through the lids.
2. Comparison of retrobulbar resistance in the two orbits: this is easily done by simultaneous thumb pressure against each globe through the closed lids (Fig. 3-6).
3. Tactile evaluation of the orbital rims: rarely a linear fracture or bone mobility resulting from fracture will be revealed by careful palpation and comparison of right and left orbital rims, even when such defects do not appear on x-ray films.

Fig. 3-6. Tactile comparison of retrobulbar resistance in the two orbits by simultaneous direct thumb pressure against each globe through the closed lids.

4. The usually clean finger ophthalmologist should also remember the value of diagnostic palpation of the zygomatic arches through the upper buccal mucosa by sliding his thumbtip laterally and upward from the canine fossa of the maxilla. The examiner's thumb should be insinuated pulp tip outward within the bony arch; this position also is of assistance later in elevating a depressed or tripod fracture of the arch.

C. Ophthalmoscopy for:
1. Venous congestion indicating impairment of return blood flow from the globe.
2. Arterial pulsations or arterial insufficiency indicating compression of the arterial supply by increased intraorbital pressure or secondarily increased intraocular pressure (compression glaucoma).
3. Striations, usually horizontal, at the posterior pole, as evidence of compression against the back curve of the globe.

D. Auscultation for vascular sounds or bruits (pp. 244-245).

E. Roentgenographic examination: standard skull views, special projections, laminography.

F. Ultrasound examination (pp. 268-280).

G. EMI scan of computerized axial tomography.

This is probably the most productive addition to diagnostic studies of ocular and orbital anatomy since the introduction of ultrasound. The head scanner, developed by G. M. Hounsfield, was introduced for clinical use in England in 1972 and in the United States in June 1973. It is a large instrument incorporating a stretcher unit on which the patient reclines with his head fixed in a soft rubber, water-filled cap. Two minute x-ray beams make linear scans of the head at intervals of 10° through a rotation of 180°. The beams of protons generate a matrix of 160 × 160 displays or 25,600 reference areas in each "cut." These "cuts" are 8 to 13 mm. in thickness. Modifications developed in 1975 at Columbia-Presbyterian Hospital make possible thinner scans of 2 to 3 mm. that show excellent detail of the optic nerve and extraocular muscles.

Detector crystals receive and register beam densities as 500 shades of white and 500 shades of black or a differential range of 1000 levels for each locus of the scan matrix. This is a far greater grey scale than afforded by conventional radiography or xeroradiography, even with the aide of substraction printing or image amplification. Each of the two dimensional printouts in grey scale yields a familiar reference frame similar to a transverse x-ray tomogram of the skull. Thus the problem of the examiner's orientation as in viewing A-scan or M-scan ultrasound displays is eliminated. Examination time is about 30 minutes in an efficient x-ray department.

The unit is exquisitely valuable in defining the optic nerves, extraocular muscles, soft tissue masses, brain infarcts, hematomas, cysts, or other tumors. It is less helpful in differentiating orbital inflammatory change as in Graves' disease or pseudotumor. In the search for neoplastic masses of the head, however, it usually exceeds all data attainable by ventriculography or pneumoencephalography, and frequently makes carotid angiography unnecessary. Lesions within the optic canal, however, may still require direct neurosurgical visualization for diagnosis. In the papilledema of pseudotumor cerebri, the EMI scanner as a single procedure offers maximum security in ruling out intracranial neoplasms.

TRANSILLUMINATION AND CONTACT ILLUMINATION

The transillumination and contact illumination methods of diagnosing structural changes in the visual apparatus have been rendered less essential by improvements in (1) binocular indirect ophthalmoscopy, especially of the peripheral fundus, (2) direct and indirect gonioscopy of the anterior chamber angle, (3) slit lamp examination of both the posterior pole and peripheral fundus with the aid of contact lenses, (4) bone-free x-ray films of the lids and anterior segment using dental film, and (5) ultrasonography with its ability to penetrate opaque media and to differentiate solid from cystic lesions.

Almost any small light of medium to moderate intensity can be used if it is fitted with an opaque collar or tubular shield to reduce the distraction of lateral light scattering. The Finnoff transilluminator, supplied in straight, angular, and extended length heads by various manufacturers (Welch Allyn, Propper, National), is a standard item for lid and anterior bulbar transillumination and can also be used as a general inspection torch. The small, curved Lancaster-Boehm (1913) transilluminator of stainless steel has a greatly reduced diameter compared to the Finnoff. The two types of minute, 1½-volt bulbs manufactured for this unit provide either end lighting or side lighting directed toward the concavity of the carrier shaft. The instrument may be sterilized for use through a conjunctival incision or for retrobulbar transillumination at surgery. Engraved markings encircle the shaft at 1-cm. intervals, so the position or depth of the bulb can be recorded during use. Both the very small diameter and the tendency for the lamps to heat render the Lancaster transilluminator unpleasant or painful when pressed deep into the conjunctival cul-de-sac. The MIRA High Intensity Transilluminator with straight and right angle probes is fitted to a 5-ft. long, flexible, fiber optic bundle and therefore yields cold light at its tip. The remote light source is 150 watts, but there is neither heat nor discomfort from the tip.

External transillumination is of differential value in examination of the *lids*, the *globe*, and the *orbit*. So-called transpupillary transillumination—a fundamental step in genesis of the ophthalmoscope—is of value in identifying opacities in the media. This is best done with a direct ophthalmoscope held a foot or two away from the pupil and facilitating coincidence of the examiner's line of vision with the line of illumination. By shifting the examiner's line of observation laterally, transpupillary transillumination is of some value in examining the coats of the eye anterior to the equator. This may reveal scleral thinning, pigment loss, cysts, staphylomas, ruptures, or intramural foreign bodies.

Intraoral or indirect light from a bright source within the mouth will, at times, transilluminate a clear cyst within the globe or orbit and differentiate it from opaque solid masses such as neoplasms or hematomata.

Contact illumination through the center of the anesthetized cornea may be done with the Finnoff illuminator or the fiber optic end tip of the MIRA instrument. Drance, in 1963, refined corneal contact illumination and designed an illuminator with a concave face that fits the central or pars optica surface. This is helpful in identifying the elusive limbal area and the proximal limit of the anterior chamber angle, particularly following mobilization of a conjunctival flap at the time of anterior segment surgery.

Transillumination of the lids from the inner surface with the aid of topical anesthesia will usually resolve any question of solid versus cystic mass in the lid and may be pivotal in ruling out or localizing a radiolucent foreign body.

Transscleral transillumination generally requires topical anesthesia. This technique is particularly essential when a pigmented lesion of the iris, the limbus, or the ciliary body is under study. Benign cystic lesions in these areas usually appeared dark in focal illumination but bright in transillumination. Eyes have been needlessly removed under the impression that such masses are malignant melanomas (the latter are opaque). Anterior scleral transillumination may be of assistance in identifying iris pigment loss, configuration of the pupil in the presence of corneal opacity, or even opaque foreign bodies hidden within a cataract. Difficulties of light positioning and irregularities of scattering make transillumination progressively less accurate in more proximal portions of the globe. Observation through the pupil of such transillumination, however, may reveal opaque (solid) masses beneath a retinal detachment or clear cysts in more peripheral sites. An extension of this technique is the Osmond (1954) combination of 12-volt transilluminator and annular diathermy electrode. This is available as a separate unit or adapted to fit major Keeler ophthalmoscopes. It may be employed at surgery to aid in localization of retinal holes during ophthalmoscopy. Similarly, for office indirect ophthalmoscopy, scleral depressors are available (Univis) with cool, fiber-optics illumination for the gadgeteer.

When there is gross reduction of vision to the level of poor light projection or questionable light perception, transscleral transillumination can elicit entoptic observation of the retinal blood vessels in the presence of a large hyphema, mature cataract, or dense blood staining the cornea. If retinal function is retained behind such opacities, the intelligent patient may describe a very helpful "map" of branching vascular shadows throughout his retinal area. This gives better geographic data with much less equipment and time than is involved in electroretinography.

INSTRUMENTAL REFRACTIVE SCREENING

Refractometers or optometers have gone through approximately a century of development, but in North America have largely been superseded by refinements of retinoscopy and cycloplegic examinations. Aside from automated objective refractors, there are four major instruments currently marketed, the Kuhl-Rodenstock, (1922-1927), the Hartinger (1937), the Arnulf-Essilor Retinofocometer (1952), and the Topcon. Basically each requires clear media and use of the retina as a diffusing screen from which reflections of incident light are manipulated. With the Kuhl-Rodenstock and Arnulf-Essilor instruments, the examiner determines a correcting lens power to obtain a "best focus." The Hartinger and the Topcon operate by the more exacting focusing system of "coincidence"; this permits a vernier adjustment and reading by the superior aligning capability of the examiner's eye rather than less critical resolving power. A continuing problem is control of accommodation. This does not bear on the aphakic and absolutely presbyopic individuals. In general, however, cycloplegia affords better baseline accuracy with these instruments.

Fixation systems and setting of the instrument to an appropriate working distance have been difficult, but the Kuhl-Rodenstock instrument ingeniously focuses a luminous ring on the iris, which generally positions the instrument at the correct working distance. Most American examiners have declined these relatively large table top instruments, favoring the simplicity and maneuverability of the hand-held streak retinoscope.

Although the Rodenstock, Hartinger, and Topcon refractors have not gained popularity in the United States, they have kept alive an interest in such technique particularly in Europe. Following World War II increasing interest in automation, refinements of servo loop mechanisms, and miniaturization of

computers laid the groundwork for automated objective refractometry. From the early and mid 1950s, technologic developments in the United States and England produced relatively crude infrared optometers.

In the United States, Aron Safir, M.D., of New York in cooperation with Bausch and Lomb technicians brought forth the B & L Safir Ophthalmetron (patented in 1964), which operates from infa-red imaging on the retina. The instrument is actually a far point retinoscopic scanning device that makes 720 scans per second progressing throughout 180° in 3 seconds; thus registering a curve plotted on 2160 retinoscopic evaluations. These are computer converted to conventional notations as spheres, cylinders, and axes. This instrument, as well as the following two, utilizes basically three subsystems that (1) monitor the alignment of the instru-

Fig. 3-7. Safir B & L Ophthalmetron in use showing examiner verifying ocular alignment and prepared to actuate examination by push-button control with his right hand. (Bausch and Lomb.)

ment, (2) present a target stimulus, and (3) measure the derived imaging (Fig. 3-7). A second infrared objective refractometer based on servo-retinoscopy is the 6600 Autorefractor of Acuity Systems, Inc., McLean, Virginia, developed by Tom Cornsweet, Ph.D., Alan Rider, and Stephen Garden, Ph.D.

These two instruments operate on different retinoscopic assumptions, and the 6600 is even larger than the Safir Ophthalmetron, which can be placed on a conventional examining table. The Acuity Systems 6600 is a floor pedestal unit of considerable rectangular bulk and forced air cooling (Fig. 3-8). Averaged measurements are recommended. Maximum myopic readings are about 9 D and maximum cylinders are about 5 D.

A third instrument of this type is a further computerized and miniaturized Dioptron produced by Coherent Radiation of Palo Alto, California (Fig. 3-9). Programming to reduce intertest variability prolongs readout time to about 30 sec. to 1 min.

Minimal operational needs for these instruments are a patient who can remain quiet and fixate for a few seconds to a minute, a generally clear cornea, little or no nystagmus, a pupillary diameter of 3 mm. or more, no or mild cataractous changes. The instruments offer advantage in examining illiterates, the deaf, those people with limited mentality, and those people who are poor responders in the objective and subjective steps of refraction.

Aside from difficulties in designing nonaccommodative visual stimuli, the longstanding problem of the near reflex as a patient brings his head toward or into any instrumental device tends to affect the spheri-

Fig. 3-8. Infrared, Auto Refractor 6600. (Acuity Systems, Inc., McLean, Virginia 22101.)

Fig. 3-9. Dioptron infrared refractor. (Coherent Radiation, Palo Alto, California 94304.)

cal results. In many examinations of my own eyes there has been vigorous reassurance that I have more than a diopter and a half of accommodation at age 53, but a vexing spread of plus values. This problem is generally minimized in cycloplegic examinations. Most users thus far espouse the Ophthalmetron and similar optometers as affording baseline equivalents of retinoscopy that usually need subjective refinement and verification. Multiple readings and discarding of unusually deviant printouts increase accuracy.

These complex and expensive machines have "individualities." Generally, alert technicians of high school graduate level learn to operate them in a few hours and become attuned to their problems or forthcoming malfunctions. Office technicians enjoy their operational role with suitable patients and providing data that are as near final as possible. Patients are pleasantly relieved of worri-

some subjective decisions and unfortunately impressed by the sound and light of the system. Continuing refinement suggests that these may become near total refracting instruments for large numbers of patients, but particularly the aphakes and the clear media cycloplegic individuals. Groups of examiners, family practitioners, or primary care physicians should anticipate the incorporation of automative refraction as a future office screening routine. This, in more modern complexity, calls back images of general practitioners several decades ago who frequently used trial cases in their general practice along with the full spectrum of medicines and treatments of the day (Safir, 1972).

MALINGERING, EXAGGERATION, AND HYSTERICAL LOSS OF VISION

Unexplained reductions in acuity or inconsistencies between subjective and objective findings raise serious concern of exaggera-

Fig. 3-10. Hand-held Kotowski Visumeter with motor-driven oscillation of grating light pattern projected on the fundus. Choice among three pattern sizes (0.1, 0.3, 0.7) will elicit some opticokinetic response even in eyes with limited acuity. (Oculus Optikgeräte, Dutenhofen, Federal Republic of Germany.)

tion, malingering, or hysterical illness. Some apprehension accompanies all disease and, in somatically oriented individuals, tends to produce exaggeration of symptoms in presence of visual loss. Reassurance and careful objectivity usually will quickly separate those who are exaggerating or benignly aggrandizing complaints, as contrasted to the malingerer who is seeking secondary gains such as insurance compensation, avoidance of military service, or excuse from labor. The malingerer is willful and often wily, rather than simplistically distressed as is the exaggerator. Quite differently, the hysterical patient unknowingly deceives himself; he may at first seem unduly indifferent, but is usually intolerant of penetrating or challenging questions and extended examinations. The malingerer, on the other hand, tends to be more evasive or may affect inability to comprehend test procedures.

The patient's own description and manner-

isms often indicate in which of the three areas he falls. Though an hysterical individual may present with functional total blindness, the malingerer usually does not elect such overwhelming visual simulation. It is easier for the malingerer to simulate unilateral or partial visual loss. For those claiming total blindness, sudden strong focal light or physically menacing gestures usually elicit avoidance response. Swinging mirrors, opticokinetic tapes and rotating drums generally evoke irresistible oscillation of the eye in the malingerer though not in the true hysteric nor the individual with organic cortical blindness. A well-schooled or skilled malingerer may occasionally fix his gaze above an opticokinetic stimulus or "look through" the movement, but this is rare. In such circumstances, the motor driven Visumeter ophthalmoscope by Oculus Products (Fig. 3-10) gives an "irresistible" grating pattern of light oscillating across the fundus that produces some opticokinetic response in even a partially sighted eye.

The tests for feigned, unilateral visual loss are based on quickness and cleverness of the examiner in manipulating the constancies of visual physiology. Bruce Miller has classified the array of tests for malingering into those based on constancies of (1) the visual angle, (2) fixation, (3) diplopia, (4) chromatic separation, (5) fogging, (6) polaroid alterations, (7) major amblyoscopic reversing, (8) binocular visual field charting.

The simplest of such tests are based on the visual angle as in reading a conventional Snellen wall chart. Thus, if a patient can read only 20/100 letters at the conventional testing distance of 20 ft., he can be walked half way down the test lane to the chart and should promptly progress to the 20/50 line. Failure to do so suggests fraudulent reporting. The same technique can be used at the tangent screen where physiologically, the outer isopter, the blind spot, or a field defect plotted at one meter should appear twice as large when plotted at two meters. For the patient to report similar sizes at 1/2, 1, or 2 m. is malingering. Another simple maneuver at the tangent screen is to tilt the patient's head 30° off the vertical; with correct reporting, there should be a slightly lesser shift of about 25° in the blind spot or a field defect.

The *displacement test* using a 4 to 6 diopter prism, as in the technique of Von Noorden or Marshall Parks, produces a normal compensatory movement in the *opposite* eye if a claimed monocularly blind eye beneath the prism has fusional capacity.

Fixation tests using the 4 to 8 diopter prism with a focal light usually function as well in claimed partial visual loss as in claimed monocular blindness. In a reading variation, the examiner simply slips a tongue blade into a vertical position midway between reading material and the patient's eyes (Javel-Cuignet Test) while he is reading aloud; with significant visual loss in either eye the patient will hesitate or shift head position to see around the blade. With both eyes open and functioning well he can progress across a line of type without hesitation.

The advent of Polaroid discs, which can be quietly rotated in either cell of a trial frame, give very unalarming test procedures. A Polaroid disc is fitted at axis 90 over one eye and 180 over the other eye. A third or rotary disc in front of the normal eye is inserted in the same axis as the primary Polaroid filter. With both eyes open, the patient is instructed to read test lines and then silently one Polaroid disc is rotated to occlude the normal eye. Such unobtrusive manipulation usually catches the patient off guard, unless he is schooled in rapidly closing either eye in an alternating fashion to keep up with the examination.

Tests with colored lenses (Snellen red/green glasses) using red/green test letters that can be perceived only through the same colored filter are hazardous. The examiner must be certain that he has a precise hue match of color in the test letters and filter in the spectacles. Traditionally the word FRIEND has been used with the three letters F I N in one color, and the alternating letters R E D in another color. Thus the patient would read F I N or R E D if either eye were blind and would read F R I E N D if both eyes were sighted.

Many variations of all of these tests can be evolved and have been described. Inconsistency on the part of the malingerer is the most revealing finding, whereas hysterics tend to be very consistent on reexamination.

Diagnosis must be established by subtle, quick, and unoffensive steps. The final diagnosis must not be arrived at by exclusion, but must be positively determined with data that can be explained to nonmedical third parties. It is preferable not to review the findings of such testing with the patient, but rather to use these as a basis for planned therapy, consultation letters, or testimony (Miller, 1972).

INSTRUMENTAL VISUAL SCREENING

As yet there is no machine substitute for the direct questioning, the skill, and the penetrating analysis of a knowledgeable examiner in either preliminary or definitive examination. Such an individual may perform superbly with minimal or relatively primitive equipment such as a simple Snellen chart and an ophthalmoscope. On the other hand, economy and maximum distribution of care are often efficiently served by nonprofessional screening done by trained volunteers or school, industrial, and highway employees prepared exclusively for such work. A parallel is seen in the teams of X-ray technicians who take preliminary chest x-rays in tuberculosis detection campaigns or office assistants who perform urinalysis in diabetic screening.

Such public health visual screening should be organized and directed by professional personnel skilled in eye diseases and their detection. Very productive screening can be accomplished with quite simple accessories such as a Snellen chart and a flashlight. Instrument manufacturers, however, market a series of variously complex equipment particularly directed to school screening, industrial preemployment evaluations, and driver licensing. Increasing educational, insurance, and safety calls for such procedures, plus the growing population involved, have created significant personnel and instrument markets. At times such programs have yielded a series of instrumentally derived numbers without fully established significance or relation to seeing functions.

Mass visual screening, like objective screening, has been particularly sought by primary educators, military services, and transport licensing agencies. Both mechanical screening prototypes and projection equipment (slides or ciné) have been generally adequate in identifying a cutoff range. They are less accurate, however, in correlation with pathology or unusual circumstances. Individual testing equipment* based on opticonystagmus or interference fringe patterns generated by lasers promise greater accuracy than the mass screeners.

Most of these instruments are outgrowths of the simple stereoscopes such as those developed by Brewster and by Wheatstone in 1838 with their pairs of stereoscopic or disparate targets. In the second half of the nineteenth century pairs of disparate pictures or stereophotographs became very popular for home amusement viewing. Early students of visual physiology turned to mathematically and physiologically designed pairs of printed stereograms with which to study quantitative aspects of binocularity (Stereocomparator of Tourcade, 1900).

An element of automation by self-administration and self-pacing of the test steps has been introduced by Tracor Medical Instruments† in their P. W. Johnston Vision Screener (Series RV-123). This 13-pound table-model unit is based on the three basic requirements of the Massachusetts Vision Test. It screens (1) by use of the "tumbling Snellen E" for simulated distance acuity that may be switched for either 20/30 or 20/40 level, (2) for vertical and horizontal heterophoria by use of a red ball which, as presented to one eye, should be within a green field seen by the other eye, and (3) for hyperopia at the +1.75 or +2.25 diopter level, again by switch selection. The examiner ex-

plains the basic test procedure to the subject and then needs only to monitor the examination, which proceeds automatically at the rate established by the subject pressing "Yes" or "No" buttons for each test. In testing large numbers of subjects, the candidates may be identified by use of numbered tokens inserted in the Yes-No control box.

A Tracor model with a more extensive and complex series of targets including central acuity levels, stereoacuity, and fundamental color recognition is available for industrial use. Model RV-123PN is specifically designed for driver testing programs. It has a horizontal form field attachment that may be inserted at the top of the ocular end of the screener, and a night vision simulator (Fig. 3-11).

The following instruments are currently marketed for visual screening programs or "battery tests" and are designed to be operated by nonprofessional workers after brief instruction.

1. American Automobile Association, N.W. Washington, D.C. 20006
   Driver Evaluator No. 3574 (Federal Stock No. 6910-597-9651)
   The Driver Evaluator is a rugged welded-steel, table-top unit requiring about 13 ft. of available room length to simulate a 20-ft. test distance with a mirror at 10 ft. It provides four tests:
   a. Letters for Snellen acuity notation from 20/100 to 20/13
   b. Near range depth judgment
   c. Horizontal form field
   d. Recognition testing of basic traffic control lights of red, amber, and green
   A fiber case is available for protection during transportation.
2. American Optical Corporation, Safety Products Division, Cleveland, Ohio
   Sight Screener (Model 18010A)
   The first of this series was introduced in 1946 and its numerical findings adapted to Hollerith form reports. Though generally similar to other instruments for this purpose, the Sight Screener differs by using Polaroid double-printed vectographs for targets rather than relying entirely on the Brewster stereoscope principles of viewing horizontally juxtaposed stereograms through base-out prisms. Case is made of cast aluminum and total weight is 22 lbs.
3. Bausch and Lomb, Inc., Rochester, New York 14602
   Under the general trade name Ortho-Rater, Bausch and Lomb introduced its first screening instrument of this series in 1943.

---

*Takata Ophthalmic Instruments Co., Ltd., Tokyo, Japan; (Retinal Visual Acuity Tester EA 250) or Optical Science Group, Inc., San Francisco, California.

†Austin, Texas 78721.

Fig. 3-11. Johnston Tracor Vision Screener designed for driver licensing and industrial examination. Horizontal arc for form field screening attaches above the ocular end to the left. (Tracor Medical Instruments, Austin, Texas 78721.)

Master Ortho-Rater

The Master Ortho-Rater is a self-contained unit with all target slides mounted internally on two manually controlled rotating drums, presenting seven far point tests on one drum and five near point tests on the other. Checkerboard patterns of alternating light and dark squares are easily understood regardless of educational attainment or reading ability. Results of these twelve tests are hand-recorded on a Hollerith-style card, noting gross color screening, central acuity using right eye, left eye, and then both eyes at near and distance, and instrumental representations of vertical and horizontal phorias for near and simulated distance. A Perimeter attachment is available as an auxiliary mounting on the headrest to assess form recognition in the horizontal only. Table space of 10×25 in. is covered by the instrument and it easily adjusts from 23 to 30 in. in height to accommodate the test subject.

Bausch and Lomb also distributes a School Vision Tester and Driver Vision Tester on bases identical with the Titmus T/O Vision Tester.

4. Good-Lite Company, Forest Park, Illinois 60130
The Good-Lite Company, which has produced many durable, simple, and portable illuminated test charts, introduced in 1968 a modification of the remote-controlled Green's Illuminated Vision Charts, under the name Insta-Line Chart. This utilizes a 10-ft. space and can test acuity against crowded (linear) versus isolated optotypes. Standard phoria screening at 6 prism diopters in or out and 1.5 prism diopters up or down is included. This unit, like the A.A.A. Driver Evaluator, avoids the instrumental or proximity factor inherent in completely contained table-top devices.

5. Keystone View Company, Meadville, Pennsylvania 16335

M. R. A. Sherman in conjunction with E. A. Betts developed in 1933 a pioneer line of screening equipment for school use under the name Telebinocular. In the mid- and late 1930s this was modified for industrial use and made more durable. All Telebinoculars are of open construction between the oculars and the stereogram targets. This enables the examiner to monitor the tests under his direct view and to point out areas on the target when he wishes the examinee's attention at a particular point. All models avoid mirrors and have completely interchangeable targets that are produced in a large and varied series. Simple design permits essentially no possibility for internal mechanical jamming or failure. Four models are available:

a. Ophthalmic Telebinocular: most versatile and complex of the line
b. Keystone Orthoscope: lighter and simpler but affording similar measurements as Ophthalmic Telebinocular
c. School Visual Survey Telebinocular: all plastic and less complex than the preceding models
d. Driver-Visual Survey Telebinocular: plastic and of same basic design as others but supplied with highway-type targets and horizontal form field attachment

6. G. Rodenstock Optische Werke, Munich, Germany
Rodenstock Vision Screener R5 for Children

The Rodenstock Screener is a small, light, and plastic-encased instrument of simple Brewster stereoscope principles. It was designed in close cooperation with Dr. C. Cuppers of Giessen. Target pairs are printed on flat discs inserted at the base of the machine at the back. Illiterate Es are used for visual acuity measurement in five gradations. The phoria test is a dot within a rectangle allowing 1 prism diopter of vertical imbalance up or down and 3 prism diopters of exophoria or 1 of esophoria within the established screening limits. Stereoacuity is tested with groups of three Punch and Judy figures; three test settings present one figure out of plane with the other two by 360, 240, and 120 seconds of arc.

Rodenstock Vision Tester-R9 Rodatest

The Rodenstock Rodatest was developed in the mid 1950s by Dr. H. Schober from the basic stereoscope design. Nine pairs of targets are mounted on one drum and viewing conditions may be modified by interposing varying lenses and diaphragms on a second drum. Visual acuity is evaluated by modified Goldmann optotypes (squares subdivided into four smaller squares composed of dots of two different diameters) through ten gradations. Dissimilar targets presented to each eye in the form of a modified Maddox wing are used for rough quantitation of phorias at near and simulated distance. Six sets of stereograms are designed to quantitate stereoacuity from 720 to 22 seconds of arc. Color testing is specifically excluded in favor of more consistent targets that can be made from pigments rather than by transmitted light. The unit is suitable for industrial screening.

7. Titmus Optical Company, Petersburg, Virginia 23803

T/O Vision Tester

The T/O Vision Tester is a lightweight (17 pounds), high impact resistant plastic unit of stereoscopic design with a relatively large drum carrying twelve sets of test slides or stereograms. These may be presented by manual rotation or by push-button controlled electric motor drive. A large number of additional test slides are optional (stereoacuity, color, subnormal vision, peripheral fusion, Massachusetts Vision Test, Michigan Pre-School Test, Driver's License and Traffic Signal Recognition). A horizontal form field perimeter with scale (Model 67) attaches to the top of the Tester.

Titmus Biopter Visual Skills Testing Instrument (Models N104 and N109)

These are minimally expensive, simplified, open construction stereoscopes. They utilize hand-inserted stereograms. A simple scoring sheet presents easily noted findings at a glance. These are probably the least expensive of all screening devices and carry the same accuracy achieved with basic printing of any stereogram. The only electrical connections are for illumination.

8. Carl Zeiss, Jena, German Democratic Republic (East Germany)

Rapid Vision Tester

The Rapid Vision Tester is a heavy, electric motor–driven unit. Stereograms are presented on a drum. Acuity is measured by checkered square patterns. Phorias are measured at 40 cm. and at simulated distance.

Zeiss Stereoscope

The Zeiss Stereoscope is an extremely simple, open-construction instrument without an illuminating system. Stereograms are designed for children and adults. The instrument is also usable orthoptically as a home training instrument.

All of these screening devices must be considered as auxiliary and yielding only partial information that necessitates interpretation and assessment of significance. An intelligent secretary, clerk, or nonprofessional operator, however, can obtain with such equipment preliminary leads that are of value, particularly in mass surveys of industry where thousands of individuals may be involved or in driver licensing programs where millions of people are examined. The nature of patient performance in this test situation is such that overestimation of ability tends not to occur. An inherent source of distress, however, lies in overdetailed numeric findings or instrumental suggestion of deficiency when no significant abnormality exists. A problem of overreferral that tends to discredit the best intentioned surveys or public health programs may be created. Therefore screeners must be used within predetermined ranges of reporting and with planned retesting in borderline cases or uncertain results before considering that such subjects have valid need for more detailed consultation.

No reassurance can be given concerning glaucoma, which is one of the most serious and frequent causes of progressive visual loss in our more mature population.

Table-top compactness, portability, generally self-contained design, potential for multifaceted testing, and results presented in seemingly specific numbers lend attractiveness to these units, particularly for public health workers and mass survey planners. They do not, however, establish ocular diagnosis and can, in the absence of proper patient explanation, be permitted to give a false sense of security to individuals passing the tests.

"The resolution of visual acuity in terms of geometry is to ascribe an unjustified simplicity to a complex and obscure psychological problem."

W. STEWART DUKE-ELDER, 1944

REFERENCES

Guide to the Evaluation of permanent impairment, Chapt. VII: The visual system, pp. 93-101, Chicago, 1971, Am. Med. Assoc.

Keeney, A. H., and Duerson, H. L.: Near vision test card with revised and collated notation, Am. J. Ophthalmol. **46**:592-594, Oct., 1958.

Keeney, A. H., Zaki, H. A.: Role of the bony orbital walls in nonaccommodative, nonparalytic horizontal strabumus, Arch. Ophthalmol. **57**:418-424, Mar., 1957.

Miller, B. W.: A review of practical tests for ocular malingering and hysteria, Survey Ophthalmol. **17**: 241-246, 1972.

Ryan, S. J.: Diagnostic tests employed in macular lesions, Survey Ophthalmol. **17**:94-100, 1972.

Safir, A.: Automatic measurement of the refractive properties of the eye, Med. Res. Eng. **11**:12-20, 1972.

Spencer, P. J., and Ensell, F. J.: Comparison of visual acuity tests and viewing condition interactions, Aerosp. Med. **44**:1290-1294, 1973.

Walker, M. B.: Treatment of myasthenia gravis with physostigmine, Lancet **1**:1200, 1934.

Examination of the pupils

Ben P. Houser, Jr., M.D.

GENERAL PRINCIPLES

Examination of the pupils is not difficult, but attention to detail is imperative. Fundamentally, the pupils constrict (c) in light or in near regard and dilate (d) in darkness or in remote fixation, but subtle variations of these basic responses often aid in neuro-ophthalmic diagnosis. As in all physical examinations, normal ranges must be appreciated in order to identify pathologic variations. Responses of the normal pupil vary with basic room illumination, degree of accommodation, age, refractive state, and other factors.

Evaluation of pupillary responses requires a small flashlight as the basic instrument and in some cases a slit lamp for the fine beam to elicit hemianopic pupillary responses. For the practitioner, the large, expensive, and time-consuming infrared pupillography equipment is not necessary. Most pupillary diagnoses can be made with light and an occluder, plus a few topical drugs.

The most important of the reflexes of the pupil are outlined in Table 1. The light and near reflexes must be preliminary parts of every eye examination.

Pupil is derived from the Latin *pupilla* meaning a little girl. As described by Trevisa in 1398, pupil refers to the tiny image of oneself seen reflected from the mirror-like surface of the cornea of another person's eye. Because the cornea is convex, reflections from its surface create reduced and virtual images. When these appear central in relationship to the cornea, they seem to overlie the pupil, which is actually an aperture in the iris.

The pupil usually appears black because of the nonluminous interior of the globe. It may, however, appear as luminous red if the observer's visual axis is slightly off the patient's visual axis and a separate illuminating source is correspondingly to the opposite side of the patient's axis. The pupil appears white (leukocoria) if a pathologic opacity (e.g. cataract) fills the pupil or a retrolental mass (e.g. retinoblastoma, cyclitic membrane, etc.) blocks the retrolental transmission of light.

Because of magnification of the cornea by its action as a convex lens, the underlying

Table 1. Summary of basic pupillary reflexes

Reflex	Stimulus	Reaction
Light	Light	Bilateral miosis
Near	Accommodation, convergence	Bilateral miosis
Orbicularis (Westphal-Piltz)	Forced closure of lid	Unilateral miosis
Vestibular	Caloric stimulation	Bilateral mydriasis (hippus)
Cochlear	Tuning fork	Mydriasis following brief miosis
Trigeminus	Touching cornea	Miosis following brief mydriasis
Psychosensory	Psychic and stimulation of any sensory nerve	Bilateral mydriasis
Vagotonic	Inspiration, expiration	Mydriasis, miosis

iris details and pupillary diameter appear about ⅛ larger than their actual size. Depth of focus is inversely proportional to pupillary diameter being about 0.01 D at a diameter of 8 mm. and increases to 5 D at 0.2 mm.

ANATOMY

Both the sympathetic and parasympathetic divisions of the autonomic nervous system exercise efferent influences on the pupils. In general, parasympathetic stimuli constrict the pupils by contracting the sphincter muscle in response to light and accommodation. Sympathetic stimuli dilate the pupils by contracting the radial dilator muscle of the iris. Both the sympathetic and parasympathetic systems are in constantly shifting balance. Thus the "resting" size of the normal

pupil is never absolutely static but fluctuates continuously by a minute amount of physiologic hippus, plus alternate dilatation with inspiration and constriction with expiration.

Anatomy of the light reflex pathways

The anatomic pathway of the light reflex (Fig. 4-1) begins in the percipient cells of the retina where apparently specialized rods and cones absorb the light stimulus and initiate electrochemical impulses along the neural path. In the optic nerve these afferent fibers are geographically located in the peripheral or outer aspect. The fibers originating from the nasal hemiretina cross in the chiasm in a distribution similar to related visual fibers. Fibers from the temporal hemiretina traverse the chiasm un-

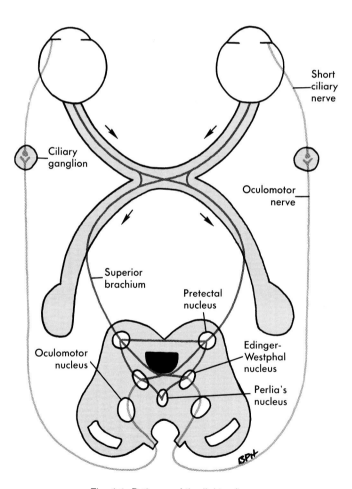

Fig. 4-1. Pathway of the light reflex.

crossed. All these fibers continue in the outer layers of the optic tract. Slightly anterior to the lateral geniculate bodies, they leave the tract and reach the tectum of the midbrain by way of the superior branchium conjunctivum. Synapse occurs in the pretectal nucleus. The fibers then proceed to the Edinger-Westphal nuclei of both sides through the posterior commissure and anterior to the aqueduct of Sylvius. The efferent arc begins at synapses in the Edinger-Westphal nuclei. The efferent fibers then continue posteriorly through the oculomotor nuclei to join the oculomotor nerve. These pupillomotor fibers synapse in the ciliary ganglion and then proceed as postganglionic fibers via the short ciliary nerves to the sphincter muscle of the iris.

Anatomy of the near reflex pathway

The near reflex pathway (Fig. 4-2), though parasympathetic, is controversial. The reflex is an inseparable triad of convergence, accommodation, and miosis. The most probable origin of the near reflex is in the visual cells of the retina, and the pathway is similar to the light reflex path back to the posterior third of the optic tract where the light reflex fibers leave. The near reflex fibers continue with the visual fibers along the geniculostriate radiation from the lateral geniculate body to the occipital cortex. The near reflex fibers then radiate to the frontal oculomotor centers, where they become part of a mass reflex that is mediated through the corticotectal tracts to the oculomotor nucleus.

The portion of the nucleus concerned

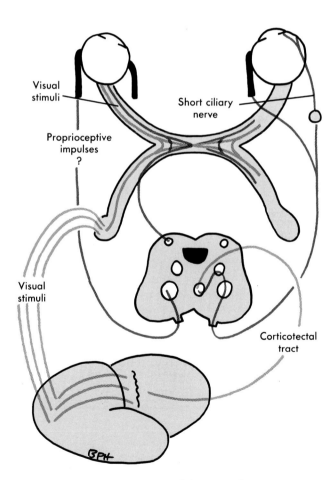

Fig. 4-2. Pathway of the near reflex.

with the near pupillary response is unknown. Perlia's nucleus apparently controls the convergence aspect of the reflex. The near reflex efferent fibers then share a common path with the light reflex fibers along the oculomotor nerve. Probably the fibers destined for the pupillary sphincter first synapse in the ciliary ganglion, or there may be a discrete path separate from the light reflex. This assumption is based on the preservation of the near pupillary reflex after ciliary ganglionectomy. The final common path is along the short ciliary nerves to the sphincter and the ciliary muscle.

Anatomy of the sympathetic pathway

The anatomy of the *sympathetic* pathway (Fig. 4-3) is fairly well established. The afferent impulses come from many sites, notably the cochlea, the skin, and the higher cortical centers of emotion. These arcs are complicated but seem to end in the hypo-thalamus, which apparently is the highest brain center involved in sympathetic control. The preganglionic fibers from the hypo-thalamus collect as a tract passing through the pons and medulla into the intermedio-lateral bundle of the spinal cord. The fibers controlling pupillary dilation leave the cord levels T_1, T_2, and T_3 (designated as Budge's area). The fibers collect into the thoraco-cervical sympathetic trunk and proceed to the superior cervical sympathetic ganglion where the first synapse occurs. Postganglionic fibers (Fig. 4-4) travel along the branches of the carotid artery to enter the globe with the long ciliary nerves to the dilator muscle of the iris. Some fibers pass through the ciliary ganglion without synapsing and enter the globe in the short ciliary nerves with the parasympathetic fibers. Both the sympathetic and parasympathetic fibers converge at the area of the superior orbital fissure (Fig. 4-5), through which they pass

Fig. 4-3. Preganglionic sympathetic pathway.

Thalamus

Superior cervical sympathetic ganglion

Pons

Upper thoracic cord

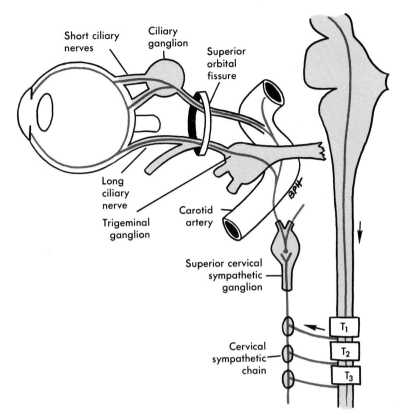

Fig. 4-4. Schema of sympathetic pathway.

Fig. 4-5. Convergence of sympathetic and parasympathetic pathways at the superior orbital fissure.

as the final common pathway of the efferent pupillary system. Lesions at the orbital apex may produce confusing pupillomotor signs by interfering with both systems in their close proximity. For this reason, disease of the eye itself sometimes has an unpredictable effect on the pupil, depending upon balance of the sympathetic and parasympathetic input to the iris muscles.

PUPILLOMOTOR VALENCE OR POWER

The concept of pupillomotor "valence" or "power" helps to evaluate pupillary responses. Each eye has a given pupillomotor power. The size of both pupils in the resting state is determined by the eye that exerts the greater pupillomotor power, providing the motor or efferent pupillary pathways are intact. For example, a lesion of the optic nerve will decrease the pupillomotor power of the involved eye. In the resting state, however, the pupils of both eyes will be equal since the uninvolved eye produces a pupillomotor power that floods the midbrain and is equally distributed and returned to both eyes by way of the efferent pathway. Therefore pupillary inequality in

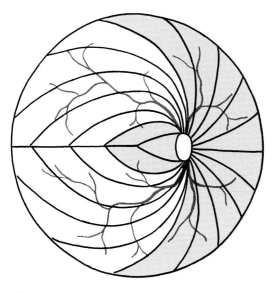

Fig. 4-6. The macular and perimacular areas have the strongest pupillomotor "valence." The nasal hemiretina has a stronger valence than the temporal hemiretina.

the resting state usually suggests a lesion of the efferent pupillary pathway.

Interestingly, a pupillomotor "valence" also exists in the retina (Fig. 4-6). The macular and perimacular areas have the strongest valence. The nasal hemiretina has a stronger pupillomotor valence than the temporal hemiretina. The practical corollary is that similar retinal areas should be stimulated by the test light if the eyes are to be compared. If the nasal retina of one eye receives a bright light and the temporal retina of the fellow eye is stimulated by the same light, the test situation is not bilaterally equal.

TECHNIQUE OF TESTING

Preliminary inspection of both pupils should be made in the resting state in normal room illumination. While the patient is fixating at distance, note the size, equality, regularity, color of irides, and the presence of synechiae. Light response should be elicited while having the patient fixate at distance in average room light. A dark room may be used if this is the examiner's normal testing situation. Standardization in testing is important for follow-up and comparisons at later dates.

A small collimated light should be moved from the periphery to shine upon the posterior pole of the eye at a distance of about 8 in. The patient should be advised not to fixate on the light but to maintain distance fixation. The direct response is noted and the fellow eye observed for consensual response. The light is then shifted to stimulate the posterior pole of the fellow eye and the observations are repeated. The pupils should be checked for rapidity of response, magnitude of constriction, and ability to maintain constriction. Fatigue of constriction under direct light is a subtle sign of decreased pupillomotor power.

The light should be alternately moved from one eye to the other to compare the pupillomotor power of each eye. The direct and consensual constriction of the pupils should normally be of equal magnitude. If in the alternate light testing (often called the "swinging light" test) one pupil dilates slightly when the light is moved to it from the fellow eye, this eye has less pupillo-motor power than the fellow and a lesion of the homolateral optic nerve should be suspected.

A fine beam of light such as from a slit lamp is needed for testing hemianopic pupillary responses. Even the narrowest slit beam is somewhat inaccurate since the ocular media disperse the light and all retinal areas receive some light. However, in frank lesions the results are positive and helpful in the diagnosis and localization of hemianopic pathology. The nasal and temporal hemi-retinas are alternately stimulated by a fine beam of light. The magnitude of constric-tion is noted and the results are weighed in view of the fact that the nasal hemiretina normally produces more pupillomotor power than the temporal hemiretina. This test is of particular value in chiasmal hemianopia where the normally stronger nasal hemi-retinal fibers are destroyed and have no pupillomotor effect.

The near response of the pupil is usually tested binocularly since convergence is part of the reflex. Accommodation is essential and is probably the initiating stimulus. The patient first fixates binocularly at a distance and pupillary diameter is noted. The pa-tient then fixates on an accommodative target approximately 6 to 8 in. from the eyes; this should not be a light since the light reflex may be stimulated. Again, the pupils should be compared for diameter, equality, and ability to maintain miosis. The degree of convergence should also be noted. In monoc-ular individuals the reflex is elicited in the same way despite the absence of con-vergence. It is often possible to elicit the reflex in blind patients or in those with very limited vision if the patient can be made aware of a near object such as his own finger or if the tip of the patient's nose is touched.

A comparison between the magnitude of the light and of the near responses of the pupil should always be made. Normally, the amount of miosis should be about the same or slightly more with the near reflex, particularly if there is forceful accommoda-tion.

Patients presenting with a miotic, appar-ently fixed pupil should be observed after 1 hour in a dark room. The ability of a small pupil to dilate in the dark is a helpful, diag-nostic sign, particularly in the differentiation of an Argyll Robertson pupil from an Adie's myotonic pupil. Adie's pupil will frequently dilate after a protracted period in the dark while the Argyll Robertson pupil will not.

The sympathetic system is not usually tested specifically in examination of the pupils. The patient should be observed for associated sympathetic signs such as a wid-ened palpebral fissure, pupillary dilatation, appearance of exophthalmus, sweating, flush-ing, hair condition, and iris color. Abnor-mality in these areas suggests increased sympathetic activity.

Sympathetic stimulation will produce a large pupil on the same side as the lesion (see p. 81). Conversely, sympathetic loss will produce a homolateral miotic pupil and other classic signs of Horner's syndrome. Amphetamines, cocaine, and similar drugs dilate the pupil through action on the sym-pathetic system. Anxiety states, with auto-nomic imbalance, will also produce large pupils because of the sympathetic domi-nance.

SPECIFIC PUPILLARY REFLEXES NOT ASSOCIATED WITH LIGHT OR NEAR

The orbicularis reflex (c), so-termed by Westphal and Piltz in 1920, is a homolateral constriction of the pupil on attempted forced closure of the lids against resistance of the examiner's fingers. It is present in about 80% of people and demonstrates integrity of the peripheral efferent pupillary pathway. The mechanism of the reflex has not been determined but it is important in validating Argyll Robertson pupils. A normal orbicularis reflex eliminates the efferent path as a site of the lesion. A false positive orbicularis reflex may appear if the patient converges.

The vestibular (d → hippus) *and cochlear* (c → d) *reflexes* probably represent over-flow of caloric, rotational, or acoustic stim-uli from the vestibular area of the midbrain and pons into the sympathetic pupillary dilating system. They are of little significance in ophthalmic disease but may at times assist in examination of the efferent pathways.

The trigeminus reflex (d) can be of practical value in verifying questionable peripheral efferent pupillary pathways. Touching the cornea will produce prompt mydriasis followed by miosis. The path of the reflex is uncertain, but most evidence indicates that the afferent trigeminal fibers stimulate the oculomotor nucleus by connections in the midbrain.

The psychosensory reflex (d) is easily observed in patients in cases of anxiety, hysteria, or fright. The reaction probably represents generalized sympathetic overlay. Bumke (1904) described the pupillary dilation in catatonia, and Redlich (1922) described reaction with intense muscular effort. The reflex is sometimes tested by pricking the skin or forcefully flexing a joint.

The vagotonic reflex (c, d) has a direct relationship to respiration with a slight dilatation on inspiration and a slight constriction on expiration. This is accentuated in pathologic breathing of hyperventilation and Cheyne-Stokes respiration.

PARASYMPATHETIC SYSTEM
Afferent tract

Optic nerve (Fig. 4-7). With a lesion of one optic nerve or of the nerve fiber layer of one retina there is a typical pupillary impairment. Both pupils exert specific pupillomotor power, and the size of both pupils is determined by the eye with the greater pupillomotor power. In the resting state the pupils are usually equal since the normal eye is controlling pupillary size. In 1904, Marcus Gunn described an abnormal response of the pupil in a case of ipsilateral retrobulbar optic neuritis. With uniform ambient light, covering the normal fellow eye produces dilation of both pupils. Consensual response to light of the affected eye is normal. Direct light to the involved eye while the sound eye is covered, however, produces ipsilateral dilatation greater than in the resting state, indicating decreased pupillomotor power of the involved eye. The

test may also be done without covering the fellow eye, but then the dilatation is of less magnitude since the normal eye is producing some pupillomotor effect. The reaction to near is normal. This type of response may occur with any lesion of the optic nerve such as:

1. Optic neuritis of any cause
2. Vascular accidents of the nerve
3. Tumors of the nerve and orbit
4. Trauma

Optic chiasm (Fig. 4-8). Sagittal division of the optic chiasm produces bitemporal hemianopia and similar interruption of the decussating nasal pupillary fibers. The hemianopic pupillary reactions are technically difficult to elicit because intraocular scatter of light stimulates the entire retina, particularly the macula. However, with a fine beam of light from a slit lamp, the bitemporal hemianopic pupillary response can often be observed. In each eye, light from the temporal field produces less pupillary constriction than light from the nasal field. When this test is positive it is often striking, but apparently normal pupillary responses do not rule out hemianopia.

Common causes of this pupillary response are the causes of interruption of the chiasm as outlined below:

A. Tumors
  1. Pituitary
  2. Meningioma
    a. Sphenoid
    b. Tuberculum sellae
    c. Olfactory groove
  3. Craniopharyngioma
  4. Third ventricle tumors
B. Aneurysms
  1. Internal carotid artery
  2. Junction of anterior cerebral and anterior communicating arteries
  3. Anterior cerebral
C. Infections
  1. Arachnoiditis
  2. Meningitis
    a. Syphilis
    b. Tuberculosis
    c. Others
D. Others
  1. Trauma
  2. Demyelinating disease (rare)

Text continued on p. 71.

Fig. 4-7. Marcus Gunn pupil. A, The anatomy of the pupillary system as seen from behind. The impaired right optic nerve retards the direct pupillary reflex. Midbrain is bilaterally flooded with the stimuli, therefore the consensual response is normal. The typical clinical findings are seen in B.

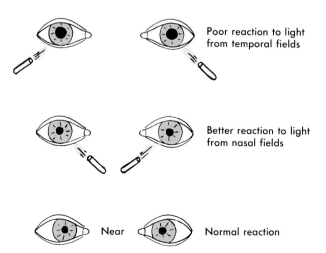

Fig. 4-8. Midline lesion of the optic chiasm. The nasal hemiretinal pupillary fibers are interrupted at the chiasm. Light directed from the temporal fields produces less pupillary constriction than light directed from the nasal fields.

Rest — Usually equal

Poor reaction to light from temporal fields

Better reaction to light from nasal fields

Near — Normal reaction

L   R

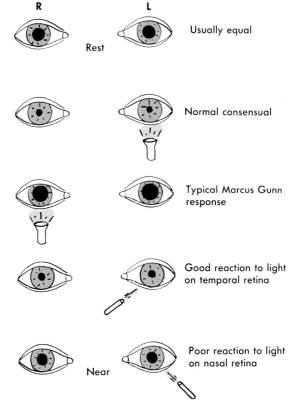

R   L

Rest   Usually equal

Normal consensual

Typical Marcus Gunn
response

Good reaction to light
on temporal retina

Near   Poor reaction to light
on nasal retina

Fig. 4-9. The anterior junctional syndrome. The optic chiasm and one of the optic nerves are involved. The right eye shows a Marcus Gunn pupil. The left eye illustrates a chiasmatic hemianoptic pupillary response.

Fig. 4-10. <u>Wernicke's hemianoptic pupillary phenomenon.</u> A lesion of the anterior optic tract will involve the pupillary fibers. Light directed from the field of the hemianopia will produce less pupillary constriction than light from the normal field (**A** and **B**). If the lesion is at the posterior limit of the optic tract the pupils will be normal (**C**).

R   L

Rest   Usually equal

Light directed from normal field produces pupillary constriction

B

Light directed from the field of the hemianopia produces a poor reaction

Near   Normal reaction

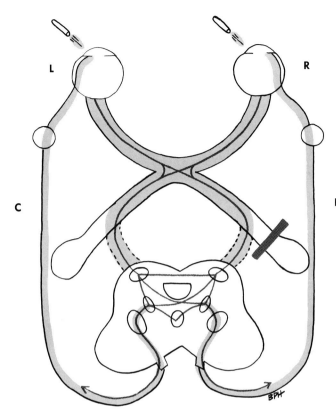

C

Fig. 4-10, cont'd. For legend see opposite page.

Anterior junctional syndromes (Fig. 4-9). The neurologic complex that constitutes the anterior junctional syndrome* often produces pupillary defects. Commonly, the lesion affects both decussating fibers of the optic chiasm and one of the optic nerves. In such cases the pupils are usually equal, and the eye ipsilateral to the involved nerve will show a Marcus Gunn response. Also, there is a poor pupillary reaction to light directed from the field of the hemianopia. The pupils react normally to near. These responses can often aid in localization of the cause of the hemianopic reaction.

The causes of this syndrome are similar to those that impinge upon the optic chiasm sagittally or posteriorly:

A. Tumors
  1. Pituitary
  2. Parasellar
    a. Meningioma of sphenoid
    b. Craniopharyngioma
  3. Third ventricle tumors
B. Aneurysms
  1. Internal carotid artery
  2. Junction of anterior cerebral and anterior communicating arteries

Optic tract (Fig. 4-10). In 1872 Wernicke first described "hemianopic pupillary rigidity." Again, this may be a difficult response to elicit but in some cases it is quite apparent. The pupils are usually equal and light directed from the field of the hemianopia produces less pupillary constriction than light from the normal field. Wernicke believed

*Temporal hemianopic scotoma in one eye and superior temporal field defect in the other from lesions at the anterior edge of the chiasm.

that this response would differentiate anterior tract lesions from those posterior to the exit of the pupillary fibers. A more posterior lesion would not affect the pupils since the pupillary fibers exit from the tract via the superior branchium conjunctivum.

Disease of the optic tract is uncommon, is characterized by incongruous field defects, and may stem from:

1. Tumors: many types, especially of temporal horn
2. Vascular accidents: of anterior choroidal artery
3. Infections: temporal lobe abscesses
4. Degenerations: Schilder's disease

Superior brachium and pretectal areas (Fig. 4-11). The superior brachium and pretectal areas are uncommon sites of clinically recognizable disease but may be the site of pathology in Argyll Robertson pupils. A lesion in this area will have no effect on visual function since it is removed from the optic tracts and radiations, but the pupillomotor input to the midbrain is blocked. However, the pathways for the near reaction from the higher cortical centers, mediated through the oculomotor nucleus, are intact. The clinical picture of the pupil in light–near dissociation as classically described by Douglas M.C.L. Argyll Robertson (1869) is:

1. Miosis
2. No reaction to light
3. Normal reaction to accommodation
4. Irregularity of the pupil
5. Unilateral or bilateral with anisocoria
6. Iris atrophy—often sector atrophy, which may account for the irregularity
7. Heterochromia iridis—secondary to the prolonged miosis and iris atrophy
8. Orbicularis reflex often intact
9. Pupil dilates poorly with atropine

The literature shows that Argyll Robertson pupils may be associated with a variety of diseases. However, in over 90% of patients with true light rigidity of the pupil the correct causative diagnosis is syphilis.

Differential diagnosis of Argyll Robertson pupils

1. Syphilis
2. Multiple sclerosis
3. Encephalitis
4. Brain tumors
5. Syringomyelia
6. Syringobulbia
7. Alcoholism
8. Diabetes mellitus
9. Trauma
10. Herpes zoster
11. Amyloidosis
12. Tuberculosis
13. Midbrain abscess
14. Midbrain hemorrhage

Many cases of true unilateral Argyll Robertson pupil (Fig. 4-12) have been reported with characteristics identical to the bilateral disease. Again, the most common diagnosis is syphilis, but herpes zoster ophthalmicus has also been associated too frequently to be coincidental. Some cases later become bilateral.

The site of the lesion has never been proved, but theoretically it would have to block all the pupillomotor input to one Edinger-Westphal nucleus.

The pathway for near is probably spared since it originates at higher levels and is only mediated through the oculomotor nucleus. Unfortunately pathologic data regarding this condition are lacking.

The failure of the pupil to react to near but its normal reaction to light may be called the *inverse Argyll Robertson pupil* (Fig. 4-13). This is very rare and is usually associated with a failure of convergence as well. Hypothetically, a lesion of Perlia's nucleus in the midbrain could produce this clinical picture. Because convergence is usually affected it is most likely caused by a cortical disease, and the failure of the near reaction of the pupil is secondary.

Efferent tract

Fixed pupil (Fig. 4-14). If the Edinger-Westphal nucleus and other portions of the oculomotor nucleus involved with the near reaction are both affected, a true internal ophthalmoplegia will develop. This is a failure of the pupil to react to light or to near and is accompanied by loss of accommodation. The condition may be unilateral or bilateral.

The local causes of internal ophthalmoplegia in the midbrain are varied:

1. Tumors: many types, primary and metastatic, including pineal tumors (Parinaud's)
2. Vascular accidents
3. Infections: encephalitis, abscess
4. Demyelinating disease: not uncommon (symptomatology in the midbrain is confusing)
5. Trauma

The pupils may also be fixed in other conditions. In midbrain lesions, the fixed pupil is usually dilated. There are other possible sites of pathology that will produce a dilated, fixed pupil.

Text continued on p. 78.

Fig. 4-11. Bilateral Argyll Robertson pupils. The pupillomotor input to the brain is blocked. The light reflex of the pupil is destroyed. The near reflex from higher cortical centers is intact.

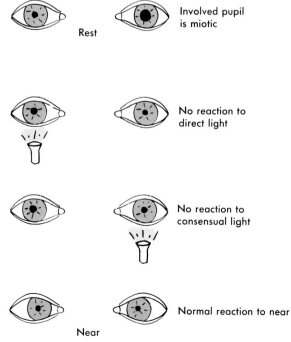

Fig. 4-12. The theoretic explanation of the unilateral Argyll Robertson pupil. The input to one Edinger-Westphal nucleus is blocked. The remainder of the pupillomotor system is intact.

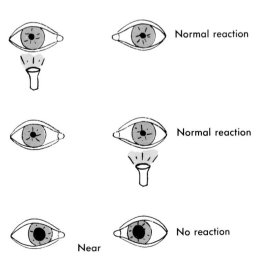

Fig. 4-13. Explanation of the inverse Argyll Robertson pupil (theoretic). A lesion of Perlia's nucleus in the midbrain could destroy the near response of the pupil and spare the light response.

Fig. 4-14. Fixed pupil. A true internal ophthalmoplegia will result if the Edinger-Westphal nucleus and the other portions of the
oculomotor nucleus, which are concerned
with the near reactions, are affected. The lids
and extraocular movements may be normal—
as contrasted to third nerve palsy.

Fig. 4-15. Oculomotor nerve palsy. A lesion of either the oculomotor nucleus or the oculomotor nerve may produce third nerve palsy. There is an internal ophthalmoplegia combined with extraocular muscle disturbance and ptosis.

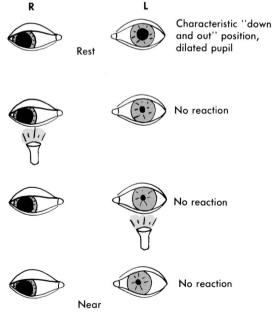

1. Oculomotor nerve
2. Ciliary ganglion: Adie's pupil
3. Short ciliary nerves: trauma, pressure of acute glaucoma, after scleral surgery
4. Eyeball: trauma, posterior synechia, use of mydriatics and cycloplegics

Miotic fixed pupils are fairly rare but may occur in:

1. Lesions of afferent arc, superior branchium, or tectum

2. Ciliary ganglion (tonic pupil)

3. Eyeball (synechia following iritis or trauma)

In general, dilated fixed pupils occur with disease of the efferent path and miotic fixed pupils occur with disease of the afferent path.

Oculomotor nerve palsy (Fig. 4-15). A lesion of either the oculomotor nucleus or of the oculomotor nerve may produce a variegated picture of oculomotor nerve palsy, in which the eye deviates "down and out" and the pupil is dilated and fixed. The differentiation of a nuclear from a nerve lesion is often difficult, and it becomes a problem for the neurologist to interpret the associated neurologic signs. The following generalities are diagnostic guidelines:

Oculomotor lesions

A. Nuclear lesions
   1. Rarely unilateral: both eyes usually have some type of disturbance
   2. Paralysis usually incomplete
   3. Pupil may not be involved
B. Nerve lesions
   1. Usually unilateral
   2. Paralysis usually complete except if the lesion is in orbit
   3. Pupil always involved to some extent

In considering oculomotor nerve lesions, the anatomy (Fig. 4-16) of its course offers four differing areas that can harbor discrete pathology: (1) en route to the cavernous sinus, (2) in the cavernous sinus, (3) in the superior orbital fissure, and (4) in the orbit.

The nerve leaves the midbrain in the basilar area and passes between the posterior cerebral and superior cerebellar arteries near the junction of the posterior communicating artery. A lesion in the basilar

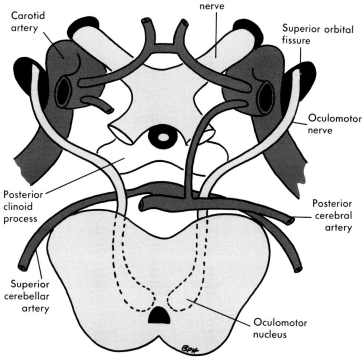

Fig. 4-16. Diagrammatic anatomy of the course of the oculomotor nerve.

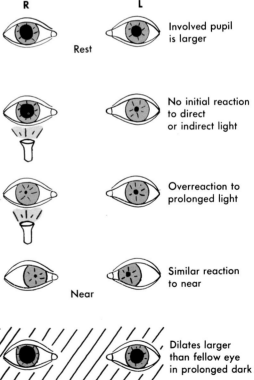

Fig. 4-17. Lesion of the ciliary ganglion (Adie's pupil). This may be confused with an Argyll Robertson pupil, but after prolonged stimulation it is found to be a tonic rather than a fixed pupil. The methacholine (Mecholyl) test (see p. 80) will help with the diagnosis.

Rest — Involved pupil is larger

No initial reaction to direct or indirect light

Overreaction to prolonged light

Near — Similar reaction to near

Dilates larger than fellow eye in prolonged dark

area will often produce bilateral signs because of the close proximity of the right and left nerves as they leave the floor of the midbrain. In this first area, the following lesions are most probable:

1. Tumors: gliomas and meningiomas
2. Aneurysms: posterior cerebral and posterior communicating arteries
3. Infections: basilar meningitis

The nerve then courses near the edge of the posterior clinoid process, where pathology usually produces unilateral signs, since the nerves are widely separated.

1. Tumors: meningiomas of sphenoid near posterior clinoids
2. Aneurysms: posterior communicating artery
3. Trauma: subdural or subarachnoid hemorrhage

The oculomotor nerve subsequently enters the cavernous sinus close to the trochlear, abducens, and trigeminal nerves and the carotid artery. Lesions within the cavernous sinus often produce oculomotor nerve palsy but with associated signs of damage to contiguous nerves and vessels.

1. Tumors: pituitary, meningiomas, metastatic, nasopharyngeal
2. Aneurysms: internal carotid artery
3. Infections: meningitis, cavernous sinus thrombosis
4. Others: carotid-cavernous fistula

The nerve continues to the superior orbital fissure and passes through to the orbit. In the orbit the oculomotor nerve divides into a superior division to the superior rectus and levator muscles and an inferior division to the medial rectus, inferior rectus, and inferior oblique, which in turn supplies the root to the ciliary ganglion. Pupillary signs in orbital disease are confusing because of the proximity of the anatomic structures. It is almost impossible to predict pupillary reaction from disease in the orbit because of the diffuse nature of the common pathology seen.

1. Tumors
2. Hemorrhages, trauma
3. Infections

All of the preceding lesions are destructive in nature and produce palsy of the nerve.

However, there can be irritation of the oculomotor nerve characterized by sudden spastic miosis and lid retraction often followed by mydriasis and ptosis. This is seen early in the course of a massive insult such as meningitis, subdural or subarachnoid hemorrhage, and rapidly expanding aneurysms.

Ciliary ganglion (Fig. 4-17). Further along the efferent pupillary path is the ciliary ganglion. Disease of the ciliary ganglion can produce a myotonic or Adie's pupil. Both structural and neuropharmacologic changes can cause Adie's pupil. The disease is usually unilateral and primarily affects young women. The typical myotonic pupil is larger than the fellow pupil. On initial stimulation the pupil does not react to direct or consensual light, but after prolonged illumination the pupil slowly constricts, then overreacts. There is a similar reaction to near. Dilation in the dark is also slow, but eventually it is of greater magnitude than the normal eye. The classic work of Scheie (1940) demonstrating the Adie's pupillary response to dilute (2.5%) methacholine (Mecholyl) has helped to differentiate Adie's pupil from the Argyll Robertson pupil with which it may be confused.

Argyll Robertson pupil	Myotonic pupil
Constricted	Dilated
Bilateral	Unilateral
No reaction with 2.5% Mecholyl	Constriction with topical 2.5% Mecholyl
Poor dilatation with atropine, cocaine	Prompt dilatation with atropine, cocaine

Sympathetic system

Horner's syndrome (sympathetic inhibition) (Fig. 4-18). The sympathetic system may be either stimulated or inhibited by a variety of lesions along its pathway. The classic picture of sympathetic inhibition is the syndrome of ptosis, miosis, and anhidrosis described by Horner in 1869. The pupil is reactive to light and accommodation, although the reactions are hard to observe because of the small pupil. A Horner's pupil usually will not dilate in the dark. Other significant signs in Horner's syndrome are seen in the following chart:

Horner's syndrome (ipsilateral sympathetic destruction)

1. Miosis (not pinpoint)
2. Usually unilateral
3. Normal reaction to near but difficult to observe
4. Narrow palpebral fissure
5. Ptosis
6. Enophthalmos (apparent, not real)
7. Anhidrosis and hypothermia of the same side of the face and neck
8. Brittle and dry hair
9. Heterochromia iridis (especially in infants; lighter iris on affected side)
10. No dilatation in the dark

Horner's syndrome may be caused by many different lesions between the hypothalamus and the globe along the sympathetic pathway.

Etiology of Horner's syndrome

1. Pons: tumors, hemorrhages, infarcts, syringomyelia
2. Medulla: tumors, hemorrhages, syringobulbia
3. Cord: tumors, hemorrhages, trauma
4. Mediastinum: lung, esophageal and tracheal lesions, aneurysms
5. Neck: trauma (birth, postoperative), lymphadenopathy, aneurysms

The clinical picture produced by most of these lesions is similar, but associated neurologic findings may lead to the etiologic diagnosis. For example, Raeder's paratrigeminal syndrome presents a partial Horner's syndrome along with weakness of the jaw muscles and pain in the face and orbit of the same side. The lesion is often a tumor or aneurysm in the region of the trigeminal nerve and the carotid sympathetic plexus.

Claude Bernard's syndrome (sympathetic stimulation) (Fig. 4-19). A typical picture of sympathetic stimulation is produced by an irritative lesion along the sympathetic pathway. The symptom complex was investigated by Claude Bernard in 1869. The eye has a characteristic appearance of lid retraction and mydriasis, usually unilateral. The pupil reacts to light and near but not fully. The precise localization of the irritative lesion is often difficult, since there are

Fig. 4-18. Horner's syndrome. Typical ptosis and miosis will result from interruption of the sympathetic pathway to the eyeball. Usually the extraocular movements are intact.

Characteristic ptosis and miosis

Rest

Slight reaction

Slight reaction

Slight reaction

Near

No dilatation in dark

Fig. 4-19. Claude Bernard's syndrome. If the sympathetic path to the eye is stimulated, the physiologic opposite of Horner's syndrome will result. Claude Bernard's syndrome is usually shortlived since the stimulation often progresses to destruction and a Horner's syndrome.

no consistently helpful clinical tests. Associated signs of the syndrome often help in the diagnosis:

Claude Bernard's syndrome (sympathetic stimulation)

1. Usually unilateral
2. Mydriasis
3. Wide palpebral fissure
4. Flushing of the same side of the face
5. Hyperhidrosis of the same side of the face
6. Appearance of exophthalmos (not measurable)

There are many possible etiologies of the condition, but few pathologic specimens have been available to demonstrate the causes.

Etiology of sympathetic irritation

1. Occasionally pontine and medullary tumors and hemorrhages
2. Usually apical lung lesions: infections, pneumothorax

REFERENCES

Bumke, O. C.: Die pupillenstörungen bei Geistes und Nervenkrankheiten, ed. 2, Jena, 1911, G. Fischer.

Davanger, M.: An analysis of the forces determining the size of the pupil, Acta. Ophthalmol. **50**:183-187, 1972.

Goodlaw, E., Moshin, H. L.: The pupil-importance in the optics of the visual system. Part 1. Clinical data, Am. J. Ophthalmol. **49**:226-233, 1972.

Gunn, R. M.: Retrobulbar neuritis, Lancet **2**:412, 1904.

Harriman, D.C.: Pathological aspects of Adie's syndrome, Adv. Ophthalmol. **23**:55-73, 1970.

Horner, F.: Ub. eine Form von Ptosis, Klin Monatsbl. f. Augenh. **7**:193, 1869.

Jagerman, L. S.: Hering's law applied to the near reflex, Am. J. Ophthalmol. **70**:579-582, 1970.

James, J. L., Nigam, M. P.: Pupillary autonomic functions in heterochromia iridis, Arch. Ophthalmol. **89**:291-292, 1973.

Koff, R. H.: Bibliography and classifications of the literature of pupillary response, Waltham, Md., 1972, Whittaker Corp.

Loewenfeld, I. E., Friedlaender, R. P., McKinnon, P. F.: Pupillary inequality associated with lateral gaze, (Tournay's phenomenon), Am. J. Ophthalmol. **78**:449-469, 1974.

Newsome, D. A., Loewenfeld, I. E.: Iris mechanics. II., Influence of pupil size and details of iris structure, Am. J. Ophthalmol. **71**:553-573, 1971.

Redlich, E.: E. Durch kräftige und anhaltende Muskelkontraktion ausgeloste Erweiterung der pupille, Ztschr. f. Augenh. **19**:171, 1908.

Robertson, Douglas M. C. L. Argyll: Four cases of spinal miosis with remarks on the action of light on the pupil, Edinburg Med. J. **15**:487, 1869.

Scheie, H. G.: Site of disturbance of Adie's syndrome, Arch. Ophthalmol. **24**:225, 1940.

Schwartz, B.: Syphilis and the eye. Baltimore, 1970, Williams and Wilkins.

Semmlow, J., Stark, L.: Pupil movements to light and accommodative stimulation: a comparative study, Vision Res. **13**:1087-1100, 1972.

Smith, M. B.: Handbook of ocular pharmacology, Acton, Mass., 1974, Publishing Sciences Group.

Thompson, H. S., Newsome, D. A., Loewenfeld, I. E.: The fixed dilated pupil: Sudden iridoplegia or mydriatic drops? A simple diagnostic test, Arch. Ophthalmol. **86**:21-27, 1971.

Weintraub, M. I., Ribner, J. A., Gallagher, B. A.: Transient internal ophthalmoplegia. Arch. Ophthalmol. **86**:595-598, 1971.

Wernicke, C.: Hemianopische pupillen-reaction, Virchow's Arch. f. Path. Anat. u. Physiol. **56**:397, 1872.

Major disease areas

The cornea and the sclera:
slit lamp and keratometer

PRELIMINARY INSPECTION

In every special area of examination, just as in the initial examination itself, a brief preliminary inspection must precede more critical and refined steps. The examiner should first note the lids for their texture, correct apposition to the globe, and position of the lacrimal puncta to furnish proper drainage of the precorneal tear film. Chronic infection in the lid borders should be noted for (1) production of irritation, (2) bacterial toxins damaging to the corneal epithelium, and (3) possible source of infection following any surgery. The amount and type of secretions on the lid borders or discharging down the cheek should be recorded. Just as important, note should be made of the *absence* of apparent tearing when the patient primarily complains of this. Clarity or injection of the conjunctiva in its bulbar, cul-de-sac, and palpebral divisions should be recorded for its relation to corneal health. Finally the brightness and clarity or gross vascularization and scarring of the cornea itself should be noted.

Thus the examiner should *not* first turn to the slit lamp without a preliminary flashlight inspection. Examination in direct daylight and the search for orderly reflection (catoptric image) of a windowpane from the corneal surface are too crude to merit any time except in underdeveloped areas of the world or in field conditions where ophthalmic equipment is not available.

Inspection in collimated or narrowed light such as from a penlight now replaces the older examination in "diffused illumination," just as the ever-present slit lamp itself now replaces the former inspection in "oblique illumination." The use of a spectacle-mounted loupe is helpful in preliminary inspection. The intermediate level of the old hand-held or portable slit lamps should be deferred to the full-scale table-based slit lamp, with the one recent exception of the new portable Kowa hand-held apparatus (Fig. 5-1),* which is valuable for mobile units or ophthalmic surveys under field conditions. Gross lesions are noted mentally from this light and loupe inspection.

SLIT LAMP EXAMINATION
Initial steps

The next step is the slit lamp examination. Of the valuable and ubiquitous instruments in ocular diagnosis, certainly the ophthalmoscope (1851) and the slit lamp (1911) are the most fundamental. Without exception, at least one modern model of each must be intimately familiar to every individual who examines patients (or sighted laboratory animals) for visual study or ocular evidence of structural and systemic disturbances.

Of all the laureates who have received the Nobel Prize in medicine and physiology since its inception in 1901, only three have been acknowledged for work directly in the visual field. The first of these was Allvar Gullstrand of Stockholm (1911) for his work in the dioptrics of the eye and his fundamental development of the slit lamp. Since 1911 there have been numerous refinements, enhancements in the illuminating system, and increased mechanical flexibility of the apparatus. Every

*Kowa Company, Ltd., Chuo-Ku, Tokyo 103, Japan.

Fig. 5-1. Kowa hand-held portable slit lamp affords 10× and 20× magnification; preselected slit widths are 0.1, 0.2, 0.8 mm.; weight is 1,700 gm. Also available as Kowa SL-2 with fiber optics, zoom lenses (5 to 20×), and continuously adjustable slit width of 0 to 10 mm.

modern model of the slit lamp, however, is based on the principles of the original Gullstrand instrument. The Haag-Streit 900 is a worldwide standard of optical and mechanical excellence. The incorporation of a tiltable illuminating system adds to its flexibility.

All biomicroscopes designated as slit lamps have two basic components: (1) an illuminating system and (2) a stereoscopic and microscopic observational system. These may be coupled or locked together at any advantageous angle or they may be, less commonly, used in optical coincidence. Alternately the two components are free from one another and the angulation frequently altered during examination to attain optimal display of details.

Before any slit lamp is brought into operation it is essential to ensure that several maintenance steps are observed. Mirrors and lenses must be kept free of dust with lens paper. The individual oculars of the biomicroscope should be focused for each eye of the observer with interpupillary distance adjusted. The proper bulb must be properly centered in its housing, and a spare bulb should always be kept with the instrument (plus a few others routinely kept in the office supply closet). Optimal efficiency is served if the slit lamp is brought to the patient in the principal examining chair without relocating him. Hydraulic, motor-driven, or counterbalanced systems are available for such mounting. When the convenience of a wall mount is used, it is essential (as with a projector chart) to be certain the wall is free of building vibrations.

Reassurance concerning sanitation is imparted by lifting off the topmost paper on the group of disposable chin pads just before the patient puts his head into position. If the patient must be moved to a nearby instrument

Fig. 5-2. Cotton-tipped applicator technique of elevating upper lid without pressure for slit lamp examination. Zeiss photoslit lamp is shown.

table, the examiner should step behind the patient's stool to ensure its not sliding backward. He should also extend one hand in front of the foreheadrest so that the patient does not bump his eye while sitting down. The headrest is adjusted to a convenient height for the patient, and the examiner accommodates himself to this position.

Some difficulty may be experienced in holding the lids open for corneal examination, particularly elevation of the upper lid for upper pole examination. The lid may be elevated with the thumb of the examiner's hand on the side of the eye under examination. A more delicate technique, however, is the use of a sterile cotton-tipped applicator to lift the lid by gentle rolling of the applicator tip from the side (Fig. 5-2). This avoids undue pressure on the eye and also avoids contamination of or by the examiner's fingers.

A patient with nystagmus should be examined under least magnification and positioned with appropriate face turning or tilting of his face to approach the nystagmus null point. Commonly this is in levoversion or dextroversion. If ocular oscillations still preclude needed detailed examination, as in foreign body removal, the Warburg Eye Immobilizer will dampen residual movement. This is a handle-mounted, scleral flange contact lens with the corneal section removed. After administering a topical anesthetic, the lens is pressed as needed against the bulbar conjunctiva serving as a fixation shell (Warburg, 1969).

Where both hands are needed, as in lid retraction and foreign body removal, the Weaver Chin Control as adaptable to the Haag-Streit, Mentor, and similar scopes, facilitates the maintenance of precise focusing (Fig. 5-3).

Initial focusing should be done with an intermediate working magnification of about 16×. In the Haag-Streit instrument this is best done by keeping the high power oculars (16×) in place and the changeover level con-

Fig. 5-3. J. H. Weaver Control of slit lamp observation arm by examiner's chin, shown attached to Haag-Streit 900 instrument. (Charles D. Bell Company, Westville, New Jersey 00093.)

trolling the objective at low (1×) power. When greater magnification is desired the objectives can be revolved within their holder to 1.6×, yielding a magnification of 25×. On the Zeiss instruments, the rotating drum can be advanced to 25× and rarely to 40× parfocal objectives, all of which are contained within a dust-free housing. Zeiss 100/16 has straight or inclined binocular tubes (but *without* convergence) and offers five powers of magnification from 6 to 40×. Manual or motorized zoom lens systems are available. The Mentor slit lamp, an effectively simplified design patterned after the Haag-Streit, offers three powers of magnification, 10, 16, and 25×.* Illumination should be kept below the maximum (5 or 6 volts rather than 7.6 volts on the Haag-Streit), which will prolong bulb life about fivefold and be better tolerated by the patient.

*Codman and Shurtleff, Inc., Randolph, Massachusetts 02368.

Illumination techniques

Examination is classically possible in seven slit lamp illuminating techniques:
1. Diffuse illumination
2. Direct (focal) illumination
3. Retroillumination or transillumination (direct or indirect)
4. Specular reflection
5. Indirect or proximal illumination
6. Scleral scatter
7. Oscillatory illumination

Diffuse illumination utilizes a wide illuminating slit slightly out of focus. It is a more stationary refinement of the preliminary penlight technique, making easily available the greater magnifying range of the microscope (Nikon zoom of 7× to 35×). This affords general localization of larger lesions on the cornea and orientation for more detailed techniques.

Direct or focal illumination is the most generally useful technique. It is achieved by critically focusing the narrowed beam onto the cornea from the right or left, depending on the examiner's habits and personal preference. The line of observation through the microscope can be adjusted from the infrequently desired complete coincidence (in most instruments) through an angular displacement up to 90 degrees.

The light, when sharply focused on the cornea, creates a brightly illuminated parallelepiped, with its anterior face corresponding to the precorneal tear film (closest to the side from which illumination is directed). The posterior face corresponds to the endothelial surface of the cornea and is in horizontal position nearer to the line of observation. Between these two curved faces are three normal lines of discontinuity anteriorly and two posteriorly.

The bulk of the depth between the surfaces is occupied by the stroma, which normally has a somewhat variable relucency. Under high magnification the stroma reveals a few delicately branching nerve fibers. A beautiful optic section of cornea is "cut" as the parallelepiped of illumination is narrowed and observed through an increased (45 to 90 degrees) angular displacement between the light and the line of observation. As the beam is narrowed the total intensity of illumination decreases, and therefore it may be necessary to increase lamp voltage during this step. Depth of lesions can be critically determined in such a narrow section. With higher magnification (18× to 25×) the three anterior lines of discontinuity are distinguished as (1) the precorneal tear film, (2) a darker or more optically transparent epithelial layer, and (3) the brighter or more relucent Bowman's membrane. Deep or posterior to the stroma can be seen the more relucent layer of Descemet and the less distinct endothelial line. This latter line of discontinuity is difficult to visualize in optic section without maximum magnification and illumination; it is more revealingly studied in specular reflection.

Retroillumination (less aptly called transillumination) is achieved by directing the light beam onto an opaque or reflecting surface (such as the iris, a lens opacity, or the posterior capsule) while focusing the microscope on the nearer tissue under study. The irregular reflection of light is particularly advantageous in bringing out corneal vacuoles, corneal bedewing, endothelial precipitates, or corneal blood vessels. Subtle fingerprint and dot dystrophies in the anterior cornea are best seen in this illumination. When the light can be returned from a lens opacity or even the posterior capsule, this affords the best method of studying iris atrophy or loss of the pigment epithelium; such changes may be inapparent with diffuse or focal illumination. In the lens this may aid definition of small opacities and subcapsular vacuoles.

Color values are generally different in retroillumination than in direct illumination. Thus a minute blood vessel in the corneal stroma appears light gray in direct illumination but much darker when seen in retroillumination. The same is true of endothelial precipitates, asteroid bodies, and many opacities in the vitreous.

In further refinement of this technique, a lesion may be visualized by *direct* retroillumination (when it is precisely in the path of the reflected light) or by *indirect* retroillumination (when it is to one side of this path and therefore viewed against a darker background). This helps to differentiate opaque bodies by their obstructive properties from vacuoles or cystoid lesions that are refractive or dispersive. The former are centrally dark at all times, whereas the latter may appear light in their centers under direct retroillumination but change to bright crescentic edges under indirect retroillumination.

Specular reflection is the most critical of the various techniques and is the prime method for studying the endothelium. Specular reflection on the normally mirrorlike anterior corneal surface is a dazzling reflection and glare to direct ophthalmoscopy, particularly when the pupil is small. When focusing critically on the front corneal surface, this glare area (limited to a small portion of the parallelepiped) may be exploited in a narrow beam to reveal minute anterior corneal pits (concavities) or excrescences (convexities) far too small to be seen in diffuse light.

With the illuminating beam directed on this anterior specular reflection, the endothelial or posterior face of the parallel-epiped must be suitably narrowed and medially displaced to avoid overlapping the anterior face. The focusing level of the microscope is then advanced the depth of the cornea to bring into clear view the somewhat darker and slightly golden endothelial surface just medial—or toward the observation line—from the line of illumination. The useful area illuminated in specular reflection is so circumscribed and critical that the reflected rays of light may center into only one of the two objective lenses of the corneal microscope. Therefore many observers, when utilizing specular reflection, prefer to close the nondominant eye, simplifying the focusing of the microscope and conducting this part of slit examination monocularly.

The normal mosaic-like pattern of the large endothelial cells is generally regular and slightly yellowish in tint. Hassall-Henle bodies are evident in the periphery of most adult corneas as nonreflecting areas or dehiscences in the mosaic. When these also involve the central area of the endothelium, this indicates the presence of the very common guttate corneal dystrophy. To examine various areas of the cornea within the circumscribed area of specular reflection, it is usually quickest and easiest to have the patient redirect the position of his eyes so that successive sites can be brought under focus.

Indirect (or lateral or proximal) illumination is obtained by focusing a fairly small beam adjacent to the feature under study and moving the line of observation to a wide angle from the line of light. Translucent deposits, foreign bodies, or similar small lesions stand out as darkened or shadowed areas in brighter surroundings. Proximal illumination through the cornea, rather than the sclera, is the best technique to reveal early marginal changes such as limbus girdle of Vogt or band keratopathy. (This same technique is used with the ophthalmoscope to bring out subtle details in the fundus that would be "washed out" by the brilliancy of direct illumination.)

Scleral scatter utilizes the principle of indirect illumination by specifically focusing the light on the limbus and gaining a large amount of internal reflection and dispersion within the cornea. With properly incident light and a cornea of normal transparency, the entire limbal area seems to light up as a faint halo. Medium rather than high magnification is first used in the corneal microscope, and minute changes in normal corneal relucency or minute lesions are detected as they obstruct or diffract the otherwise uniform light pattern. Under scleral scatter corneal lesions generally appear larger than they are, and subsequent to their identification and localization by this technique they should be studied with higher power and direct illumination.

Oscillatory illumination with a small range of movement under moderate to higher magnification gives alternate direct and indirect illumination and creates changing shadows. This may reveal pinpoint defects in the cornea (also aqueous, lens, and retrolental space) that might otherwise be washed out by more static and diffuse illumination. This also conserves the photosensitivity of the examiner's foveal cones and facilitates his own ability to resolve minute details.

Specular microscopy

Specular microscopy was introduced by Maurice in 1968 as an experimental laboratory tool, but is adaptable to clinical use at about 200× magnification, and is suitable for photographic recording. This nearly brings the magnification of histologic light microscopy to clinical analysis of corneal endothelial disease in vivo. Slightly simpler ophthalmic microscopes or binocular prism magnifiers are manufactured for general examination and macrophotography of the anterior segment (Ernst Leitz GMBH Wetzlar, Germany). These generally do not afford true slit illumination, coincidence of illuminating and observing systems, nor examination in and beyond the deep vitreous.

Measurement of thickness or depth (pachometry)

For sequential studies of corneal disease that may lead to thinning (keratoconus, congenital glaucoma, marginal ectasia, high myopia) or thickening (chronic inflammation, endothelial dystrophy, disciform disease, hyaline degeneration, phthisis bulbi), it is helpful to have an accurate record of thickness. At times, precise measurement of anterior chamber depth or lens thickness should be noted and accomplished by the same instrumentation used to measure corneal thickness. Early measurements of this type were derived to establish optic constants of the eye, but there is more practical need for anatomic measurements in relation to disease. Many techniques have been recorded, from refined tricks of inspectional estimation by Vogt,* to ocular micrometers, to complex photographic systems.

The simplest technique is that of direct or subjective slit lamp estimation of a thin optic section viewed at an angle of about 60 degrees. The slit beam length should exceed half the corneal diameter in order to afford comparison of central and peripheral thickness. Normally the central cornea appears slightly thinner than the peripheral cornea, and the maintenance of this relationship suggests an absence of pathology. Significant thickening involving the deep stroma almost invariably creates some wrinkling in Descemet's membrane as the inner curvature is flattened. Actually a lessened amount of Descemet's membrane and endothelium is needed to cover this surface.

A more quantitative method of estimating corneal thickness under the slit lamp is to place a corneal contact lens of known thickness on the eye. This constitutes a reference measurement in the slit beam, and corneal thickness is gauged accordingly.

Systems of corneal measurement are generally based on either the apparent optic depth or the real anatomic depth. Direct optic measurements using a microscope fitted with the Ulbrich calibrated drum (1914) suffer from disadvantages induced by movements of the patient's eyes, refractive distortion, and changes in the observer's accommodation. Anatomic measurements are calculated from optic measurements by formulas based on the average refractive power of the cornea and, in case of anterior chamber depth, the aqueous. High-frequency ultrasound with standoff transducers offers a new type of reliability in real measurement.

Two recent instrumental refinements have been evolved by Professor W. Jaeger of Heidelberg, Germany (1952), from the astronomic technique of *doublement* utilized by von Helmholtz. These are practical, compact, and efficient slit lamp attachments manufactured by Haag-Streit. Either apparatus is mounted with a single screw atop the eyepiece in the position also used for a camera attachment on the Haag-Streit slit lamp. A single (right) ocular is used; this must be fitted with a $10\times$, split-image eyepiece. Two depth-measuring attachments of different ranges are manufactured. No. 1 measures up to 1.2 mm. for corneal thickness, and No. 2 measures up to 6 mm., as needed for anterior chamber depth.

The principle of measurement is based on doubling by two plano glass plates located edge to edge in front of the right objective and dividing the reflected light entering the microscope. The lower plate is fixed, but the upper plate can be rotated around a vertical axis by turning the scale segment of the device. A vertical diaphragm slit in an arm extending to the left of the measurement device reduces illumination to a thin knife of light and also ensures the predetermined angulation of 40 degrees be-

---

*The Vogt technique of estimation (1930) is based on $20\times$ magnification and halving the apparent width of the illuminated optic section because of angulation between the light beam and the line of observation. Thus with an assumed real corneal thickness of 0.6 mm. (Vogt actually erred on the high side with an assumed central corneal thickness of 0.8 mm.), the apparent width of the illuminated section would be $0.6 \times 20 \div 2$ or 6 mm. He would then mentally divide this apparent section into units of 1 mm., corresponding to actual distances of 0.1 mm., for localizing the distance of alterations in the cornea.

tween the line of observation through the right ocular and the slit lamp beam.

In use, the microscope and slit lamp are firmly coupled at a 40-degree angulation. The objective magnification lever is set to 1×. The slit must be projected perpendicularly to the surface of the cornea at the point of observation with the scale segment set in the zero position. The slit lamp is focused at the apparent center of the distance to be measured. Observations are made monocularly through the right ocular only. The scale segment is rotated to the left or up the scale, thus rotating the upper glass plate until the split images are positioned so that the measuring points coincide. This should be repeated a few times for consistency and then the value recorded.

For measuring the corneal thickness, the scale segment is moved until the anterior corneal or epithelial line in one image is brought into precise alignment with the posterior corneal or endothelial line in the other image. For measurement of anterior chamber depth, it is first necessary to establish the corneal thickness with attachment No. 1 and then, with attachment No. 2, to measure the anterior chamber depth from the reference point of the anterior cornea to the anterior surface of the iris or lens. Corneal thickness is subtracted to give the optic depth of the chamber.

Corrective tables (No. 1 and No. 2) must be used to derive linear measurement from the observed optic figures. Corneal thickness is normally less in the central area (.50 to .52 mm.) than in the periphery (.68 to 1.10 mm.) and both increase slightly till full ocular growth is achieved in the mid 20's. Peripheral corneal thickness, however, tends to decrease in each decade of life after age 50, ranging downward from .68 to .52. All of these values follow a Gaussian distribution. Refractive error probably has no significant effect on corneal thickness.

Stromal thickness tends to increase in most wearers of hard or methacrylate contact lenses. More recent evidence suggests similar changes should be expected in soft contact lens wearers over months and years.

Though worrisome, this probably does not represent potentially debilitating pathology unless accompanied by mild or recurrent epithelial edema.

VITAL STAINING OF THE CORNEA AND CONJUNCTIVA

Because the cornea and conjunctiva are both essentially transparent, minute breaks or losses of tissue are often difficult to identify even with moderate magnification. Surface staining becomes of great practical importance in diagnosing epithelial loss and impairments as with abrasions, foreign body injuries, ultraviolet damage, exposure drying, or tear deficiencies. Sodium fluorescein is by far the most practical and widely understood stain. It is used preferably in individual, sealed, dry, sterile paper strips rather than the solutions of years gone by, which were notorious for their growth of *Pseudomonas aeruginosa*.

Where there is a break, a scratch, an avulsion, or an area of devitalization in the corneal epithelium, the immediately underlying Bowman's membrane stains bright green, clearly demarking the extent of defect. Even if no breaks are being sought, the use of fluorescein to stain the precorneal tear film is an asset in thin optic sections to estimate uniformity and thickness of the epithelium, which appears as a dark or nonrelucent band between the green-tinged precorneal film line and the brightly relucent underlying Bowman's glass membrane. In staining for subtle or early corneal lesions, the tip of the sterile, dry strip should be moistened with saline and gently touched to the conjunctiva rather than the corneal surface. Faint iatrogenic staining may be imparted by no more than touching the cornea with the impregnated paper strip.

In deep stromal ulceration it should be remembered that Descemet's membrane will not take fluorescein stain, though the stroma does absorb the dye. If excess stain remains in the conjunctival sac for several minutes, it may penetrate the intact epithelium and create a greenish flare in the aqueous. Very subtle staining is often seen better in short wavelength illumination, such as by inserting a cobalt glass filter (Wratten C) in front of the light source.

In injuries or chemical insults involving both the cornea and the conjunctiva, it must be remembered that fluorescein staining in areas of conjunctival epithelial loss will appear yellowish rather than green.

The next most valuable dye is probably a 1% aqueous solution of rose bengal, which keeps indefinitely. This has disadvantages of slightly greater irritability and a tendency of some distress to the patient for pinkish staining of the conjunctiva, lid borders, or even the lid skin that may persist for an hour or two. This dye is particularly valuable to demonstrate early areas of epithelial desiccation from tear deficiencies as in Sjögren's disease. A drop of topical anesthetic should be instilled first and then a small drop or glass rod application of the rose bengal made above the upper limbus. This promptly spreads throughout the lacrimal lake and should be flushed with sterile saline or irrigating solution. If allowed to pool in the inferior cul-de-sac, some punctate rose staining will occur even in normally moist eyes. Positive findings are indicated by fairly intense punctate staining throughout the corneal epithelium and bulbar conjunctiva. Rose bengal is quite different from fluorescein in that it stains mucous and dead or degenerating cells.

Many other dyes of the aniline and methylene blue families have been used largely as investigative tools or to aid in demonstration of corneal nerves. These may be quite irritating and are not of practical clinical importance.*

CORNEAL SENSITIVITY

Sensitivity to pain, touch, or pressure in the superficial cornea is quite high and many-

*Alcian blue 0.25 to 1%; tetrazolium 1%; trypan blue 0.1 to 1%; Bromothymol blue 0.2%; Fluorexon 2%.

Fig. 5-4. Gross quantitation of corneal sensitivity to cotton wisp advanced laterally and beyond field of view.

fold greater than in skin areas. This sensitivity is particularly reduced by lesions in the ophthalmic division of the trigeminal nerve and by the frequent invasion of herpes simplex virus. At least a gross qualitation of corneal sensitivity is therefore clinically important and can be achieved (Fig. 5-4) simply with a teased-out wisp of cotton a few millimeters longer than an ordinary cotton-tipped applicator. The patient should be instructed to look to the opposite side from the eye being tested. The examiner gently keeps the lids separated with the thumb and forefinger of one hand (to avoid undesirably contacting a lash) and then brings the cotton in from a lateral position, nearly parallel to the plane of the iris. This avoids the patient seeing the approach and making a

visual avoidance response. When normal sensation is present, a lightly applied touch to either cornea should evoke (1) a blink reflex, (2) slight discomfort, and (3) increased lacrimation.

Quantitative tests of sensitivity were evolved in the past century by such devices as the graded von Frey hairs, but they have been superseded by the more stable and reproducible instruments based on durable nylon threads (Puglisi-Duranti, Boberg-Ans, Olah and Szarbo, Cochet and Bonnet). A simple and practical esthesiometer is that of Cochet and Bonnet* based on a single nylon filament (Fig. 5-5). The instrument is held like a pencil with the examiner's index

*3, Rue d'Edimbourg, Paris 8, France.

Fig. 5-5. Cochet and Bonnet's corneal esthesiometer in actual use with extended nylon filament directed perpendicularly into center of cornea. (Luneau and Coffignon, Paris 8e, France.)

finger on the knurled wheel of a rack and pinion mechanism that adjusts the exposed length of nylon. The longer the exposed filament, the less the pressure required to bend it. The tip of the filament is brought into perpendicular contact with the area of cornea to be tested, and initially a moderately long (40-mm.) extension of filament is used. The minimum amount of force is applied to cause a just visible bending of the filament. If no sensation is evoked, the filament is progressively shortened until the patient senses the contact. Sensitivity is then recorded as the length of filament. Immediately after use the filament should be completely drawn into the body of the instrument to protect it from accidental damage. Reading of filament length in millimeters (5 to 60) may, as in the reading of an indentation tonometer, be converted by nomograms to contact values of milligrams per square millimeter.

Sensitivity of the cornea varies greatly in different areas and is highest in the thin optic center. Generally the sensitivity falls progressively from the center to the limbus, but it also is lower in areas of less frequent exposure. Thus the horizontal meridian tends to show greater sensitivity than the vertical, and the lower cornea is more sensitive than the upper, but these variations are only of small percentage difference.

CONTACT LENS DIFFERENTIATION OF VISION IMPAIRMENT BY OPACITIES VERSUS IRREGULARITIES

Visual impairments from corneal lesions are caused both by scars or opacities and by irregularities in the surface curvature. The latter is often underestimated in its amount of contribution to total visual reduction. In the presence of modest to even gross opacities in the stroma, vision may be surprisingly good if the epithelial surface of the cornea is smooth and unaffected. An immediate guide is afforded in noting the regularity of the slit lamp light reflection from the epithelial surface. When such reflections are undistorted, acuity may be well preserved even though it is difficult for the examiner to visualize iris details. The more crippling role of surface irregularities may be evaluated with a suitable diameter, plano strength, trial contact lens in place. For this type of trial refraction 1 drop of topical anesthetic should be used—assuming the patient is not in the habit of wearing contact lenses—and then the lens generously moistened with a wetting solution before insertion. Conventional refraction over such a lens in place may yield markedly improved vision, even in the presence of seemingly significant opacities.

CORNEAL CONFIGURATION

Any suspect abnormality found on preliminary inspection and slit lamp examination should be followed by progressively detailed studies. These generally advance through size estimates, curvature estimates, Placido techniques, and quantitative surface measurements.

Corneal dimensions

Viewed from the front, the cornea is slightly elliptic, with its horizontal diameter a little greater than its vertical. Estimates of corneal size render valuable clues to the overriding handicap of microphthalmos or the destructive bulbar enlargements of congenital glaucoma. These two disturbances in size are more frequent and of weightier prognostic importance than the relatively infrequent identification of microcornea or megalocornea, with or without megalophthalmia. The latter structural and optic deviations from normal have refractive and genetic implications but are safely diagnosed at leisure or with the aid of many subtleties of refractional and ultrasonic gear.

Clinical accuracy in corneal measurement cannot extend beyond 1.0 or 0.5 mm. because of (1) the difficulty in defining or identifying limbal limits, (2) irregularities of limbal scleralization, (3) impracticalities of bringing a ruler or caliper into close approximation or contact with the cornea, and (4) restiveness on the part of pediatric patients, where such measurements are usually most important.

Just as the total eyeball increases much less (about threefold) than the entire body (about twentyfold) from birth to maturity, so the cornea shows very little size enlargement compared to the rest of the globe during this period. Most of the 1 or 2 mm. of postnatal corneal enlargement occurs during the second 6 months of life, and essentially all of it is achieved by the age of 2 years.

The horizontal corneal diameter is the most accessible and therefore the most frequently measured and specified. Normally this is 11 to 12 mm., whereas the vertical corneal diameter, like each of the diameters in the female, is slightly less. This is caused by greater scleral overlap at the vertical than at the horizontal corneal poles. Critical measurement of corneal diameter is not only restricted by vagaries of anatomic landmarks but is clinically far less important than measurement of intraocular pressure, which can be done with high accuracy and which identifies the sinister causative mechanism of corneal enlargement in early life. Small, hand-held, single-tube penscopes or eye gauge magnifiers* are available with built-in metric scales or graticules to facilitate diameter measurements. In use these superimpose the image of the cornea on the scale at the focal length of the lens and afford more repeatable, if not more accurate, measurements than does unaided visual inspection. A vernier scale available with the Haag-Streit slit lamp also affords a high degree of linear accuracy.

Horizontal diameter of 10 mm. or less may indicate simple microcornea or the more crippling hypoplasia of micropthalmia. A horizontal diameter of 12 mm. or more suggests the distending and destructive effects of congenital glaucoma, which affects the entire globe; the simpler megalocornea (macrocornea), which is clear, bilateral, non-

progressive, and almost exclusively found in males; or else the rare and progressive thinning throughout the cornea designated as keratoglobus.

Topographic inspection is often assisted by (1) lateral examination aligning the observer's view in the plane of the iris to delineate better any abnormalities of curvature (the relatively frequent keratoconus or the progressively more rare megalocornea, keratoglobus, and cornea plana) or (2) inspection from above while the eyes are rotated downward. In this maneuver, the upper lids are retracted with the thumb and forefinger of one hand and the lower lid borders are brought to rest over the horizontal midline of the corneas. The use of the opaque lid border to outline the transparent cornea aids identification of gross disturbances in the anterior surface. Sharply forward or conic angulation as revealed by this technique is referred to as Munson's sign of keratoconus.

Corneal curvature
Normal values

The anterior corneal surface has a radius of curvature (7.6 to 7.8 mm.) slightly shorter than does the rest of the globe. This is particularly marked in the visually important optic portion, which is limited to approximately the central 4 mm. The transitional and peripheral zones are somewhat flatter (longer radius of curvature) though still more acutely curved than the sclera.

The posterior corneal curvature, on the other hand, is steeper, particularly in the central portion where the radius is about 1 mm. less than that of the overlying anterior corneal curve. Thus the high dioptric power (+44 to +46 diopters) of the cornea is actually a magnificently compensated base curve lens. The apposition of these dissimilar curves is associated with a normal central thickness of about 0.5 mm. and peripheral or limbal thickness slightly exceeding 1 mm.

Optic measurements of the anterior corneal surface are more important in the total refraction of an eye than are the measure-

---

*Western Optical Co. (WO-1005A), Seattle, Washington 98109; Zeiss Jena (60-24-23) Keratometer, Jena, German Democratic Republic.

ments of the posterior corneal curve. Both are now increasingly important in prescribing for contact lenses.

The anterior curvatures are easily measured and have received much attention since introduction of Placido's disc of concentric circles (1882) and the application of the old French astronomic measuring principle of doublement* by Louis Javal. This Parisian engineer turned physician devised the first practical keratometer (less aptly called "ophthalmometer") in 1881. Enduringly, the instrument has rightly borne his name and that of his distinguished ophthalmic student, Hjalmar Schiøtz of Norway.

Keratoscope or Placido's disc

Placido's disc can be made in many diameters and gives topographic mapping of the cornea over a wider area than is achieved

by Javal-Schiøtz keratometer readings. Currently the most useful and popular model is the self-illuminating, power-handled Klein (1958) keratoscope (Fig. 5-6).* Minor irregularities in reflection of the illuminated rings near the corneal center or particularly distorting the horizontal axis suggest early keratoconus. In use, the observer looks through a small diameter plus lens (usually +6 diopters) in the center of the illuminated disc and approaches the patient's eye at the focal distance of this lens (about 3½ in.) until optimal clarity of the reflected image is obtained. The observer then notes the location or degree of distortion as he and the patient maintain fixation through the center of the instrument. To study peripheral areas of the cornea beyond visualization in this primary fixation, the patient is instructed to shift his fixation to a specified edge of

*Servington Savary, 1743; Pierre Bouger, 1748; John and Peter Dolland, 1754.

*Manufactured by Keeler Optical Co., London, England, W1M 6DS.

Fig. 5-6. Klein-Keeler keratoscope made on principle of Placido disc of concentric circles. This instrument is self-illuminated. Reflected images from the corneal surface are seen as the observer looks through the center condensing lens.

the examining disc opposite the corneal area to be studied. This provides (1) a fixation point for the patient and (2) a standard displacement distance that facilitates accurate comparison of corneal areas at later dates. The simple Donaldson photokeratograph based on the Placido principle affords the derivation of an exact radius of curvature at any point by a graph applied to an original photograph. Elegant and expensive photokeratoscopes* are also available for recording such topographic mapping, but they are not necessary for good clinical practice.

Keratometry

Keratometry is the instrumental measurement of corneal curvatures, which for clinical purposes is confined to the anterior surface. It is not ophthalmometry or optometry (though many instruments have been and are marketed under the names "ophthalmometer" or "optometer"), because it does not include measurement of the posterior corneal curvature, lenticular curvatures, and linear distances within the globe that are components of the total dioptric system of the eye. These are measured in summation by retinoscopy, total refraction, or allegedly with instruments such as the Hartinger, Rodenstock, or Topcon Refractionometers.

Unfortunately the term "keratometer" is sometimes applied to small instruments sold in the aim of more accurate measurement of corneal diameter (p. 96). They may also be used from a lateral position as a vertometer or distometer to measure linear distance between the corneal apex and the back surface of a trial spectacle lens.

Keratometry is based upon (1) the convex mirror characteristic of the cornea, which reduces the size of a reflected object in direct relation to its radius of curvature,† and (2)

the astronomic technique of a double-image micrometer or "heliometer" for measuring short arcs (angular distances) in the celestial system. Both in the history of astronomy and in practical optics, this measuring system is one of the most accurate ever devised. The illuminated objects used to obtain the double reflections have traditionally been called "mires" from the French astronomic term meaning "meridian marks." Basic components of the instrument are (1) a pair of illuminated mires that can be positioned at precise distances apart on a rotatable arc, (2) a doubling or Wollaston birefringent prism, (3) a compound telescope for observing the reduced images of the mires, and (4) a sturdy base to hold the components and provide rest points for the face of the patient. Literally dozens of modifications have been produced under a corresponding array of eponymic designations. Many of the modifications have concerned configuration of the mires. Demands of corneal contact lens fitting in the last decade have revived usefulness of the keratometer, which ordinarily is not a helpful portion of visual or refractive examination. Many table- or suspension-mounted production models are available.*

In use the eyecap of the observing telescope is first adjusted for the focus of the observer and the height of the chinrest adapted to the patient. Each eye is examined singly, the right eye first. The opposite eye is occluded. The patient and telescope are leveled so that the patient can fix on the reflection of his own eye (in some instruments a fixation light) in the objective lens axis. The examiner then aligns and focuses the optic axis of the instrument on the corneal center with the aid of cross hairs or concentric rings. Focusing of the mires is done by both rotation and adjustments in distance to

---

*Soper PhotoMont; PEK Mart III and Compu-Graph (1970) Wesley-Jessen, Chicago, Illinois 60603.

†Thus if the radius of curvature is long (or the corneal surface flat), the image of the mire will appear larger. If the radius of curvature is relatively short (or the corneal surface steep), the image will be proportionately smaller.

*Bausch and Lomb, Rochester, New York ("Keratometer"); Carl Zeiss, Oberkochen, Germany ("Ophthalmometer"); American Optical Corp., Buffalo, New York ("AO-CLC Ophthalmometer"); Zeiss Jena, German Democratic Republic ("Ophthalmometer"); and Haag-Streit, Berne, Switzerland ("Javal-Schiøtz Ophthalmometer"). The last two instruments use the three-step mires of the original French design.

bring their sharp image on the principal corneal meridian. The mires are then brought into apposition (on the principal corneal axis or meridian) in accordance with the manufacturer's design of the contact points. The radius of curvature in millimeters may be read from the dial and the meridian or axis similarly noted from another dial. The entire component of mires and telescope is then rotated on its axis 90 degrees to read the second axis of the cornea. The adjustment in mire setting to achieve apposition on this axis gives the secondary radius of curvature.

If the two mires are at identical positions on each radius, there is no anterior corneal astigmatism; if they are not equal, the difference between readings on the two axes measures the anterior corneal astigmatism.

The Bausch and Lomb keratometer, developed before World War II, has long afforded significantly greater precision in reading by supplanting the initial "step" configuration of mires (as in the Haag-Streit Javal-Schiøtz instrument) with coincidence or superimposition targets.* These use the more sensitive *aligning* power rather than *resolving* power of the eye. The Bausch and Lomb mires, unchanged for more than a third of a century, are circles with a pair of minus signs just outside one diameter and a pair of plus signs just outside a second diameter at right angles to the first. A focusing or reference circle appears centrally, with an identical circle for the horizontal meridian to one side and a third identical circle for the vertical meridian positioned 90° away. As soon as the aligning cross hairs are adjusted to maximum clarity near the center of the focusing circle (optical axis of the instrument coincident with visual axis of the patient) the instrument is locked in position.

Fig. 5-7. Bausch and Lomb Keratometer Mires as seen when the center of the focusing circle is brought into adjustment with the optical axis of the instrument coinciding with the visual axis of the patient. The instrument is then locked into position.

*Based on the 1908 Sutcliffe, one-position keratometer with ring mires.

Fig. 5-8. Bausch and Lomb Keratometer Mires as seen when the horizontal plus signs are brought into continuous and unbroken line by rotating the telescope. The principal meridian of astigmatism can now be read directly and no further rotation is needed.

Fig. 5-9. Bausch and Lomb Keratometer Mires as seen after the horizontal measuring drum has been rotated to superimpose the two plus signs. The power reading for the horizontal meridian may now be taken.

The focusing circle appears doubled (Fig. 5-7) until the keratometer is in proper focus. The examiner then concentrates on the horizontal plus signs bringing these into continuous and unbroken line by rotating the eye piece or telescope (Fig. 5-8). The principal meridian of astigmatism can now be read directly and no further rotation of the instrument is needed. The horizontal measuring drum is then rotated to superimpose the two plus signs at which time the power reading for the meridian is taken from the drum (Fig. 5-9).

Lastly the two adjacent minus signs must be superimposed first by refocusing the keratometer and then turning the vertical measuring drum on the right; the reading for this vertical meridian is taken from the drum. Only with a spherical cornea will both principle meridians, the plus and minus signs, be in focus at the same time.

This instrument has long dominated the North American market and its high accuracy is attested to by the adoption of this mire system in the Topcon "ophthalmometer." Also in 1972* the American Optical Corporation "CLC" keratometer was introduced as an improved, one-position instrument with coincidence focusing of similar pattern; its range is from 35 D (9.6 mm. radius) to 60 D (5.6 mm. radius). A fixation light movable to 5 mm. on either side of center gives a 10 mm. zone for topographic analysis.

All keratometers actually measure radii of anterior corneal curvature in millimeters. Many instruments, however, have imprinted on them conversion values (Tabo scales) suggesting approximate dioptric powers of these radii. This is based on a presupposed refractive index of 1.3375 in the human cornea, which may be either basically imprecise or inaccurate in terms of the eye under study.

There is some inherent inaccuracy in converting keratometric readings to dioptric values, and it is manifestly foolish to convert these figures to corrective cylinder strengths for spectacles. Unfortunately, a "Javal rule" and a "Javal table" exist that seek to incorporate an average figure for posterior corneal astigmatism with the anterior corneal reading and then adjust this resultant for forward displacement of 14 mm., presumed to be the average distance from the back of a spectacle lens to the front of the cornea. This is of such limited accuracy that it should be abandoned. Another limitation of keratometry is that readings embrace limited corneal areas of only 2.5 to slightly less than 4 mm., which is in proportion to radii of curvature measuring between 6.3 and 9.5 mm. A single pair of keratometric measurements therefore cannot encompass all the variously curved areas of corneal surface from central to limbal.

Topogometers or toposcopes

Because the Javal-Schiøtz keratometers measure only in a restricted zone of about 2.5 to 4 mm. and because the keratoscope of Placido gives a qualitative rather than quantitative reading, there is clinical need for geographically fuller measurements of anterior corneal topography. This is particularly indicated in prescribing contact lenses.

Topogometers are scaled and usually illuminated instruments* often attaching to a keratometer to extend accurate readings from the limited keratometric area throughout both central and peripheral portions of the cornea. With such aid it is possible to map the separate locations of the geometric, visual, and apical centers of the cornea. Of these three, the visual center (on the visual axis) can usually be measured satisfactorily without assistance of a topogometer. Around the apical center there can be identified a *limiting margin* or imaginary line that circumscribes the steepest curvature and beyond which is the progressively decreasing curvature of the *transitional zone*, leading to the flatter scleral curvature.

The Soper Topogometer (1963)† is particularly designed to clamp onto the large

---

*Replacing the old and less accurate Micromatic instrument.

*Volk-Conoscope, Toposcope.
†Manufactured by the Topogometer Co., Houston, Texas 77027.

Fig. 5-11. Soper Topogometer attached to B & L Keratometer seen in patient's view. Note illustrative displacement of fixation light down and to patient's right.

Fig. 5-10. Soper Topogometer attached to B & L Keratometer as seen from the examiner's view. Horizontal and vertical scale readings to measure decentration of fixation are marked in subdivisions of 0.1 mm. Each sliding arm can be moved a maximum of 7 mm. in either direction. Measurements are in chord length. (Courtesy of The Methodist Hospital, Texas Medical Center, Houston, Texas.)

cylindrical end of the Bausch and Lomb keratometer or Topcon OM-1 just in front of its light housing. It consists essentially of a central fixation light assembly (with switch box and transformer that attach under the keratometer chinrest) and graduated vertical and horizontal decentration scales, each fitted with sliding indicator arms. In use, the sliding arms are initially positioned at zero on both the horizontal and vertical scales, and the patient's eye is directly aligned on the fixation light. This base situation is the same as when the eye is sighting directly

on its image for visual center or visual axis readings without the topogometer (Fig. 5-10).

Subsequently the patient continues to maintain alignment on the fixation light. The corneal curvatures are systematically measured at decentrations of 0.5 to 1.0 mm. as the fixation light (and therefore the visual center) is moved by the sliding arms on the vertical and horizontal scales from the optic axis of the keratometer. After making readings at the visual center, the steepest corneal point or apex is sought and recorded both in millimeters from the visual center and in "K" (keratometric) readings. The horizontal and vertical meridians to each side of the visual center should be surveyed and the "K" readings recorded at significant decentrations, such as the limiting apical margin where flattening first appears. This should be noted by millimeters of decentration in the four principal meridians from the visual center. Measurement of the mean apical curve, plus important plotting of the apical diameter, and corneal diameter (by localization of the "keratometric limbus") greatly assist in fabricating both central and peripheral posterior curves of a contact lens. (Fig. 5-11).

TOPOGRAPHIC DIAGNOSIS

The anatomic position of defects and disease in the cornea often gives a specific clue to causative diagnosis. The immediate accessibility of the cornea makes this an easily apparent and recorded localization. The conspicuous, gross topographic considerations of the cornea are those of the frontal or presenting aspect, which is divisible into: (1) limbal, marginal, or peripheral area (superior, inferior, interpalpebral, medial, or temporal), (2) transitional or midzone, (3) central or pars optica, (4) interpalpebral (visible segments of the limbal, midzone, and central areas as exposed between the lid borders), and (5) total. Topographic classification should also be made, particularly with the aid of the slit lamp, in relation to the layer or depth of involvement: (1) epithelium or anterior layer, (2) Bowman's zone, (3) combined epithelium and subepithelium, (4) stroma (anterior, mid, or deep), (5) Descemet's zone, (6) endothelium (mesothelium), and (7) posterior surface (as keratic precipitates, epithelial down growths, or translucent strands).

The most common corneal culprit in the United States today is the contact lens. The wearer should be examined once or twice a year (and lenses inspected and cleaned on similar schedule). Smaller lenses with increased accuracy and simplicity of fitting lull wearers through early stages of irritation. Slit lamp examination using scleral scatter (p. 90) may reveal early epithelial haze (edema) before epithelial erosion or staining. Loss of uniform fluorescein layering beneath the contact lens heralds discomfort and pressure erosions. This is particularly serious with apical defects from a lens that is too flat.

Limbal, marginal, or peripheral area
Limbal areas generally

The limbal area is the initial site of Mooren's chronic serpiginous ulcer with its pain, relentless progression, characteristically undermined border, and predilection for the elderly. It is also the site of bilateral and symmetric marginal ectasia or gutter dystrophy, which tends to progress slowly and symmetrically to 360-degree involvement; irritative symptoms are minimal. Fuchs-Terrien marginal dystrophy is an age-related collagen disease with usual onset in the mid 40s and occurring in this site. Most of these processes seem to be ischemic reactions or vascular insufficiency diseases and, hence, merit careful attention to both local vascular supply and systemic arterial occlusive disease.

The common marginal or catarrhal ulcers generally are superficial, small, and usually separated from the limbus by a narrow area of less affected cornea. These may be related to infectious conjunctivitis or to allergic mechanisms. Fuchs' superficial marginal keratitis, which tends to be bilateral and appear after midlife, is more painful, serious, exacerbative, and complete in its encirclement of the corneal periphery. Either of these disease processes may coalesce into the visually destructive *ring ulcer* or a pyogenic deep stromal *ring abscess.*

The malignant changes of epitheliomas and intraepithelial epithelioma (Bowen's disease)—essentially unknown in the central cornea—almost invariably begin here.

Interpalpebral limbus (medial and lateral limbus)

The common white *limbus girdle of* Vogt occurs in the interpalpebral limbus. This delicate, lattice-like marking in Bowman's zone appears in the medial and temporal limbus, usually without symptoms and with no clear cornea between it and the limbus. It appears symmetrically and in increasing percentages of the population with advancing age. Rarely, it seems to be associated with early band dystrophic changes beginning in the interpalpebral corneal periphery and carrying an involutional prognosis. More often band keratopathy begins its untoward course in these areas and extends horizontally across the cornea with pathognomonic, dark round holes at Bowman's level.

In parts of the world where onchocerciasis is endemic, the punctate keratitis associated with this *thread worm* usually begins its intermittently progressive course here.

Superior limbus

The superior limbus is practically the specific site for vascularization and pannus formation destroying Bowman's membrane in trachoma and leprosy. It is also the site for corneal manifestations of atopic processes such as vernal catarrh or neurodermatitis marked by Trantas points. By definition, it is also the site of superior limbic keratoconjunctivitis.

Vertical (superior and inferior) limbus

The age-related stromal deposits of arcus presenilis, arcus senilis (gerontoxon), or arcus lipoides first appear at the upper and lower near-limbal areas separated by a narrow rim of clear cornea (lucid interval of Vogt) from the limbus. Over many years, these arcuate deposits tend to extend in annular fashion, uniting medially and temporally to form a *circulus senilis*. There tends to be relationship to both familial incidence and hyperlipemia in various fractions. Lesions are generally symmetric in the two eyes.

Transitional or midzone

The transitional ring of the cornea can be identified by its curvature, which is flatter than that of the central or apical portions, but it generally is a subordinate or secondary area both in optic or disease consideration. It is commonly involved with dystrophies or other primarily central corneal disturbances that progress more widely. It is the site of copper accumulation in the deep cornea, which is known as the Kayser-Fleischer ring of Wilson's hepatolenticular degeneration. This is a familial and progressive disease of the cerebral cortex and basal ganglia developing in late childhood or the early decades of life with the striking and symmetric, colored corneal rings that begin near the limbus and progress centrally over a distance of 2 to 4 mm. The ophthalmic examiner

is frequently the first to identify this etiologic mechanism in a poorly coordinated patient or even before systemic signs are identified.

Salzmann's nodular degeneration, which tends to be unilateral and following previous keratitis, predominantly involves this area through the anterior half of the cornea.

The very rare primary calcareous degeneration of Axenfeld spreads through a similar area of the cornea involving Bowman's zone and the anterior stroma, with similar distribution in both eyes.

Scalloped or map-like opacities associated with cryoglobulinemia involves the deep stroma in this area of the cornea.

A crescent of rose bengal staining in this area of a contact lens patient indicates pressure from the intermediary lens curve and calls for modification of the inner lens surface.

Central area or pars optica

The central area of the normally avascular cornea is the furthest removed from the nutritive limbal vasculature and is a vulnerable site for many dystrophic changes and destructive invasion by bacteria and fungi (*Diplococcus pneumoniae, Pseudomonas aeruginosa*, diplobacillus of Petit, *Actinomyces, Candida albicans*). Anteriorly, this is the site of Cogan's microscopic cystic epithelial dystrophy, which has a predilection for healthy adult females. Neutrotropic keratopathies, evidenced by corneal anesthesia, generally begin in the central epithelium with clouding or vesiculation and commonly extend with superficial excavations throughout the cornea. The central area may also harbor the rare superficial reticular dystrophy of Koby, which causes painless and progressive loss of vision.

Mosaic degeneration or "crocodile shagreen" is almost exclusively limited to Bowman's membrane in its central part; it causes progressive visual loss that may be relieved by lamellar keratoplasty.

Somewhat more deeply in the corneal stroma, central lesions are represented by Groenouw's granular dystrophy (type I), lattice dystrophy, and hereditary crystalline dystrophy, which is very slowly progressing and nonirritative. Rarer affections in this area are the central speckled dystrophies of François and Neeten.

In the deep stroma, the localized and nonsuppurative thickening of disciform keratitis follows an irritative course of nearly a year or longer. In the deepest layers of the cornea, dystrophies tend to be widespread rather than axial. Blood staining, however, resulting from hyphema and glaucoma is generally most dense in the central area and is uniformally preceded by some damage to the endothelium.

Interpalpebral area (visible segments of the limbal, midzone, and central areas)

The interpalpebral area of the cornea, again by definition, is the site of *exposure keratitis* of various types. It is particularly affected by actinic trauma (actinic keratitis) from welder's arcs or other sources of ultraviolet rays that are destructive to superficial cells. Chemical contaminants in the atmosphere similarly create identifying patterns of damage because the lids shield the upper and lower poles of the cornea. The usually unilateral, torpid, or sluggish lesions of Dimmer's nummular keratitis just under Bowman's membrane tend to be largely in the interpalpebral area and without conjunctivitis. Similarly, the more conspicuous changes of Sjögren's keratitis sicca affect the exposed interpalpebral area and the inferior corneal pole.

Meesmann's juvenile dystrophy, consisting of myriads of minute punctate opacities in the epithelium, appears in this area usually during the first 2 years of life. The vertical poles at the cornea are usually spared, and the painless, autosomal dominant process causes little visual loss until late life.

Total corneal involvement

Some of the incapacitating dystrophies and diseases that begin in the central portion spread widely throughout the cornea. Groenouw's macular dystrophy type II, seen less frequently than type I, is one of these beginning in the first decade of life, with clouding and surface irregularity in the cen-

tral area. The process, however, rapidly spreads through all layers and the total area of the cornea, so that by the third or fourth decade there is major visual loss. The disease is an autosomal recessive trait marked by reduced corneal sensitivity and recurrent attacks of irritation and light sensitivity.

Fatty degeneration or corneal xanthomatosis, which occurs bilaterally in adult life, is often associated with increased serum cholesterol and ultimately affects all layers of the cornea.

The ring-like dystrophy of Reis and Bucklers principally distorts and destroys Bowman's membrane, with recurrently painful episodes beginning about the age of 5 and continuing through the second decade of life. Irregular mottling and opacification progress in subsequent decades with marked reduction in corneal sensitivity and in vision.

Lattice dystrophy of Biber, Haab, and Dimmer usually begins in childhood or early adult life with irregular linear opacities in the anterior stroma. The process may particularly involve the central area but spreads through the midzone and often through the periphery. Useful vision may be lost by the age of 40 in association with the increasingly dense opacities.

Keratoconus with its noninflammatory apical thinning usually affects the central area progressively from early adolescent life. It tends to spread through the midzone. Hemosiderin arcs in the epithelium frequently outline the base of the conical area and may form the incomplete Fleischer's ring, which appears as a dirty yellowish green color.

THE SCLERA AND ITS DISTURBANCES

"Do not shoot until you see the white of their eyes."
LEGEND OF THE BATTLE OF BUNKER HILL, JUNE 17, 1775

The sclera or the "white of the eye" derives its name from Galen's introduction of the Greek word meaning "hard." The sclera is a dense, largely inert, and almost acellular supporting coat of the globe. It is composed of elongated fibers that in turn constitute interlacing fiber bundles and lamellae. Their chemistry is predominantly collagenous, though some elastic fibers are found in the periphery of the fiber bundles. The role of the sclera is generally a passive one in local and systemic disease as well as in response to injury. Disorders of the sclera are comparatively rare, and primary diseases of the sclera are exceedingly rare. In common with the completely avascular lens and the normally avascular central cornea, but in sharp contradistinction to the vascular transition zone of the limbus, primary scleral neoplasms are essentially unknown.

Examination of the sclera must avoid easy confusion with disturbances of the overlying *bulbar conjunctiva,* the loosely fibrous and vascular *episclera,* and the fibroelastic condensation known as the *fascia bulbi* or *capsule of Tenon.* Within a few millimeters of the limbus, all of these anatomic layers tend to fuse with the sclera so that anatomic and pathologic differentiations are clinically less significant. Posteriorly, however, they may be separately involved in disease alterations, though inflammations often rapidly involve all the contiguous structures.

An important anterior landmark is the *external scleral sulcus,* which is just proximal to the limbus and which serves as a guide for anterior segment incisions. More important diagnostically is the corresponding *internal scleral sulcus,* whose posterior margin projects forward as the *scleral spur.* Gonioscopically this is seen as a whitish ring into which the anterior edge of the darker ciliary body normally inserts. The internal scleral sulcus is not specifically identified on gonioscopy because of the overlying trabecular meshwork.

The sclera varies widely in thickness at different areas within a normal eye, with changes of age, with physiologic differences among individuals, and with pathologic alterations. The thinnest and weakest area of the sclera is the posterior foramen, spanned only by delicate fibrils of the *lamina cribrosa* in order to permit exit of the optic nerve fasciculi. Here is where the increased intraocular pressure of glaucoma first causes pathologic distension. The sclera is also normally thin (about 0.3 mm.) in the areas proximal to insertion of the rectus muscles.

Beyond the age of 50 there is a widespread and increasing incidence of symmetric thinning and hyalinization just anterior to the horizontal rectus muscle insertions. These are asymptomatic and translucent *senile hyaline plaques* that permit the underlying darkness of the choroid to show through. The overlying bulbar conjunctiva is not involved and the plaques are only of cosmetic concern.

Another physiologic finding that occasionally misleads the unwary examiner is the presence of intrascleral nerve loops of Axenfeld (1902), which appear as two or three small dark spots beneath the bulbar conjunctiva 3 or 4 mm. from the limbus. These are branches of the long ciliary nerves that usually carry with them a few pigmented chromatophores from the suprachoroid or the cellular inner layer of the sclera, known as the lamina fusca sclerae. They are nearly always located superiorly and disclosed on elevation of the upper lid where they might be mistaken for foreign bodies. They occur rarely in other quadrants, and nearly always their true nature is confirmed by the presence of a single small blood vessel radiating from them.

Myopia in its progressive and higher degrees is commonly associated with scleral elongation and thinning that can be verified by ultrasound biometry. At times this may be visualized along the equator of the globe as increased transmission of the dark blue choroidal color through thinned sclera.

In logical extension of this alteration, the sclera may present serious pathologic stretching or ectasia diffusely or in localized portions. Outward movement of the underlying choroid and ciliary body into such areas creates the ominously dark *staphylomas* of adult life, which may cause retinal detachment or even perforation of the globe. Such staphylomas when present anteriorly or as intercalary lesions (between the iris and ciliary body) are more viciously progressive than are similar defects at the equator.

Inflammatory disturbances of the sclera generally represent collagen systemic diseases of obscure origin and should be provisionally described by their morphology as: diffuse or brawny scleritis, deep scleritis, nodular scleritis, anterior scleritis, annular scleritis, sclerokeratitis, necrotizing scleritis, posterior scleritis, scleromalacia perforans, and so on. More superficially there may be nodular episcleritis or episcleritis fugax. More posteriorly there may be sclerotenonitis or tenonitis with its painful effects on attempted rotation of the globe. Rarely there may be true pyogenic or bacterial scleritis from extension of similar enophthalmitis or exogenous agents ranging from the common *Staphylococcus* and *Streptococcus* to the granuloma-producing organisms of tuberculosis, syphilis, or leprosy.

In the presence of suspect pyogenic infections, attempts should be made at identification of organisms by smears and cultures.

Masses appearing as granulomas in the sclera or on the scleral surface may at times be extensions of intraocular malignancies such as malignant melanoma of the choroid, which is the most common intraocular malignancy. This usually represents advanced and neglected disease with preceding visual loss and growth through the small scleral emissary channels that normally transmit nerves and vessels. The basic diagnosis is clearly suggested by ophthalmoscopic discovery of a large single or multilocular dark tumor mass within the eye. Ultrasound will show a solid pattern of irregular echoes throughout such a mass.

Pigmentation or color changes in the sclera present accentuated values because of its normally alabaster white coloration. The inertness of the sclera precludes it from early participation in most diseases accompanied by biologic staining. Jaundice is commonly associated with yellow coloration over the white of the eyes resulting from bile pigment deposits. Careful examination with the slit lamp reveals that such color changes, like those of argyria or silver staining, are overwhelmingly confined to the bulbar conjunctiva and are merely rendered more conspicuous by the white scleral background. This is confirmed by noting that the maximum amount of discoloration is located peripherally or in the fornix areas rather than in the near limbal region. "Scleral jaundice" is a misnomer.

Blue sclerotics represent a congenital and hereditary abnormality of the sclera and other connective tissue. The sclera has increased translucency and may at times be thinned, causing the blue color of the choroid to show through uniformly. This is not a pigmentary abnormality. The anomaly is associated in a high percentage of patients with multiple fractures, deafness, and joint dislocations.

Ochronosis (congenital alkaptonuria) is indicated by bilateral and generally symmetric patchy deposits of yellow greenish pigment in the interpalpebral sclera and episclera. Associated darkening and discoloration in the cartilage of the pinnas and the nose is seen in the third or fourth decade of life (though it may appear either earlier or later) and tends to be progressive. This usually causes no visual difficulty.

REFERENCES

Bourne, W. M., and Enoch, J. M.: Optical principles of the clinical specular microscope, Invest. Ophthalmol. **15**:29-32, 1976.

Donaldson, D. D.: A new instrument for keratography, Arch. Ophthalmol. **88**:425-431, 1972.

Hanna, C.; Fraunfelder, F. T., and Sanchez, J.: Ultrastructural study of argyrosis of cornea and conjunctiva, Arch. Ophthalmol. **92**:18-22, 1974.

Javal, L., and Schiøtz, H.: Un ophtalmometre pratique Ann. d'ocul. **86**:5, July-Aug., 1881.

Warburg, M.: Eye immobilization for slit lamp examination of patients with nystagmus, Acta. Ophthalmol. **47**:781-783, 1969.

CHAPTER 6

Ocular motility and strabismus

Ocular motility examining techniques encompass study of both the sensory (afferent) components and the motor (efferent) components. Therefore ocular motility is actually a subdivision within the neuroophthalmic examination. This embraces afferent pathways along cranial nerves II (visual and pupillary) and V (corneal, conjunctival, and lid sensitivity). Efferent pathways are along cranial nerves III (oculomotor), IV (trochlear), VI (abducens), and VII (facial). Examining routines and techniques are identified by legions of literature and enormous eponymology, reflecting inherent inadequacies in the peripheral approach (muscles, tendons, and fascia) to what is far more frequently a central problem (vision, binocularity, fusion, and motor control). This attack via the end-organ has perforce characterized strabismology from the birth of modern ophthalmic study up to the findings of recent decades from investigations into electromyography, electroencephalography, better sensory diagnostics, and developmental neurology of lower primates.

Many diagnostic tests duplicate or overlap in their spheres of usefulness. In general, the simplest and most physiologic maneuver should be selected to minimize introduction of abnormal or instrumental conditions. Thus the Bagolini striated glass is preferable to the multiple Maddox rod because it maintains more usual or physiologic conditions for vision.

PRELIMINARY GENERAL INSPECTION

Preliminary general inspection in the area of ocular motility presupposes the examiner's full understanding of ocular and orbital anatomy and should note (1) activity pattern of the patient (hyperkinetic pattern in children, head-nodding in infants, aimless movements of the mongoloid patient), (2) normal versus abnormal head and cervical spine positions (usual freedom of cervical motion, contracture of a sternomastoid muscle, ankylosis or deformity of the spine), (3) gross positioning of the eyes (apparently normal versus internal deviation, external deviation, and so on), (4) presence of chronic ocular movements (pendular nystagmus in severe congenital impairments of vision, jerk nystagmus in central and vestibular lesions, vertical nystagmus in subtentorial lesions, random movements of blindisms), (5) position of the lids (protective ptosis in acquired diplopia, levator impairment associated with localized muscular dystrophy involving the superior rectus, lid lag in hyperophthalmic Graves' disease).

PRELIMINARY OCULAR INSPECTION

Preliminary ocular inspection in the primary position of gaze (direct or straight ahead) establishes the following points.

Usual positioning of the face and head. Position of the head should be checked for normal attitude versus chin-lifting in elevator paralyses, face-turning in abducens palsy, and head tilt in oblique impairment.

Anatomic characteristics of the orbits influencing strabismic appearance (pseudostrabismus). The factors influencing pseudostrabismus include facial or orbital asymmetry, hypertelorism simulating exotropia, epicanthus simulating esotropia, small interpupillary distance also simulating esotropia, traumatic deformities, disturbances of tumors or possible tumors, enophthalmos following orbital floor fractures, and vertical asymmetry stimulating vertical imbalance. Diagnosis of small defects in facial configuration and documentation of growth changes in these details are helped by simple linear measurements with a millimeter ruler. Ordinarily the intercanthal distance should be less than half of the interpupillary distance.

Angle kappa. Much of preliminary ocular inspection is based on observation of the corneal light reflex, the reflection of the examiner's inspection light held in front of the patient. The corneal light reflex (reflection) generally appears on the shiny cornea of the normal eye in its visual or fixation axis. For practical clinical purposes the visual or fixation axis is the principle visual line that extends from the object of regard, through the corneal light reflex, to the fixating portion of the retina (normally the fovea). The examiner must estimate the angle formed between the visual axis and the apparent pupillary center or pupillary axis. This is usually designated as *angle kappa.* Rarely are the visual and pupillary axes the same, at which time angle kappa is zero.

When the corneal reflex is slightly nasal to the pupillary center or pupillary axis, the angle kappa is positive.* A positive angle kappa of 3 to 5 degrees may be physiologic in emmetropia, whereas higher degrees of angle kappa are seen in hyperopia. Light reflex temporal to the pupillary axis, which may be seen in myopia, is called negative angle kappa.

Positive angle kappa tends to simulate

---

*Of the series of angles in strabismometry, angle kappa (between the visual axis and central pupillary line) is the most important (Landolt, 1878). This is a familiar and practical approximation of what in more precise terms is the angle between the optic and fixation axis (angle gamma) at the center of rotation, but the optic axis is essentially impossible to locate clinically. Academic minutiae in definition of the optic axis (the theoretic line through the centers of curvature of all refracting surfaces), the visual axis (line from fixation point through nodal points to the fovea), and the fixation axis (line from the fixation point to the center of rotation) have led to theoretic and insignificant clutter of the literature with designations such as angle alpha (angle at the anterior nodal point between optic and visual axes) or the less familiar angle lambda of Glenn Fry (a clinical expression for angle kappa).

slight divergence or exodeviation, while negative angle kappa may simulate slight convergence or esodeviation.

Angle kappa, for practical clinical purposes, is adequately measured by the examiner's estimation. More precise measurements may be made, if desired, objectively in degrees on an arc perimeter or subjectively in a major amblyoscope using slides with horizontally aligned targets at 1-degree intervals. Usual practical needs of measurement are served by the examiner's direct visual estimation of the distance between the apparent pupillary center and the corneal light reflex seen in monocular fixation. Normally the right and left angles kappa are essentially equal unless there is marked anisometropia. Thus if loss of fixation ability precludes measurement of angle kappa in one eye, it may be estimated from measurement in the isometropic opposite eye.

Estimation of fixation. Gross estimation of the fixation pattern of each eye to a stimulus such as a small light bulb or for young children a small animated toy or squeaker (Fig. 6-1), is made with both eyes open. A spectrum of other fixation devices includes small closed loop, rear-projection movies, and expensive ($200) electronic "Watchits" of serial light displays.* One of my favorites is the flat disc, ¼ watt "night light" that may be plugged into any standard electrical wall outlet without mechanical suspension and costs 50¢ at any hardware store.

Fixation may be:
1. Normal, centric or foveolar, and binocular
2. Normal but influenced by significantly positive (simulating exodeviation) or negative (simulating esodeviation) angle kappa
3. Unilateral
4. Eccentric (caused by strabismic amblyopia, macular lesion, displaced or ectopic macula)
5. Alternating
6. Absent or nonfixing, as in a blind eye

In the cooperative adult and older child

---

*Ocutron Company, Shaker Heights, Ohio 44122.

Fig. 6-1. Electrically activated and illuminated remote fixation devices to attract attention of child. Foot control illuminates eyes and activates components of each toy. (Made by Jenkel-Davidson House of Vision, San Francisco, California 94119.)

showing the second through the fourth types of fixation as estimated by the corneal light reflex, it is often helpful to clarify these patterns by Visuscopic or Projectoscopic measurements of fixation targets projected on the fundus (p. 117).

Evaluation of deviation. Gross evaluation of deviation of the eyes from parallelism is observed objectively by the position of the corneal light reflex.

Cover test for each eye to detect heterotropia

The simple qualitative cover test is a refinement in observations of the corneal light reflex and should be the examiner's first, and almost automatic, maneuver following preliminary inspection. With a fixation light in one hand and facing the patient frontally for careful observation of the corneal light reflexes, the examiner brings an opaque cover, held in his other hand, over one eye. The test presupposes fixation ability in each eye. If the *uncovered* eye makes a movement of redress or realignment to the fixation light, this eye has been deviating (in a direction opposite to its movement of realignment) and

is now taking up fixation. If a deviating eye is covered, there will be no movement of the fixing eye. Therefore the test must be applied to each eye in turn while the fellow eye is under observation. An accommodative target or stimulus must be used in near range testing.

If there is no movement of either eye while *uncovered*, there is good binocular balance (relative orthophoria) or anomalous retinal correspondence of the harmonious type.

The test is more critical and diagnostic in near than distance range, but it is preferably recorded also with the aid of a fixation light at least 20 ft. away, because some deviations appear only at distance. Though the test is useful at every age, small deviations of a few prism diopters or so may not be detected and will require further diagnostic refinements of the subjective type, which are generally not possible until the age of 4 or 5 years.

This cover test may also be executed in each of the other eight cardinal positions of gaze to elicit deviations not apparent in the primary position. It may be used to separate *primary deviation* (that of a squinting eye while behind the cover or while it is not fixing) from *secondary deviation* (that of a nonsquinting eye while behind the cover or while the paretic eye is forced to fix).

Cover-uncover test to detect heterophorias

The cover-uncover test is an immediate extension of the cover test, predicated upon fixation ability in each eye. However, attention is given here to the covered eye *as* the cover is removed, rather than to the uncovered eye. In this test the cover serves to disrupt fusion and thereby a heterophoria or latent tendency to squint may be revealed by deviation of the eye under cover.

Each eye is tested separately. Careful observation is directed to the eye as its cover is removed. If the eye under cover has not deviated, relative orthophoria is present; if the eye moves in recovery of fixation, heterophoria is present. For example, if the eye moves outward to fixate as the cover is removed, an esophoria is present; if the left eye moves downward to fixate, then a left hyperphoria is present. Again, though applicable at all ages, this rather primitive dissociation procedure may miss small heterophorias, particularly in the vertical direction, but these can be elicited in patients older than 5 or 6 by subjective tests such as the Maddox rod test (p. 121).

Estimate of rotations

"Just what to look for almost defies description and there is no substitute for experience."
RICHARD SCOBEE, 1947

Techniques

Just as soon as the estimates of fixation and gross evaluation of deviation have been made, the examiner assesses the rotational ability of the eyes. Required equipment consists only of a fixation light, an occluder (often most easily the examiner's hand), and a near or accommodation target carrying print or small figure details.

Quantitation of rotation is usually done by one of three techniques: (1) visual approximation based on the Hirschberg estimate of corneal light reflex displacement, (2) mea-

surement of the fixation field based again on position of the corneal light reflex but with more precise localization on an arc perimeter, or (3) prism cover neutralization test. The first method is obviously most simple, appealing, and rapid. It fails to quantitate minute degrees of deviation, but such specificity in a variable and fatigable neuromuscular feat is of doubtful validity. The arc perimeter adds more critical evaluation in units of approximately 5 degrees and may also be used to standardize the selected distance from the primary position for reproducible positions in which to measure. This is far more time consuming than the Hirschberg estimate and requires a quiet and attentive child.

The orthoptically traditional and venerated neutralization of deviation in the cardinal positions with prism and cover yields specific numbers in terms of a few prism diopters. Such measures usually have their significance eroded by (1) vagaries in patient attention and effort, (2) influence of fatigue or medical factors, (3) mechanical difficulty in keeping the back surface of the prism perpendicular to the visual axis, (4) alterations in prism strength by tilting, (5) manual problems of properly holding horizontal and vertical prisms when both are needed, and (6) compounding errors in each of these items as the need for prism strength exceeds 20 or 25 diopters. The comic term "FFP" test (fist full of prisms) was born with reason.

Diagnostic positions

In addition to preliminary ocular inspection in the primary or straight-ahead position of gaze, the other eight *principal* or *diagnostic* positions of gaze must be utilized. This evaluates each of the twelve extraocular muscles in the six specific directions of their maximum action (right, left, up and right, down and right, up and left, down and left) and in the two functionally important positions of straight up and straight down.

Versions

Versions are conjugate or yoke movements of the two eyes executing gaze directions in response to normally equal innervation (Hering's law, 1879). These are commonly evaluated first as the patient fixes with his nondeviating or preferred eye, if one is preferred. The patient is asked to follow, or with small children hopefully to be attracted to, a small inspection or fixation light. This enables the examiner to gauge the position of the eyes by maintaining a close watch on the corneal light reflexes, rapidly alternating his own observation from the patient's right to left cornea. The primary position of gaze is straight ahead with remote fixation.

Versions are commonly designated (1) dextroversion (right gaze), (2) levoversion (left gaze), (3) supraversion (straight-up gaze), and (4) infraversion (straight-down gaze). These move the eyes into "secondary" positions. A "unitized" name is not available for the equally important oblique rotations of gaze: (5) up and right, (6) down and right, (7) up and left, and (8) down and left. These move the eyes into "tertiary" positions. It is necessary to examine in each of these positions. If the corneal light reflex on either eye appears to slip forward of the visual axis in the direction toward which rotations are being tested, then that eye is not rotating fully with its fixating fellow eye.

After testing with the preferred or nondeviating eye fixing (to quantitate the *primary* deviation), an attempt should be made to repeat these same eight rotations with the nonpreferred or deviating eye fixing (to quantitate the *secondary* deviation). To achieve this, it may be necessary to cover the preferred eye briefly or even intermittently. In comitant, nonparalytic, or older and compensated paretic heterotropia, the primary and secondary deviations will be essentially the same. In paretic heterotropia, secondary deviation (of the nonsquinting eye) will exceed primary deviation. Where only small and uncertain inequalities exist between amounts of primary and secondary deviation, intermittent cover helps to bring out these measurements.

Cycloversion. The two types of cycloversions (dextrocycloversion and levocycloversion) are named by the rotation of the upper

corneal poles. Torsional concomitant squints or cyclotropias are exceedingly rare, usually difficult to quantitate, and may escape detection unless special studies are made on a major amblyoscope.

On the basis of supranuclear lesions there may be gaze impairments related to the type of version stimulus. Thus versions in response to *command* may be impaired by a lesion in the descending pathway from the midfrontal convolutions. Versions in response to *attraction* may be impaired by lesions in less well-defined pathways from the occipital lobes. Versions in response to *following* apparently represent the lowest level of internuclear coordination and may persist in the absence of both command and attraction versions.

A and V patterns. Particular attention should be given to variations in amount of horizontal heterotropia on execution of versions straight upward (supraversion) and straight downward (infraversion). For standardization in evaluation of these two important diagnostic positions of gaze, it is desirable to make the upward measurement about 25 degrees above the primary position and to make the downward measurement about 35 degrees below the primary position. Normally there is a slight tendency for increased convergence in infraversions and a slightly greater tendency to increased divergence in supraversion. Measurement of A and V patterns at distant fixation eliminates accommodative components that may confound diagnostic findings at near. To do this, the examiner tilts the patient's face upward or downward to obtain, respectively, depression or elevation of gaze while maintaining fixation on a small light source at least 20 ft. away. Near testing of an esodeviating patient in these positions should be with an accommodative target to bring out maximum overconvergence. Similarly, to elicit the maximum cosmetic deviation when testing an exodeviating patient, a nonaccommodative target or light should be used.

The A or V pattern may be present with or without horizontal deviation in the primary position. Strong V esotropia in downward gaze may be accompanied by habitual chin-tucking, particularly in the reading position, to avoid the convergent area. Significance probably should not be attached to variations with horizontal position in supraversion and infraversion unless a difference of at least 15 or 20 prism diopters is found with V esodeviation or V exodeviation. Similarly there should be a difference of at least 10 prism diopters in establishing A esodeviation or A exodeviation.

The A or V pattern, with or without horizontal deviation in the primary position, must be identified because of symptoms it may produce, compensatory chin-tucking or chin elevation that may be used by the patient, and difference in surgical correction that may be required. A and V patterns will commonly be found in association with disturbances of the oblique muscles, which will require correction in their own right. Thus the inferior oblique muscles, which act as abductors in upward gaze, tend to decrease esotropia or to increase exotropia in supraversion if these muscles are overacting (or if the superior oblique muscles are underacting). When specific abnormalities are not present in the oblique muscles, it may be necessary to correct these patterns by supraplacement or infraplacement of the horizontal recti, according to the precise diagnosis established. In general these patterns will be found to be symmetric and therefore require symmetric surgery. Supraplacement or infraplacement of the horizontal muscles in recession correction will be in the direction where most correction is desired. Thus in a V esotropia without oblique muscle defects, it is usually indicated to combine the recession surgery with infraplacement.

Observation should be made for antimongoloid slant (outer canthi downward) of the interpalpebral fissures, because this is frequently associated with V pattern.

Vergence

Vergences are disjunctive or disjugate movements in which the two eyes move in opposite directions. Clinically the most significant, the most demanding, and the most easily measured are the horizontal vergences: divergence and convergence. These relate to two major and frequent motility problems, divergence excess and convergence insufficiency. The first, a common disturbance in children, should be evaluated by directing the patient to remote fixation by looking out a window at a landmark several miles away. This effect is enhanced by the brightness of a sunny day and is significantly masked by examination in a dimly lighted room at a test distance of 20 ft. or less. Measurement is best accomplished by noting the position of the corneal light reflexes.

Convergence should be measured at the reading distance of about 13 in. by determining the near point of convergence (NPC). It is essential to use a finely detailed target commanding the patient's focusing effort in the near range. The patient must wear his distance spectacle correction. Convergence is usually increased by (1) tonic factors, (2) accommodative efforts, (3) the proximal stimulus (nearness to an object), and, in some people, (4) voluntary effort.

The NPC is influenced by the interpupillary distance, requiring less convergence effort when this distance is small and more when it is large. Theoretically, therefore, the NPC should be measured from a convergence base line that connects the centers of rotation of each eye. For practical purposes this baseline is equal in length to the interpupillary distance when the eyes are in the primary position, but it is located about 13 mm. posterior to the corneal apices. Measurements made from the nasal bridge should therefore have added to them an amount to compensate for the height of the bridge anterior to the corneas, plus the additional 13 mm. In clinical testing, a small accommodative target is advanced toward the patient along a ruler edge (Prince, Duane, Gulden, Foster) extending from the bridge of the nose. The examiner watches both eyes of the patient for the first evidence of one breaking from convergence (moving laterally); this represents the NPC. An intelligent patient may also be instructed to report the moment the target appears to double; this will confirm the measurement.

Generally, each eye adducts similarly in

Fig. 6-2. Technique of measuring horizontal prism vergences with near fixation targets suspended on bridge of examiner's spectacles. Risley rotary prism is held horizontally to measure base-in or base-out prism power.

response to convergence stimuli. The NPC should be expressed in millimeters and is significant primarily when interpreted in the light of age, refractive errors, and horizontal imbalance. As a rule of thumb, the NPC is normally less than the near point of accommodation for the single emmetropic (or corrected) eye and about equal to the interpupillary distance.

Analysis of vergences should also note and record the infrequent vertical divergence when present. These are right sursumvergence (right eye higher), sometimes called positive vertical divergence, and right deorsumvergence (right eye lower), sometimes called negative vertical divergence. Near versus distance fixation generally has no effect on vertical vergences. In conjunction with change from distance to near, or from primary position down to the reading position, there may at times be significant cyclovergences. If the upper corneal poles rotate nasally, this is incyclovergence (conclination or adtorsion), and if the upper corneal poles rotate laterally, this is excyclovergence (disclination or abtorsion). Infrequently, this is important in the presence of a high cylindric refractive correction, which must be prescribed at different axes in separate pairs of glasses for distance and near use. Cyclovergences and cyclotropias can be best measured with the major amblyoscope but can also be quantitated with the Maddox double-rod procedure (red and white Maddox rods with the ribs placed vertically before each eye while looking at a bright light source).

Prism vergence, or ability to maintain single binocular vision against increasing prismatic obstacles (base-out for convergence, base-in for divergence), is another quantitative measuring technique. However, it is largely an abnormal or instrumental hurdle and may relate more to comfort factors in sustained near work than to precise diagnostics in motor aspects of fusion (Fig. 6-2).

Ductions (active and passive)

Ductions are monocular rotations evaluated in each of the six directions of maximal action corresponding to the six extraocular muscles. The fellow eye must be occluded to minimize any inhibitional palsy from that eye. Ductions are generally less diagnostic than versions because each muscle has approximately 100 times more strength than is needed to move the globe (Lancaster, 1941). Thus, a significant number of muscle bundles may be knocked out, and ductions still appear fairly normal. Measurement may be made by estimation from the corneal reflex or by perimeter arc determination of the fixation field. Such fixation fields are of significance primarily in comparison with those of a fellow eye.

Active ductions on command or following provide limited information and need not be done routinely, but passive or forced ductions with forceps under topical or general anesthesia are of highly specific value in differentiating an innervational paralysis from a mechanical obstacle to rotation (such as an adherent superior oblique tendon sheath or incarceration of an inferior oblique in an orbital floor fracture).

In planning surgical procedures for reoperations, the analysis of rotational limitations on forced duction is often crucial to successful correction. Similarly, as the planned surgery is executed at the table, reevaluation of forced ductions will indicate the effectiveness of the procedure or the necessity of additional steps. If the surgeon cannot rotate the globe in forced ductions following a corrective intervention, certainly the patient will be unable to do so.

To test forced ductions in most adults, a topical anesthetic must be instilled several times. The patient is instructed to look in the direction to which the eye under examination is to be moved. A toothed forceps is used to engage the conjunctiva and episclera near the limbus, and effort is made to rotate the globe by direct mechanical action. Generally children will not tolerate this procedure. Many adults will complain of discomfort, and usually a small conjunctival hemorrhage remains for a few days at the site of forceps application.

Forced ductions are more easily and reliably performed under general anesthesia, which excludes voluntary eye movements and eliminates pain. Under these conditions firm fixation can be made with the forceps into the tendinous insertion of one of the rectus muscles. Alternatively, pressure can be exerted with the broad portion of a squint hook into the conjunctival cul-de-sac in line with the direction of action of the muscle under examination. This also tends to produce a series of small conjunctival hemorrhages in the area of pressure application.

Recording rotations

Methods or schema of recording rotations are almost as numerous as the population of strabismologists. A simple diagram should be part of every record and should indicate increased or decreased functions in the nine diagnostic positions. Specifically, quantitative notations in degrees or prism diopters should be emphasized in the primary, the straight-up, and the straight-down positions. The older record systems that omitted straight-up and straight-down positions were oblivious to the A, V, and X components that enter so many cases of heterotrophia. Therefore they should not be used.

Amblyopia

Amblyopia is an abnormal sensory deficit, predominantly of macular vision, occuring in childhood prior to 9 years of age, and commonly resulting from efforts to avoid diplopia in the presence of heterotropia. Classically it is considered to be derived by two mechanisms: (1) cortical inhibition or (2) retinal nonuse (exanopsia). It is without morphologic evidence in the globe. It is limited largely to photopic vision (cone function) and yet may be accompanied by very little reduction in color discrimination. For unexplainable reasons it is particularly demonstrated in the "crowding phenomenon" where central visual acuity is seen to drop in proportion to the crowding of letters together on a line. Thus, the examiner may miss early or mild degrees of amblyopia if single or isolated letters are used in the testing.

For working purposes amblyopia may be classified into the following four functional types:

1. Strabismic or suppression amblyopia: impairment of acuity in one eye of a patient with strabismus or a history of such imbalance previously, particularly the eso deviation type.

2. Refractive or anisometropic: poor vision in an eye associated with differences in re-

fractive status between the two eyes usually greater than 2.5 diopters. This is associated with differences in retinal image size and lends to preferential use of the more nearly emmetropic eye.

3. Congenital amblyopia: poor vision associated with true congenital strabismus or developmental arrest of the globes as seen in high hyperopia usually above +6 diopters.

4. Organic amblyopia: visual impairment in an eye without morphologic defects or anisometropia but possibly associated with birth trauma or macular hemorrhage at birth. In contradistinction to the first three types, neutral density filters in the presence of organic amblyopia usually cause further distinct reduction in acuity.

Quantitative measurement of the degree of deviation

Fundamentally, reliance in establishing diagnoses should be based on objective procedures in preference to tests requiring subjective responses or participation. Although precision is an inherent element of all scientific measurements, practicality and true understanding dictate the level of exactness to be sought. Thus the width of a prism is not measured in inches nor the power of spectacle lenses in tenths of a diopter. Similarly, at surgery, the insertional line of an extraocular muscle cannot be measured in tenths of a millimeter from the limbus. Because of hour-to-hour and day-to-day variability in most strabismus, and because of the influence of attention, concentration, and relaxation, it is misleading to measure most deviations in units of less than 5 degrees and a waste of time and effort to measure in units of less than 5 prism diopters. Valid exceptions, however, exist in Visuscopic measurements of eccentricity of fixation, or prism measurements of small deviations in the primary position.

The *Hirschberg estimation* (1875) of the angle of deviation, based on the position of the corneal light reflection from an inspection (fixation) light held at the near or reading distance (33 mm.), is a sheet anchor measure used particularly in young children or uncooperative patients. This requires attention and fixation ability in at least one eye. Estimates are based on simplified geometry of the cornea, equating each millimeter on its surface with slightly more than 7 degrees or 15 prism diopters. Thus displacement of the corneal light reflex to a position just beyond the limbus equals about 45 degrees (90 prism diopters) of deviation; displacement of the light reflex midway between the corneal center and limbus equals about 20 degrees (40 prism diopters) of deviation. Though not precise and prone to miss deviations under 7 degrees (1 mm.), this may be the best or only method usable in infants, toddlers, or hyperactive children. In deriving Hirschberg figures, it is necessary to correct for a large angle kappa or for a small "physiologic" positive angle kappa that simulates a small exodeviation or obscures a small esodeviation.

The *Krimsky measurement* (prism reflex test, 1943) derives the prism power needed before the fixing eye (apex in the direction of duction) to induce yoke movement of the opposite eye, which moves its corneal light reflex from an eccentric to a centric location. This requires attention and ability of the patient to fixate with his preferred eye, but it is advantageously independent of any fixational capacity of the other or deviating eye. Findings are slightly more precise than with the Hirschberg method, but they require the back surface of the prism to be kept perpendicular to the line of fixation. Results are progressively less precise as high amounts of prism are required. Measurements for distance are imprecise because the examiner's face, which should be directly in front of the patient, must be moved to one side.

The *Duane alternate prism and cover test* or parallax test (1889) combines the fusional interruption achieved by rapidly moving an opaque cover from one eye to the other while placing before one eye a prism with the apex in the direction of deviation. Beginning always in the primary position, increasing amounts of prism are placed before the deviating eye until all movements of redress or realignment are neutralized or compensated for by the prism. Mechanical difficulty in testing is reduced in deviations under 30 prism diopters by use of a Risley or Hughes rotary prism; this is held in one hand so that the thumb and forefinger operate the knurled knob, varying the prism strength from zero to 30$^\triangle$ (Fig. 6-3). Though awkwardly requiring more drawer or storage space, a prism set (1$^\triangle$ to 40$^\triangle$) or a Berens plastic prism bar* (vertical, 1 to 25; horizontal, 1 to 40) can be used for the same purpose. Small sets (5$^\triangle$, 10$^\triangle$, 20$^\triangle$) or small bars (vertical, ½ to 10; horizontal, 1 to 20), though less expensive and easier to store, often are inadequate when most needed. This test may also be extended to each of the other eight cardinal positions of gaze and may be carried out with prisms, first over the deviating eye (preferred eye fixing) and then over the nondeviating eye, to separate primary and secondary deviation.

In the study of paretic or noncomitant

* Manufactured by R. O. Gulden, Philadelphia, Pennsylvania 19117.

heterotropia, as contrasted with nonparetic or comitant deviations, efforts should be made to establish a topographic diagnosis of the level of extraocular muscle impairment. These may be divided into the following five levels:

1. Mechanical anomaly of muscle, tendon, or orbit: congenital, local neoplastic, posttraumatic
2. Muscle itself: thyroid myopathy, myositis
3. Neuromuscular transmission: myasthenia gravis
4. Peripheral neuron: neurogenic paralysis as secondary to intracranial tumor
5. Supranuclear lesions: serious central nervous system defects that may be paranuclear, internal capsular, or cortical

DETAILED MOTILITY EXAMINATION

The preceding tests are generally objective in nature and require little on the part

Fig. 6-3. Risley rotary prism held horizontally before patient's eye in position to induce 0 to 30 degrees of horizontal prism.

of the patient other than obtaining his fixation. In addition to the standard steps of examination (history, vision, refraction, fundus examination), this may be all that can be obtained from a young and restless patient. It may be an adequate working amount of information in many simple, initial, or uncomplicated patients with heterotropia. Depending, however, on the age and level of cooperation of the patient, vagaries or uncertain aspects of particular functions in the case, and personal preference of the examiner, a further series of progressively detailed examinations may follow.

Objective quantitative diagnostic measurements

These objective diagnostic measurements include primarily the identification and measurement of monocular fixation patterns and angular strabismometry.

Fig. 6-4. Visuscope by Oculus Optikgeräte combines features of direct ophthalmoscope with star test in concentric circles at 20-second separation to measure fixation patterns. Interchangeable retinoscope and transilluminator heads are available (6 volts; 6 watts).

Monocular fixation patterns

In the cooperative adult and older child, the estimates of fixation behavior based on position of the corneal light reflex often need to be refined by the ophthalmoscopic projection and localization of a macular target graticule (such as a "Linksz Star") on the posterior pole. This is indicated principally when vision is reduced or fixation is unstable. Testing is done with a modification of the direct ophthalmoscope such as the Oculus Visuscope (Fig. 6-4), the Propper (Heine) Auto Foc, the Keeler Projectoscope, or most elegantly with the recording assistance of multiple fundus photographs (Fig. 18-4).

This is a monocular test and the opposite eye should be occluded. The patient is instructed to look directly at the projected star, asterisk, small ½-degree ring, or other device being used. The examiner notes, or photographs, the position of this target in relation to the foveola on the basis of several repeated fixations. The following are the patterns of monocular fixation that may be noted and differentiated.

1. Normal centric or foveolar fixation. The target is held steadily on the foveal center. Three or four types of minute, involuntary, and physiologic ocular oscillations or tremors may be identified and recorded while a patient is holding normal and steady fixation. These should be ignored in the identification of pathology, and differentiated from nonphysiologic micronystagmus that may account for reduced acuity even in the absence of strabismus.

2. Eccentric fixation. Eccentric fixation may be parafoveal, perifoveal, or peripheral. (a) In parafoveal fixation the fixation target is off the fovea centralis but maintained within the vessel-free concavity (or clivus) of the central area. (b) In perifoveal (or paramacular) fixation the fixation target is at the far edge of or beyond the clival slope into the small vessel area. Fixation becomes progressively less steady as the target is imaged farther from the foveola. (c) In peripheral fixation the fixation target is beyond the fiber layer of Henle and beyond the luteal pigmented portions of the central area. Unsteadiness or inconsistency of fixation may extend through an area 2 disc diameters or more in size. Patients with persistent fixed esotropia of 25 to 30 prism diopters at distance and at near and using the optic nerve head scotoma or blind spot mechanism (Swan) to avoid diplopia in binocular vision do not fix the Visuscopic target on their blind spot but rather may have good monocular acuity and centric fixation.

3. Paradoxic fixation. In this condition the fixation target is in the opposite direction from the fovea to that which would be anticipated on the basis of ocular deviation. Thus an esotropic patient may fix the target temporally rather than nasally, as would be expected. This is more apt to be found after surgical corrections, after overcorrections, in spontaneous (consecutive) change of a deviation as from esotropia to exotropia, or some times without apparent cause.

Accommodative convergence/accommodation ratio (AC/A ratio)

Patients with horizontal, nonparalytic deviations should always be studied both at near and at distance fixation targets when wearing their full, distance refractive correction. In children this necessitates refraction after complete atropinization and then a suitable interval for the effects of atropine to wear off. Several factors may influence differences in degree of deviation for near and for distance. One significant though variable factor is the ratio of accomodative convergence to accommodation (AC/A ratio) in the particular patient. Convergence responses are closely linked with accommodative efforts, as illustrated by the uncorrected hyperopic individual who must exert extra diopters of accommodative effort to focus for near and far; he will generate extra convergence impulses and may show excessive *accommodative convergence* in relation to his particular AC/A ratio.

Normally the amount of accommodative convergence to accommodation varies between 3 and 5. Thus 3 to 5 prism diopters of accommodative convergence occurs with each diopter of accommodation. High ratios

tend to be associated with convergence excess or accommodative esotropia as well as myopia without strabismus. Low AC/A ratios tend to be associated with convergence insufficiency as well as hyperopia without strabismus. The AC/A ratio, however, does not depend on refractive errors, heterophoria, or heterotropia and may remain constant in an individual even through presbyopia.

Interpupillary distance also affects the manifestations of AC/A ratios, because a high interpupillary distance demands greater AC/A ratios to achieve bifoveal fixation in the near range. Conversely, narrow-set eyes need less accommodative convergence per diopter of accommodation.

In use the AC/A ratio is first assessed by measuring the deviation at distance and near with the alternate cover test. If the results are essentially the same at near and distance, the AC/A ratio for that patient is normal. Differences should be established numerically with prism neutralization of movement during the alternate cover test. Measurement at ⅓ meter calls for 3 diopters of accommodation as compared to measurements at infinity or its simulation at 6 meters. Thus, to determine the AC/A ratio, the difference in prism diopters of deviation as measured at 6 meters and at ⅓ meter is divided by 3.

The basic ratio is not altered by orthoptic exercises, prisms, spectacle correction, or bifocals. Lenses as well as miotic drugs, however, may have profound effects on the apparent position of the eyes when properly prescribed for abnormal AC/A ratios. Similarly, surgical changes in the extraocular muscles will significantly alter the findings on clinical measurement of the AC/A ratio.

Angular strabismometry

Angular strabismometry, begun by the Parisians Landolt in 1875 and Javal in 1896, has gone through countless perimetric techniques and short-lived tangent scales, tapes, anglometers, linear gauges, transparent rules, measuring bridges, pupillometers, deviometers, tropophorometers, minor amblyoscopes, and so forth. All of these have been clearly superseded by the more adaptable and flexible major haploscopes or amblyoscopes, which afford measurement of both objective and subjective angles of deviation as well as considerable analysis of the sensory components in strabismus. Such instruments may also be used to a lesser degree for orthoptic training as an adjunct to other, more major methods in treatment. These instruments include the Orthoscope and the table-top Synoptophores 2051, 2052, and 2053 with plug-in but separate electric control by Clement Clarke* and the completely integrated table and Synoptophore by Oculus Optikgeräte (Fig. 6-5).† Other generally similar table-top models are the standard No. 11 Synoptiscope and the 5000 Synoptiscope (1970) by Curpax‡ and the Troposcope by American Optical Corporation.

Several specific limitations must be recognized in the operation of an amblyoscope: (1) the artificial lighting does not approach maximum ambient conditions and may not bring out full exodeviation, (2) targets are isolated from usual background stimuli and even with maximum size slides cover only about 10° on the retina, (3) the *near* response to such instrumental structures variably reduces the effective test distance from simulated infinity toward near point, and (4) esodeviations tend to be over estimated and exodeviations tend to be under estimated in comparison to prism and cover tests.

Instruments establishing fixation points by meridians and linear distance from the primary position are valuable in obtaining reproducible measurements on subsequent examination. The Owens deviometer has been helpful for this, or the table-stand Lavat Deviometer,* utilizing double luminous points on a fully rotational axis, affords standardized measurements that may be recorded on pads of diagrammatic sheets furnished with the instrument.

*London W1H, ODH, England.
†Dutenhofen, Federal Republic of Germany.
‡Curry & Paxton, Ltd., London, England.

Dissociation tests

> "Finally, the confusion is rendered greater by the underlying fact that we do not know what we are measuring but are certain that we are measuring different things with different tests."
> STEWART DUKE-ELDER, 1949

The individual with good vision in each eye (20/40 or better), asymptomatic binocularity, and cosmetically acceptable appearance does not usually come for an ocular motility examination. Many factors such as visual fixation, the high cerebral function of fusion, and the unacceptability of diplopia are strong curbs against strabismus or ocular deviation. However, the patient complaining of ocular use discomfort, variable diplopia, poor vision in one eye, or intermittently manifest squint requires not only careful evaluation of the optic components of refraction (which may be abnormal) and the preceding preliminary inspections (which may appear normal) but also examination of the eyes while interrupting fusion or dissociating the images of the two eyes in various ways. With such testing, latent (heterophoric),

Fig. 6-5. Synoptophore, standard model, with integrated table, is shown from operator's side. (Manufactured by Oculus Optikgeräte, Dutenhofen, Federal Republic of Germany.)

*Luneau and Coffignon, Paris 8e, France.

intermittent, or subtle impairments in binocularity are uncovered, in some fashion quantitated, and then interpreted as to significance.

The major amblyoscope or haploscope is traditionally the ally of the twentieth century orthoptist in deriving rather minute numerical values in measurement of both objective and subjective angles of squint. All such measurements, however, like the photograph of one ultrasonic echo, represent only one brief moment in the course of a process that may be highly variable. Amblyoscopic figures also inevitably are distorted by the influences of such extraneous factors as instrumental convergence and the near or proximal reflex.

Classifications of objective and subjective angle measurements include test findings without and later with dissociative measures to interrupt fusion. Many methods may be employed to produce dissociation. Each yields a level or type of dissociation that is difficult or impossible to quantitate numerically but that should be designated by the name of the test method and assigned somewhat of a rank order or degree of magnitude designation. Thus the Bagolini lenses produce one of the most subtle and physiologic forms of dissociation. The stroboscopic flash-afterimage tester produces one of the most coarse and least physiologic dissociations, and its use is becoming less popular.

In general, dissociation is commonly produced by (1) complete exclusion of the field of one eye from the other, as by an opaque cover, in the cover-uncover test, (2) use of color differences between the two eyes, as in the Lancaster red-green projection test, (3) distorting one image, as with the Maddox rod test, (4) displacing one image, as with a prism of a few diopters before one eye aligned at right angles to the major direction of deviation, or (5) adding subtle markers over the usual visual fields as with Bagolini striated glass. Less commonly it is produced by polarized illumination of the test objects and Polaroid lenses at opposite angles before each eye, or dissimilar bright stimuli generating afterimages, as with the electronic flash afterimage tester. The orthoptist turns most frequently to different, partial, or fusional test targets presented to each eye through the separate arms of a major amblyoscope.

One of the most precisely quantitative expressions of dissociation is the angular measurement of stereoscopic acuity or "stereo-acuity." This may normally be developed to a very high degree (a few seconds of arc), but it is closely dependent upon visual acuity and is unrewarding to test in the presence of poor vision.

Both causative mechanics and corrective procedures necessitate measurement of deviation at near and far. Near fixation distance has generally been standardized at 13 in. or 33 cm. Distance measurements should be at a stated distance of 20 ft. or 6 meters and, for all questions of divergence excess, should be repeated while the patient is "looking out the window" or fixing on an object at least a few hundred yards away.

Differentiation may further be made between *true divergence excess* and *simulated divergence excess*. This is done after initial measurement of the exodeviation for near and for distance by occluding the dominant eye with an opaque Elastoplast patch for at least an hour. The patch is then removed and measurements of the exodeviation repeated at near and distance. Remember, however, that permission of even brief binocularity on removing the patch may reinstate strong convergence mechanisms; therefore, a cover or occluder paddle should be placed over the nonpatched eye before removing the patch.

Testing then proceeds with a routine of the alternate cover technique using an estimation of corneal light reflex position or measurement in prism diopters. If there is no increase in near exotropia on removal of the patch, this suggests a *true* divergence excess. However, if the manifest exotropia at near is increased after patching, this is a *simulated* divergence excess. Along with the weighing of other factors such as amblyopia or orbital asymmetry, the simulated divergence excess will more likely require unilateral surgery (medial rectus muscle resection and lateral rectus muscle recession), whereas the true divergence excess constitutes a more specific indication for recession of both lateral rectus muscles.

Maddox rod test

The multiple Maddox rod test (1890) still stands as the most widely familiar dissociation procedure and has been used as an official measurement in the U. S. armed services for many decades. It is applicable only in the measurement of heterophorias (not heterotropias) and is more accurate and valuable in vertical than in horizontal phorias. A relatively bright light (usually brighter than afforded by a projection acuity device) and a darkened room are necessary to achieve visualization of the line, which appears at about half intensity compared to the brighter dot seen by the eye not behind the rod.

Use is facilitated by a phoropter or major refractor that includes swing-away Maddox rods and Risley rotary prisms before the apertures for each eye. Testing should be for distance and for near. First the patient's distance refractive prescription is set in the phoropter and then the Maddox rod presented before one eye. To enhance contrast, a red Maddox rod is usually used with a white light. With both eyes open, the patient is instructed to fix on a small bright light 20 ft. away and to describe the position of the red line he sees through the Maddox rod in relation to the light. For vertical testing the bars are set vertically and the patient sees a horizontal line (at right angles to the bars of the Maddox rod). If the line appears to run through the light, there is no vertical heterophoria. If the line does not run through the light, then the Risley prism is placed over the aperture with the rod and its zero line set horizontally. Vertical prism power is introduced base-up or base-down, as needed, to move the line into coincidence with the light. The examiner may have to interrupt the image of the fixation light by briefly placing his thumb before this eye in order for the patient to attain visualization of the relatively less-bright line.

If the test is elected to estimate horizontal phorias, the rod is rotated so that its components are horizontal and the resulting line, as visualized, appears vertically. Fusional impulses, however, will affect horizontal, quantitative measurements.

Similar Maddox principles can be tried to diagnose and measure cyclodeviations by positioning a red Maddox rod vertically before one eye and a white Maddox rod, also vertically, before the other eye. For this procedure, the phoropter (or trial frame) must be aligned precisely so that both rods are in accurate vertical alignment. Again with both eyes open, the patient fixes on a bright light 20 ft. away. If there is no vertical imbalance and no cyclodeviation, the patient sees only one horizontal pinkish line—a blending of the red line from one eye and the white line from the other eye. This may be verified by placing a 3- or 4-diopter prism base-down before either eye. Two separate horizontal lines (one red and one white) will then appear to the patient. These will be horizontal and parallel if there is no cyclodeviation. If one eye tends to intort or extort, however, the line before it will appear rotated in the opposite direction to the torsional disturbance of the globe. The Maddox rod (not a prism) is then rotated by the examiner or the intelligent patient until the two lines appear parallel. The amount of cyclodeviation is read in degrees from the trial or phoropter frame. This test, however, does not differentiate between cyclophorias and cyclotropias.

Although a major amblyoscope may be satisfactory for measuring the amplitude of torsion, it allows only for measurement in the primary position and is always accompanied by its inherent near stimulus or "machine factor" of variable and uncertain test distance simulation. The Maddox rod allows clearly known test distances (the actual physical location of the light stimulus from the patient) and some latitude of excursion into the other eight principal or diagnostic positions of gaze.

Maddox rod testing may also be repeated in the near or reading range. For this measurement the phoropter is less suitable than the trial frame because it does not permit the usual downward deviation of the eyes common in near use. The refractive correction and any needed near point add should also be in place before near readings are made. Cycloplegics are, of course, contraindicated in these near measurements.

Bagolini striated glass test

A more physiologic test, presenting less instrumental disturbance in the test situation, is the examination with Bagolini lenses (1960). These are plano lenses sized for insertion in the cells of a trial frame and containing almost imperceptible striations that do not obscure visualization of the environment. They may be likened to glass that has been lightly but unidirectionally streaked with slightly oily fingers. In fact, you can easily convert the patient's own glasses to the

Bagolini type by streaking them with your fingers after rubbing the side of your nose. Point light sources visualized through these lenses appear as luminous stripes at right angles to the lines of striation. This is the same directional relationship as with the Maddox rod. Simplicity of the procedure makes reporting easy even for children, and the patient's eyes are observable throughout the test.

In use, the room light should be slightly subdued and the fixation light should not have other light sources nearby. By convention, the Bagolini lens before the right eye has its striations oriented at the 45-degree axis, and the lens before the left eye is oriented at the 135-degree axis (Fig. 6-6).

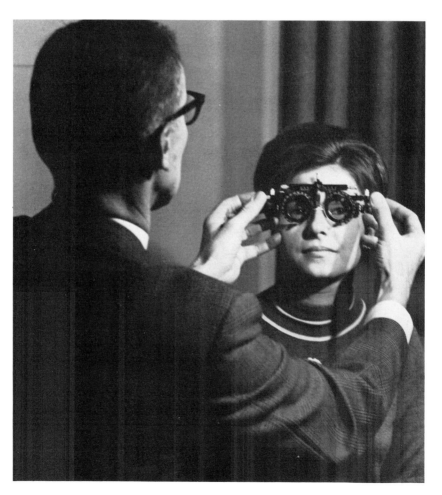

Fig. 6-6. Bagolini striated lenses being placed in position with conventional trial frame.

The patient is asked to report the position of the lines he sees. A perfectly intersecting X indicates no suppression and either no deviation or deviation with harmonious, anomalous retinal correspondence (ARC). An interruption in one line suggests foveal suppression or a macular lesion. Absence of either line suggests suppression throughout the area of conscious regard, and possibly peripheral suppression.

When a perfectly intersecting X is reported, the cover test is used on top of the Bagolini lenses to differentiate normal retinal correspondence (NRC) from harmonious, anomalous retinal correspondence (ARC). If the cover test shows no shift of the uncovered eye and if fixation is central, then NRC is present. If the cover test shows shift of the uncovered eye, then harmonious ARC is present. Unharmonious retinal correspondence cannot be diagnosed by this method.

Afterimage test

Perhaps the least sensitive or least subtle and most unphysiologic dissociation procedure is the afterimage test, developed by Hering in 1868 and further refined by Bielschwosky in 1938, to a bright light filament.* The test is unrestricted by modest limitation of acuity or opacities in the media but requires fixation ability in each eye and cooperation to describe, or preferably draw, the appearance of linear afterimages. The electronic flash, hand-held tester gives instantaneous stimulus exposure, though old, filament instruments are still available in many places in lieu of the electronic flash.

In use, the nonpreferred eye is first covered. The patient then fixes with the better eye on an opaque central marker in a horizontal light source for an electronic flash, or filament exposure of about 20 seconds. The cover is then transferred to the better eye, the light is rotated to a vertical position,

*Electronic flash, After Image Tester, manufactured by Nytronics, Inc., Kutztown, Pennsylvania. A more economical alternative can be made from a simple strobe light for a home camera; the illuminating area on the flash face should be narrowed to 2 or 3 mm.

and fixation and stimulus are held as before. The light is extinguished, the occluder removed, and the patient instructed to draw the position of the afterimages as they appear against a blank wall. The gap in each linear afterimage corresponds to the visual direction of each fovea, *if* central fixation is present. A perfect cross indicates normal retinal correspondence or deeply entrenched eccentric fixation with harmonious ARC.

When central (foveal) fixation is still retained in each eye in spite of heterotropia, the relative position of the afterimages will be displaced (outward in exotropia, inward in esotropia) because ARC is present and the two foveas no longer have a common visual direction. In the intermediate stage, designated as *eccentric viewing* (rather than the more deeply entrenched level known as *eccentric fixation*), the two foveas retain their common visual direction. Though the patient may use an extrafoveal area in casual viewing, the relative position of afterimages is displaced (NRC is present).

In full *eccentric fixation*, the visual direction and motor orientation are firmly associated with an extrafoveal retinal area, even though the patient has the sensation of looking directly at an object. In this situation, afterimages intersect precisely because of the ARC.

Major amblyoscopes present significant variability in afterimage testing and are not advised. Light intensities are generally too low to elicit stable afterimages and fixation time requirements tend to impair necessary steadiness of fixation. This is particularly true in a restive child or individual with a short attention span.

Subjective dissociation tests based on color

The subjective dissociation tests based on color as introduced by Javal in 1880 include: (1) the red glass diplopia test and tangent scale measurements, (2) the Lancaster red-green projection test (1939), (3) the Hess screen test (1908-1916), and (4) the Tschermak congruence test (1899-1903).

The use of medium-density color filters

(such as red, green-blue, and Snellen glasses) to achieve visual dissociation of the two eyes while using the same geometric stimulus has a record of usefulness in sensory evaluation from the latter nineteenth century.

The red glass test is the simplest of these procedures and is first used for subjective (diplopia) measurement of heterotropia (in which case a light- to medium-density red is used to minimize uncovering or eliciting heterophoria) with normal retinal correspondence. In use, the patient holds the red glass before his better eye while fixing on a pocket-light (Fig. 6-7) or similar light source at the intersection of the vertical and horizontal arms of a Maddox tangent scale (1890), which is marked in degrees of angular deviation for a predetermined test distance of 1 or 5 meters. With normal retinal correspondence, both foveas have a common visual direction. Therefore the linear separation of the red and white images, either in space or on the tangent scale, indicates the angular deviation. The observation of a single "pink" image indicates no deviation and no diplopia.

The test may be done in all principal positions of gaze to elicit incomitant deviations. A linear target light also enables identification of torsional (oblique) deviations.

The red glass test may also be used to estimate suppression and retinal correspondence. Here a medium- to high-density red is needed and the tangent scale is omitted. Just as for the subjective measurement of heterotropia, the red glass helps the patient identify the images from each by changing the value of one. If the red image falls on a scotomatous area, then suppression, anomalous retinal correspondence, or a local pathologic lesion may be present. To differentiate between suppression and ARC in such cases, a 3- or 4-diopter prism is placed vertically before the red filter. The red image is then vertically separated (subjectively appearing toward the apex of the prism) from the white fixation light. In heterotropia with NRC it is displaced opposite the direction of the squint. In heterotropia with ARC, the red image is aligned with the fixation light. Suppression, however, can be more reliably determined on the major amblyoscope and

Fig. 6-7. Red glass tests with filter held before patient's right eye while fixating on flashlight in left lateral position of gaze.

correspondence is better determined with the Visuscope.

The Lancaster red-green projection test is the simplest, least affected by subjective elements, most productive of diagnostic information, and easiest to interpret of all tests in this group. It may be used against any dull, dark, and homogeneous wall or with a marked tangent screen supplied for a predetermined testing distance, usually 1 meter. In use (Fig 6-8) the patient wears the red-green glasses and usually begins with red over the right eye. A red and a green torch projecting linear images are used (Foster penlight torches containing streak retinoscope bulbs beneath a focusing sleeve; larger Welch-Allyn torches with transformer-supplied light sources; or the Strabismometer,* which uses the identical red-

*Allied Ophthalmic Products Corp., Morton Grove, Illinois, 60053.

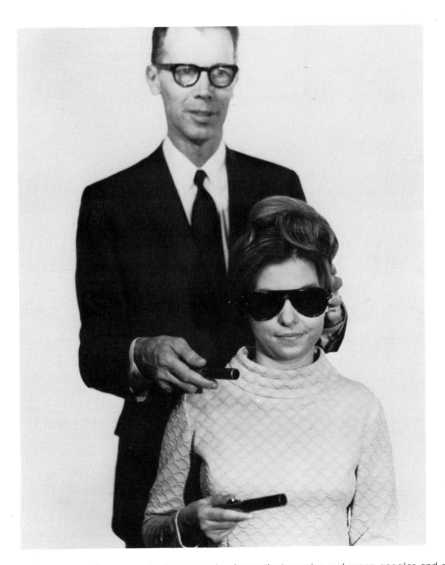

Fig. 6-8. Lancaster red-green projection tests showing patient wearing red-green goggles and responding to fixation with eye behind colored glass corresponding to examiner's colored torch. Patient's head is steadied by examiner's left hand to avoid movement during testing. Images of each torch are projected on screen in front of patient.

green principle by projecting a circle from one flashlight and, fitting the central hole in the circle, a solid disc of complementary color from the other).

Room lights are dimmed. The examiner, standing behind the patient, projects a red line on the wall or screen. The patient sees this red line (through his red lens) only with his right eye and therefore fixes with his right eye. With the green projection torch in his hand, the patient then superimposes the green slit, as seen with his left eye only, over the position he relates to the red line. Torsion and displacement of the slit directly indicate the corresponding position of the eyes (when NRC is present). When the normal eye is fixing, the primary deviation is demonstrated; when the red-green lenses are reversed, the secondary deviation is demonstrated. Deviation in each cardinal position is quickly and easily quantitated. Even small children enjoy the "game" and provide data that cannot be elicited with the more subjective red-green procedures. If neither the inexpensive Foster torches nor the expensive Welch-Allyn Lancaster or Allied sets are available, the examiner may quickly make suitable torches from a pair of flashlight pointers (or two old streak retinoscopes) by covering them with appropriate red and green cellophane.

The Hess screen (1908-1916) is an accurate, wall-mounted tangent screen made of black or gray felt with red stitching, scaled for use at ½ meter. Alignment of suspended green threads or use of a Law or similar green pointer provides the two color components. In use, the red-green Snellen (diplopia) glasses are worn and may be reversed for measurements of primary and secondary deviation. Torsional components can be identified, particularly if the linear green threads are used instead of a nonlinear pointer. The test is somewhat cumbersome and is fixed to the distance for which the screen is designed.

The congruence test of Tschermak, even after 65 years, is used very little, and less in the United States than in Europe. It requires a retroilluminated box with extend-ing opaque vertical shields for each eye. It cannot be adapted to projection devices. It presents an illuminated white cross to both eyes, a vertical red extension above to the left eye, and a vertical green extension below to the right eye. Rather than requiring red-green glasses, the projecting opaque shields secure the colored line extensions to the respective eyes. Though accurate, this test requires considerable explanation and subjective reporting not needed in other tests.

Small base-out prism test for verification in small angle esodeviation

Patients who may have small central scotomas (under 2 degrees) or who show uncertain abduction of a questionably esodeviating eye when the fellow eye is occluded may be better diagnosed and better understood by small-degree image displacement testing. Uncertainties particularly arise in small-angle esotropia and microstrabismus or following surgical correction of a larger deviation. This technique necessitates a very small fixation light that will fall within a minute central scotoma. It may be employed for near or distance so long as the the patient can follow the fixational instructions of the examiner.

A weak base-out prism—conventionally 2 to 4 diopters—is successively placed before the right and left eyes to displace the image of the fixation light temporally, but within an area of suspect central scotoma. An orthophoric individual shows an immediate binocular movement or version away from the side of the prism, followed by a slower fusional movement or duction of the fellow eye in the reverse or return direction to correct for the image displacement.

If, when placing the base-out prism before the right eye, both eyes move in levoversion, there is no foveal suppression in the right eye. If a subsequent slow fusional duction of the left eye occurs, there is no foveal suppression of this eye.

If, when the prism is placed before one eye, both eyes show a version to the opposite side, but the fellow eye makes no secondary fusional duction, then the fellow eye has a central scotoma. This is confirmed on changing the prism to this eye and noting that neither eye moves (the prism has merely displaced the image within the scotoma).

The test will thus confirm the presence of small degrees of esotropia and small central scotomas. It is not applicable in large deviations, absence of fixation ability, or established eccentric fixation.

Stereoscopic acuity or stereoacuity

Identification and quantitation of "fusion" is often confused because it entails two distinct though overlapping components: (1) the motor component or motor power, which may be quantitated over its widely variable range by prism vergence amplitude testing with rotary prisms, and (2) the sensory component of bifixation, which may be quantitated through gross tests such as the Worth four-dot test (1903) to minute measurements of stereoacuity. The somewhat crude Worth terminology of 3 degrees implying levels of "fusion" has been superseded so that his first degree is now better described as *single binocular vision* and his second degree simplified merely to *fusion*. His third degree is *true stereopsis*, which is quantitated under stereoacuity.

Stereoacuity is simply the least fractional change in depth that can be detected binocularly. This is the most precise clinical measure of sensory fusion. It is inversely proportional to the square of the distance an object is away from the eye and directly proportional to the interpupillary distance. (Thus range finders are built to increase interpupillary distance by several feet.) Because of the marked effect of distance, there is a *near range* up to 20 or 30 meters where stereopsis is accurate and critical, a *medium range* where stereopsis is poor, and a *far range* beyond 500 or 600 meters where there actually is no stereopsis. Horizontal, rather than vertical, disparities appear responsible for stereoacuity, but it is also asymptotically related to illumination levels and increases with exposure time by a factor of 4 from exposures of .004 seconds to 1 second. Beyond

this time period there is no further enhancement by additional exposure.

Instruments used to measure sensory fusion and stereoacuity,* in order of increasing precision, are:

1. Worth four-dot test for distance (1903) and the Hardy (1937) near modification for gross testing of extramacular fusion

2. Targets for either macular or extramacular fusion and stereopsis in a major amblyoscope

3. Polaroid vectograms, developed by Wirt-Titmus in 1947, which are double-printed with polarizing axes at right angles to each other (These are inspected through polarizing filters worn over each of the patient's eyes and oriented at right angles to each other.)

The Worth four-dot (paramacular) test presents one red, two green, and one white disc, usually subtending a visual angle of 1 to 1.5 degrees at 20 ft. The patient wears a matching red filter before one eye and green filter before the other. Thus the green lights are seen only through the green filter and the red light through the red filter. The normal patient will see the white light through both filters and may report it as a blend of changing red and green because of retinal color rivalry. The normal individual with normal vision in each eye may also report the white to appear predominantly red, regardless of which eye is wearing the red filter. This is because psychophysically most individuals perceive the color red as dominant to that of green. The patient with moderate to severe amblyopia in one eye will usually report seeing no lights with that eye and the appropriate two or three lights with his bet-

*The Howard-Dohlman aligning box for testing at 6 meters with two pegs separated by about 10 minutes of arc (64 mm.) is extremely crude and affords neither quantitative measurements for a strabismic patient in the near range nor correlation with performance in far ranges. It has been abandoned by civilian and military transport examiners for inapplicability. The Verhoeff battery-powered, hand-held Stereopter (1942) gives qualitative judgment of near stereopsis but does not give quantitations (Fig. 6-9).

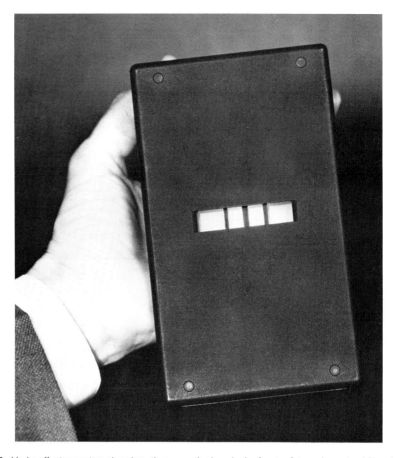

Fig. 6-9. Verhoeff stereopter showing three vertical rods in front of translucent white glass (as viewed by patient). (American Optical Corp., Buffalo, New York 14215.)

ter eye. The heterophoric or mildly heterotropic patient will often report seeing five lights, two red and three green, appearing in crossed positions with exotropia and uncrossed positions with estropia. The Hardy flashlight modification (Fig. 6-10) of this test has similar value for identification of bifixation and elementary paramacular fusion in the near range. In most instruments these dots are about 5 mm. in diameter and 20 to 30 mm. apart so that they create an image 5 to 6° in diameter when held ⅓ of a meter from the observer. The test should always be repeated with the red-green glasses reversed for confirmation. This test subtends too broad an angle to detect suppression limited to the fovea.

The major amblyoscope (haploscope) has the advantage of being able to present count-

less variations of target designs and sizes. Foveal targets should subtend 1 or 2 degrees at the most, and paramacular targets should subtend no more than 5 to 7 degress. Targets for peripheral function generally should be larger than 7 to 10 degrees. Muenzler, however, offers a penlight miniaturization of the Hardy unit for true macular testing. One mm. dots within a 9-mm. spread when held at a distance of ⅓ of a meter create a retinal image of about 0.4 to 0.5 mm. in diameter. This falls within the rod-free fovea, which is 0.5 to 0.6 mm. in diameter. Nonsuppression here indicates true bifixation but is not a quantitation of high degree of stereoacuity.* In order to grade very fine degrees

*Parson's Optical Laboratory, San Francisco, California, 94108.

Fig. 6-10. Worth four-dot test modified by Hardy for near range, paramacular fusion. Patient wears red-green Snellen spectacles as shown.

of stereopsis, however, horizontal disparity of targets in small fractions of a millimeter must be achieved. Irregularities in slide bindings and necessary clearance to lift target slides in and out of an amblyoscope exceed these differences, and therefore finer grading of stereoacuity must be done with the Wirt type of printed vectograms.

The familiar Polaroid stereoscopic fly test* is a simple and direct measure of third-degree fusion but is relatively gross and can be perceived in true stereopsis by an individual with up to 3,000 seconds (50 minutes) of arc disparity. Thus a patient with as much as 10 or 15 prism diopters of manifest exotropia in the near range may be able to visualize the Polaroid fly satisfactorily. The series of quantitative stereoacuity targets double-printed as Polaroid vectographs by S. E. Wirt are available (Fig. 6-11) in a booklet

or folder (Titmus) convenient for both child or adult patients. Polaroid spectacles are worn with the polarizing axes of the two lenses oriented 90 degrees from each other to correspond with each of the printings of the vectograph. This permits gradation of stereoacuity in a series of nine steps down to 40 seconds of arc. (The initial Wirt series went to 14 seconds of arc.)

Project-O-Chart vectograph slides are also manufactured by the American Optical Corporation with eccentric circles to measure stereoacuity to 60 seconds of arc but at far range test distance. In use, a nondepolarizing screen is necessary, and the patient wears Polaroid glasses. More critical vectographs measuring down to 15 or 20 seconds of arc can be produced, and the limits of stereoacuity with good central acuity may be measured down to a few seconds of arc under laboratory conditions.

One of the recent and rewarding diagnostic developments in strabismology has been identification of the involved mechanisms in patients with mild amblyopia whose eyes appear to be straight or who do not show

---

*Titmus Optical Co., Petersburg, Virginia, 23803. Random dot stereograms as emphasized by Bela Julesz have been adapted for less exacting tests of stereoacuity (Reinecke) Stereo Optical Co., Chicago, Ill. 60641; TNO test for Stereovision, 7 red/green plates.

Fig. 6-11. Wirt-Titmus double-printed Polaroid vectograph for quantitating stereoacuity through Polaroid spectacles. Nine sets of four rings each across upper half of left page present separations of 800, 400, 200, 140, 100, 80, 60, 50, and 40 sec. of arc (upper left to lower right).

a fixation movement of the uncovered eye when either eye is subjected to the cover test for heterotropia. A movement of realignment may or may not be apparent on the cover-uncover test for heterophoria. Clinically, such patients usually have mild to modest anisometropia (exceeding 1.5 diopters), an antecedent history of manifest esotropia that may have been approached surgically in early childhood, and peripheral fusion with amplitude if amblyoscopic examination is done. This is sometimes designated as small-angle strabismus or microstrabismus (Helveston and von Noorden, 1968). Measurement of foveal stereoacuity reveals distinct limitations but better performance than in heterotropic patients with macular suppression and worse than in those with bifixational heterophoria or orthophoria.

Thus it is diagnostically helpful in patients with straight or nearly straight eyes and with uncertain amblyopia to measure stereoacuity. High-grade stereoacuity is found only in the presence of bifixation and enhances the outlook for functional improvement. Contrariwise, very poor stereoacuity limits the prognosis for full functional restoration, particularly when the history of strabismus is from early infancy or birth.

Special tests and procedures

The examinations discussed in the preceding pages yield a satisfactory diagnosis and plan for treatment in the large majority of motility problems. The perceptive examiner culls from these procedures those most productive of diagnostic data and least fatiguing to patient and to self. Thus he should prefer the Lancaster red-green projection test to the more cumbersome Hess screen test or the old congruence test of Tschermak. He should try to avoid the gross afterimage testing of Hering-Bielschowsky. In practicality of testing he also tries to avoid the "fist full of prisms" tests, favoring rather the best analysis of corneal light reflexes by simpler means.

Yet there remain many other tests of value that the individualist will espouse and that, at times, an individual patient will require.

The Bielschowsky head-tilt test (1935) and its three-step elaboration by Parks (1958) are specifically valuable in differential diagnosis of vertical, or preferably designated "cyclovertical," impairments. The Bielschowsky maneuvers are particularly diagnostic in isolating the offending muscle requiring surgery, whether impairment is recent (without secondary contracture of the homolateral antagonist or the contralateral yoke muscle or disturbances in the antagonist of the yoke) or long standing (with such secondary changes or with loss of the distinction between primary and secondary deviation). Park's three-step procedure may be inapplicable following long-standing secondary changes or surgical interventions.

Bielschowsky head-tilt test

The Bielschowsky test is applicable only in cyclovertical paresis, where good sensory fusion or distaste for diplopia stimulate a compensatory head tilt. This is more conspicuous in oblique than in vertical rectus muscle impairment. Therefore quantitative responses noted while testing will be more marked in oblique than in vertical rectus impairment. When a superior oblique muscle is underacting, its normal incyclotorsional tone is reduced, the eye consequently is extorted by the less opposed action of the homolateral inferior oblique muscle, and the patient takes up head-tilting to the opposite side to restore verticality to the 6 to 12 o'clock axis of the involved globe. Forcibly tilting the head to the side of the palsied superior oblique (reversing the spontaneous tilt) in the Bielschowsky test increases the excycloposition; this calls on the homolateral superior rectus, which has a minor incyclotorsional component in its action, to make a compensatory contracture. A greater component of action in the superior rectus, however, is elevation. Therefore the involved eye shoots upward (positive Bielschowsky test).

If the superior rectus—rather than the superior oblique—is at fault, spontaneous or compensatory head-tilting (to the opposite side) is distinctly less conspicuous. There is theoretic depression of the involved eye resulting from unopposed action of its superior oblique. On forcible tilting of the head to the involved side, the eye does not elevate and may even show some depression. This identifies the superior rectus as the impaired muscle.

The test is also applicable in the presence of impairment of the inferior oblique and the inferior rectus muscles, which have, respectively, major and minor components of extorsion. Paresis of either of these muscles tends to permit some intorsion of the globe and to stimulate compensatory tilting of the head to the *same* side. The amount and clarity of these cyclovertical findings is less with the inferior than with the superior pair of muscles and least with the inferior rectus. Forcibly tilting the head to the opposite (uninvolved) side increases the incycloposition of the affected eye, and thus if the inferior oblique is at fault, the compensatory contraction of the homolateral inferior rectus leads to a diagnostic downward displacement of the eye.

The complete objectivity of the findings in the Bielschowsky test makes it particularly valuable to use at any age and with almost any degree of interest on the part of the patient.

Three-step test of Parks

The Parks' test, developed in 1958, is done to identify nonoperative and nontraumatic cyclovertical palsies. The tests are best done with distant fixation and good light with which to observe movement of the eyes.

Step I   Identify whether the right or the left eye is higher by direct inspection or by use of the cover-uncover test if necessary. This eliminates four of the eight muscles that can be suspect in vertical palsy. Thus if the patient has *right* hypertropia, only one of the following four muscles can be paretic: right superior oblique, right inferior rectus, left superior rectus, or left inferior oblique.

Step II   Determine whether the vertical deviation increases in dextroversion or in levoversion. This eliminates two of the remaining four suspected muscles. Thus if the right hypertropia increases in dextroversion, only one of two muscles (those now in the field of maximum action) can be paretic: the right inferior rectus or the left inferior oblique.

Step III Determine whether the vertical deviation increases on tilting the head toward the right or the left shoulder. This may be apparent in direct inspection (particularly when a superior oblique muscle is paretic) or may require alternate cover to elicit the difference. Thus if the right hypertropia increases on tilting the head to right, the paretic muscle is the left inferior oblique, and the left eye has been rotated downward by compensatory contraction of the left inferior rectus, as explained under the Bielschowsky head-tilt test.

CONCLUSION

Some component of ocular motility evaluation is an integral part of every complete eye examination. This is initiated by the leads communicated from the patient in his chief complaint. It is more specifically oriented by the ocular and central nervous system history. The examiner then progresses step-by-step from preliminary inspection through the minimum number of separate tests needed to establish either normal ocular motility or the presence of abnormality. In the presence of disorder, a reasonably quantitative anatomic and functional diagnosis must be made. The examiner who dares to pass up a small amount of acquired esodeviation in a child with a passing assurance of improvement with age will make some catastrophic errors. The otherwise silent brain tumor first evidenced by partial paralysis of one lateral rectus muscle must always be considered in either the history or the finding of convergent strabismus.

In the presence of diagnostic uncertainties, highly variable findings, or inconsistent results from different tests, the examiner may often attain valuable clarification on the basis of a reexamination or two. At times, specific instructions to a mother or a mate as to what to watch for may greatly aid an otherwise vague history.

As in the evaluation of ptosis onset, it is often helpful to obtain old photographs of the patient, beginning with the newborn nursery. This will save time otherwise spent in vague discussions, and better dating of onset can be established by resurrecting fairly good facial photographs.

There is no substitute for the penetrating history augmented by careful and searching observation of the patient. In the restless child or infant those steps that should be limited to preliminary inspection of the older individual may constitute the entire field of information obtainable. In spite of this, the examiner still must achieve satisfactory data to rule out malignant possibilities and to institute appropriately constructive programs.

REFERENCES

Franceschetti, A. T.: The AC/A ratio; Methods of determining the AC/A ratio, J. Fr. Orthopt. 3:7-32, 1971.

Hardy, L. H.: A modification of the four-dot test, Trans. Am. Acad. Ophthalmol. Otolaryngol. 42:491, 1937.

Helveston, E. M., and Von Noorden, G. K.: Microtropia: A newly defined entity, Arch. Ophthalmol. 78:272, 1967.

Hering, E.: Zur Lehre von Ortssinn der Netzhaut, Beitrage zur Physiologie, Leipzig, Wilhelm Engelmann 3:182, 1801.

Muenzler, W. S.: Combination four-dot light, Am. J. Ophthalmol. 69:1080, June, 1970.

Owens, W. C.: A fixation light for the cardinal directions of gaze, Am. J. Ophthalmol. 50:611, 1947.

Parks, M. M.: Isolated cyclovertical muscle palsy, Arch. Ophthalmol. 60:1027-1035, Dec., 1958.

Reinecke, R. D., and Simmons, K.: A new stereoscopic test (Random Dot E) for amblyopia screening, Am. J. Ophthalmol. 78:714-721, 1974.

Romano, P. E., and Romano, J. A.: Fusion: A new classification and method for determining the level of sensory binocular cooperation, Surv. Ophthalmol. 17:458-468, May-June, 1973.

Romano, P. E., and Von Noorden, G. K.: Limitation of cover test in determining strabismus, Am. J. Ophthalmol. 72:10-12, 1971.

Sanfilippo, S.: A critical evaluation of the major amblyoscope, Am. Orthopt. J. 22:54-58, 1972.

Verhoeff, F. H.: Simple quantitative test for acuity and reliability of binocular stereopsis, Arch. Ophthalmol. 28:1000-1019, Dec., 1942.

Von Noorden, G. K.: Divergence excess and simulated divergence excess; diagnosis and surgical management, Ophthalmologica 26:719, 1969.

Walraven, J.: Amblyopia screening with Random-Dot (TNO-Julesz) Stereograms, Am. J. Ophthalmol. 80: 893-900, 1975.

CHAPTER 7

Glaucoma, ocular hypertension, and hypotony

INTRODUCTION
Definitions
Glaucoma

Glaucoma is a complex of many causative disease mechanisms having a common pathologic factor of increased intraocular pressure. The disease may be acute or chronic, primary or secondary, painful or painless and may cause temporary or permanent impairment of visual fields, night vision, and visual acuity. It is one of the most frequent causes of visual loss in our older population and one that produces far too much needless impairment. Suspicion of glaucoma should be part of the perpetual set of the examiner, and diagnostic steps with this in mind should be part of *every* eye examination. Glaucoma is not only a photophobic enlargement of the globe in infants, and an excruciatingly painful crisis in angle-closure episodes, but it also is a frequent, unsuspected concomitant of maturity or an occasional subtle devil in the progressively myopic patient.

Ocular hypertension

This is a hazardous and worrisome diagnosis, in a presumably normal eye in which careful and repeated measurements of intraocular pressure indicate a level above the usually accepted upper limits of normal. Such an eye theoretically is physiologically tolerating its individual level of intraocular pressure and shows normal out flow on tonography. The optic nerve head should show no defects on serial examination, and critical study of the central visual field with 1 mm. kinetic or preferably static perimetry shows no defects. If possible, similarly careful studies of siblings, parents, aunts, and uncles should be made. If any of these have glaucoma, then the "ocular hypertensive" individual should be considered as *preglaucomatous*. Even if the family examinations are negative, greater safeguard to the patient is afforded by considering such individuals as *glaucoma suspects*. Under this heading the examiner will impose more rigorous repeat examination schedules and maintain a higher index of suspicion.

Hypotony

The presence of pathologically low pressure or hypotony is often accompanied by variable disturbances in visual acuity resulting from failure in hydrodynamic support of the refractive components of the cornea. In postoperative eyes—even many years after surgery—a small and obscure wound leak should be suspicioned and sought out by slit lamp observation while the eye is bathed in fluorescein solution (Seidel test). A wound leak may produce minute spontaneous streaming through the fluorescein or may require gentle pressure on the globe through the upper eyelid to elicit a positive Seidel sign. Other causative factors are previous destructive surgical procedures to the ciliary body (cyclodiathermy, cyclocryopexy, cyclocatholysis) or previous retinal detachment. In the presence of long-standing retinal detachment, hypotony relates to the duration rather than the area of detachment. Following buckling procedures, patients should be checked for glaucoma or hypotony every 6 months for the rest of their lives. Other systemic causes are diabetic hyperglycemia, ipsilateral carotid artery impairment, myotonic dystrophy, and systemic dehydration.

Local ocular causes are (1) measurements during wide excursion of diurnal variation, (2) abnormally low scleral rigidity as in the myope of more than −8 diopters, especially when read by Schiøtz rather than applanation tonometry, (3) choroidal or ciliary body detachment or hydrops, (4) active cyclitis, and (5) postural effect of greater pressure when patient is supine rather than in the sitting position. Elevations of 2 to 9 mm. may be recorded by applanation in the supine position, particularly in patients who have borderline intraocular pressure in the seated position.

Minimum diagnostic examinations

In every initial examination of the globe, an estimate must be made of chamber depth centrally and angle depth peripherally. This is first done as part of the inspection in focal light by directing a flashlight beam along the plane of the iris from the temporal side. If the chamber is shallowed by the iris bowing forward, only the temporal half of the iris will be illuminated and the nasal half will be shadowed. This warns of a narrow angle anatomy and calls for careful contact lens gonioscopy. Conversely, a broadly illuminated iris gives some reassuring index of safe chamber depth for pupillary dilatation with little danger of angle-closure glaucoma.

Between estimation of depth by illuminating the iris surface and by careful gonioscopy, reliable measurement of depth may be secured with the slit lamp beam. This is easily and directly done in the center of the chamber. For more critical estimation of angle depth, a vertical beam should be focused nearly perpendicular to the corneal surface and positioned as close as possible to the limbus at one of its horizontal sites. The beam must be as narrow as possible and viewed from an angle of approximately 60 degrees. The optic section of the cornea thus illuminated is used as a unit for estimating angle depth on the basis of peripheral chamber depth at the entrance to the angle (Herick, Shaffer, and Schwartz, 1969).

If the distance between the illuminated endothelial curve of the cornea and the anterior surface of the iris is equal to or greater than the depth of the corneal section seen in this slit beam, gonioscopy will always show a wide open or grade 4 angle. If the distance is only half the width of the slit beam, the angle is incapable of closure and may be estimated as grade 3. When the width is equal to one-fourth of the corneal section, this is probably a grade 2 angle and merits careful gonioscopy. If the width is less than one-fourth the slit beam, the angle is functionally a grade 1, and gonioscopy will usually confirm an extremely narrow angle.

This is an excellent premydriatic test to avoid medically induced angle-closure glaucoma. Such a simple step incorporated in routine slit lamp examination of the anterior segment will also eliminate the danger of overestimating angle depth in the presence of a plateau-type iris, where the chamber is deep centrally and most of the iris plane may be illuminated in the simple test of a flashlight beam directed from the temporal aspect. With such a plateau iris, there is danger of angle closure even though chamber depth centrally appears superficially reassuring.

Every ocular examination—even if only for a slight increase in a schoolchild's myopic correction or similar increase in a presbyopic patient's reading aid—must include an intraocular inspection for glaucoma. The prime target is the optic nerve head under ophthalmoscopic inspection. Here the basic anatomy of the nerve head and the strength of diastolic pressure constitute a twofold defense against nerve fiber atrophy induced by increased intraocular pressure. The ruddy and small nerve head with a small or no physiologic cup, as in the hyperopic eye, is most difficult to damage by glaucoma. The large disc with large cup and less capillarity, as particularly seen in the myopic eye, is more vulnerable to small increases in pressure. Systemic blood pressure, particularly at the sustained diastolic level, is important in maintaining adequate circulation to the axon fibers. Thus a drop in blood pressure, especially if diastolic, has a similar effect to that of increased intraocular pressure in creating ischemia or nutritional compromise, which damages the optic nerve fibers. Knowledge of blood pressure is of both diagnostic and follow-up importance in glaucoma. By the same token, the family physician or internist caring for a hypertensive patient who also has chronic or open-angle glaucoma should not abruptly reduce the patient's blood pressure. This may lead to glaucomatous field loss, but fortunately such changes are usually reversible. Statistically, patients with systemic hypertension resist potential damage from glaucoma better than do normotensive patients.

In any pair of eyes, suggestion of glaucomatous change or susceptibility is evidenced by (1) inequality in the size of the right and left optic cups (the larger is more likely to prove glaucomatous now or in years ahead), (2) verticalized enlargement or vertical elongation of the cup, (3) broad saucerization of the cup approaching the disc border, even in the presence of apparently good capillarity, (4) nasal positioning of the major vessels on the nerve head, and (5) angulation or knuckling of the vessels as they go over the nerve head rim into the cup.

The examiner will helpfully force himself to be more analytic about the size of the cup in the optic nerve head if he notes and records a specific cup/disc ratio expressed in decimal notation from 0.1 to 1.0. This is best accomplished on the basis of an imaginary horizontal line extending across the maximum width of the disc. If, on such a horizontal line, the cup appears to be half the total width of the disc, it should be recorded as 0.5. If the cup has almost completely involved the width of the disc, it would be recorded as 0.9. This gives a comparative value for subsequent examinations. Usually it is easy to localize the nasal edge of the cup, but difficulty is experienced in establishing the temporal limit of the cup when there is a gently sloping or saucerized configuration. Under such circumstances, the examiner should attempt to estimate a point at which the slope has come up to what would be the level of the unaltered rim or else estimate an arbitrary point near the disc border. A more adverse prognosis is suggested when the temporal extension of the cup is

directed below the imaginary horizontal line. This may be associated with nasal field defects found on tangent screen examination. For quick and comparative recording a simple diagram of two circles should be used to depict the disc border and the outer edge of the cup. Elongation and eccentricity of the cup are more clearly recorded than by word or numbers. Sloping of the disc rim can be indicated by a few radial lines, and bearing of the lamina cribrosa by drawing in a group of small circles at the appropriate part of the cup. This actually may be *better* than more elegant fundus photography, stereophotography or stereogrammetry where differences in angulation, illumination, magnification, or centering of discs on-film make serial comparisons of photographs inexact. Contrary to earlier conclusions, increased cupping has been documented to *precede* early nasal field loss and therefore the cup is a crucial focus in diagnosis.

Any of these suspect findings should be followed by corneal tonometry, preferably of the applanation type. Remember, however, that normal applanation tonometry (10 to 22 mm. Hg) may be found in the presence of disc changes, or vice versa. In either event the patient should be continued under observation at least twice a year as a glaucoma suspect. Mean value for healthy adult eyes is 15 to 16 mm. Hg and infants usually range between 10 and 12 mm. Hg.

The next step in the minimum diagnostic series is central visual field examination on a tangent screen at a distance of at least 1 meter, with a white target of 2-mm. diameter. Frequently the location of suspect alterations in the optic nerve head points to areas of probable field impairment. Careful tangent screen examination should be made for reductions in the superior nasal outer isopter, a Rönne nasal step, or Bjerrum arcuate defect. The earliest defects usually detectable are small paracentral islands of loss within 15° of fixation. These subsequently merge into a classical arcuate defect and later vertical winging of the blind spot (Seidel's sickle scotoma, 1914). If a laterally inverted nerve head is present, these defects are more likely to be found in the temporal than in the usual nasal field.

Beyond these minimum steps of (1) chamber depth estimation, (2) optic nerve head inspection, (3) tonometry, and (4) tangent screen study of the central fields, there are many other sophisticated and specific examinations that must be included in many glaucoma work-ups or the consultation examination. Knowledgeability, alertness, suspicion, and experience by the examiner, however, are frequently more valuable than many routinely performed tests of variable interpretation.

MEASUREMENTS OF INTRAOCULAR PRESSURE

A series of progressively critical techniques is available for diagnostic measurements of intraocular pressure. These are:

1. Digital palpation (tactile tension)
2. Indentation tonometry
3. Applanation tonometry
   a. Optical
   b. Electronic
   c. Pressure balance
   d. Air blast
4. Tonography
5. Provocative testing
6. Diurnal curves
7. Ballistic tonometry (viscoelastometry)

Measurements of indentation tonometry, optical applanation tonometry, and tonography are generally predicted on a clear, smooth cornea of usual configuration and resistance. The presence of scarring, thickening, vesiculation, edema, or other disturbances makes these instruments record poorly and less reliably. In such cases, experienced tactile estimation of tension or use of the Mackay-Marg or Durham instruments may be less inaccurate.

Digital palpation or tactile estimation of ocular tension

Tactile estimation of ocular tension is a qualitative method with which every physician should be familiar. It cannot begin to approach the accuracy of instrumental tonometry, but it is a substitute for quantitative methods when corneal scars, irregularities,

Fig. 7-1. Correct position of patient's downward gaze and examiner's fingers above tarsal plate for digital tonometry.

or infections preclude instruments. This technique requires experienced palpation plus instrumental confirmation on many eyes before even such coarse gradations as increased +1, +2, +3 or decreased −1, −2, −3 can be made. In emergency situations or under field conditions it can be vitally helpful. Proper diagnosis of the unconscious diabetic patient who may be in either insulin shock or diabetic coma can be pivotally assisted by palpation of the soft globe consequent to the hyperglycemia of diabetic coma.

For digital tonometry (Fig. 7-1), the patient must look down with both eyes open. In some patients the protective tendency to close the lids, causing the globes to roll upward in Bell's phenomenon, will be reduced by having the patient fixate on his own hand held at waist level.

The third and fourth fingers of the examiner's hands are rested on the patient's brow to sustain the weight of his hands. This gives maximum freedom to the pulp tips of the index fingers, which then palpate the globe *above* the tarsal plate and *above* the limbus. An estimation of fluctuation of the globe is made by alternate and light indention (not ballottement) with one finger while gently steadying the globe with the other. Tactile sensation is impaired if palpation is done through the tarsal plate. A misleading sense of undue firmness is introduced by palpating against the cornea rather than the sclera. The reverse is true of instrumental tonometry, where the normal cornea should be used for sensitivity, consistency, and maximum accuracy of reading.

Indentation tonometry

Instrument. Though many instruments and many modifications create an international history of bioengineering from 1863 (von Graefe, Donders, Gradle, McLean, and so on), by far the best standardized and critically evaluated indentation instrument is that of Schiøtz, introduced in 1905. It has undergone modest refinements of design: multiple weights (1924); convex plunger x-model (1926); Harrington scale magnification (1941); Sklar mirror scale to reduce parallax in reading, and epicycloid lever (concave upward) to reduce friction (1948); Friedenwald refined nomograms for converting scale readings to millimeters of mercury (1955); Allen (Gulden, Pilling) modification to hold the plunger in elevation prior to contact with the eye (1964); Sklar jewel-mounted plunger. The Schiøtz tonometer can be purchased from many sources for $50 to $200, including the necessary verification and certification.*

Technique. For identation tonometry, the patient should be recumbent, comfortable, and without any constrictions of clothing at the neck that may impede venous return from the jugular system and artificially increase intraocular pressure. Men often need to loosen their neckties and collars. A drop of topical anesthetic such as proparacaine hydrochloride (0.5% Ophthaine, or 0.5% Oph-

thetic) or benoxinate hydrochloride (0.4% Dorsacaine) is instilled. These short-acting agents neither burn nor soften the epithelium as does cocaine, which is contraindicated. While the reaction from this drop is quieting down, the Schiøtz instrument may be quickly checked for zero reading on the steel test block furnished with the instrument. Plunger freedom should be quickly checked with the fingertip and then the contact area of the instrument should be dry wiped on an unused tissue. The patient may be instructed to fixate a mark on the ceiling directly overhead—if there is adequate sight in a fellow eye—or to fixate a fingertip on his hand extended at arm's length above his face. The hand fixation technique is essential in a one-eyed patient or in the presence of heterotropia where a compensatory version is needed to bring the cornea under examination into a proper horizontal plane.

The thumb and forefinger of one hand hold the lids away from the eye and against the orbital rim, carefully avoiding any pressure that may be transmitted to the globe. With the thumb and forefinger of the other hand, the vertically held tonometer is brought to rest on the center of the cornea. Touching the lashes can stimulate both blink and Bell's responses and so must be avoided. Freedom of plunger in the sleeve is evidenced by rhythmic transmission of the cardiac impulse in the indicator needle. To reduce inaccuracies at low- or high-scale readings, an appropriate weight (the normal 5.5 or the accessory 7.5, 10, or 15 gm.) should be used to obtain, if possible, scale readings of 4 to 10 units. The right eye is traditionally read first and then the left (Fig. 7-2). The patient should be routinely cautioned not to hold his breath and, if he appears tense, should be asked to breathe through his mouth. A brief complimentary word as the chair back is returned to vertical or as the clinician checks the conversion table imparts to the patient a feeling of cooperative accomplishment and makes the procedure easier the next time.

Results are most appropriately expressed as a fraction, with the test weight being the denominator and the scale reading the nu-

*University Hospital of Cleveland, Department of Ophthalmology, Cleveland, Ohio 44106; Electronic Testing Laboratories, University of Tübingen, Tübingen, Democratic Republic of Germany; Physikalisch-Technische, Bundesanstalt Institut, Berlin, Federal Republic of Germany; Ross Foundation, Edinburgh, Scotland.

Fig. 7-2. Correct positioning of Schiøtz indentation tonometer vertically and directly centered on cornea of supine patient. Lids are gently retracted against bony orbital rim above and below, avoiding all pressure against globe. Sterile Tonofilm covers plunger and footplate.

merator. Many physicians and patients, however, have a more comfortable feeling in a pressure notation expressed as millimeters of mercury. Generally it is preferable to tell the patient his pressure as it is recorded. The intelligent individual appreciates this participation in the studies, and it is a help to him if he needs eye care in some foreign port at a later date.

Instrument sterilization. There is no way to achieve total and safe sterilization of a tonometer in clinical use other than to shield its operating footplate and plunger within sterile Tonofilm* so that no direct contact is made with the cornea or lids (Fig. 7-3). Such a film, affixed before each use and discarded immediately thereafter, is also an almost complete safeguard against corneal abrasion and an indispensable protection in mass screening programs. Cold sterilizing (Berens) solutions, if concentrated enough to be bactericidal and viracidal, present a caustic threat of residual chemical between the plunger and cylinder. Alcohol presents the

same threat plus ineffectiveness against certain viruses. Flaming or other heat devices (Bell, Sklar*) have been employed with occasional inadvertent coagulation calamities. Ultraviolet (Stirne, Rosner) does not penetrate the recesses between plunger and cylinder nor any waxy secretion that might remain on the tonometer. In practice, workable safety against transmission of infection is achieved by never using the instrument on a suspect or frankly infected eye, wiping the instrument clean and dry after each use, and firmly wiping the dried instrument before each use.

Contraindications to tonometry and tonography. The following conditions, which contraindicate instrumental tonometry, relate to either possibilities of infection or conditions that render the procedure inaccurate.

1. Ocular infection or discharge: suspect, frank, or resolving
2. Recent ocular injury, perforation, corneal abrasion, or chemical burn
3. Herpes on the face or lids

*Clini-Tech, Inc., Littlestown, Pennsylvania 17340.

*475° F. in seven-minute cycle.

Fig. 7-3. A, Sterile Tonofilm within clear plastic cylinder being inserted over footplate of Schiøtz tonometer. B, Tonofilm in place over footplate of tonometer. Clear plastic cylinder has been withdrawn and discarded to right. Other disposable rubber membranes are available for most indentation instruments and also the Mackay-Marg (Tonotips).

4. Corneal edema, which both predisposes to epithelial displacement and makes reading inaccurate
5. Marked nystagmus
6. Corneal distortion, thickening, stromal loss, or major scarring
7. Significant apprehension, blepharospasm, or strong Bell's phenomenon as an avoidance response
8. Constant and uncontrollable coughing
9. Endemic outbreaking of ocular infection such as shipyard keratoconjunctivitis (adenovirus type 8)
10. High myopia (for indentation only)

In each of the preceding, a carefully performed digital estimation of ocular tension is of qualitative value and should be recorded. The examiner, of course, must wash his hands after touching any infected eye.

Applanation tonometry

The introduction of applanation principles by Weber in 1867, and more enduringly by Maklakoff in 1885, followed the primitive indentation instruments of the earlier 1860s. Maklakoff's fixed force applanation rods with no moving parts had simplicity in their favor, but they were subject to considerable variation in findings dependent upon lightness or crudeness of the examiner's hand and vagaries of stains and papers with which disc-like imprints (called "tonograms") were recorded from the cornea. Though modified by Filatov and Kalfa, and later by Barraquer, they have been subject to challenge of accuracy. Posner and Inglima, in 1964, revived interest in these weights of 5, 7.5, 10, and 15 gm. (available in a "Tonomat" kit*) for home evaluation of ocular tension. Families capable of understanding topical anesthetic procedures and use of such instruments, however, may derive more exact comparative data, particularly on the same patient, by purchasing a Schiøtz tonometer for instructed, home use.

Greatest accuracy is achieved in applanation by use of a fixed area and variable force.

Optic measurement. The niceties and advantages of minimizing instrumental deformity or indentation, however, have been fostered by the applanation principle and long championed by Frederick Verhoeff, using the simple Souter (American Optical Co.) tonometer of 1916. Dr. Verhoeff would apply this variable force applanator against the anesthetized cornea of a seated patient while watching for the first distortion of a windowpane reflection on the cornea. From these Maklakoff and Souter principles, Hans Goldmann in 1954 presented unquestionably the most significant and accurate advance in tonometry of modern times.

The Goldmann applanation tonometer* can be mounted on nearly any slit lamp, though most easily of course, on the Haag-Streit 360 or 900, where it may be used as an auxiliary attachment (Model T 900) and stored in an accessory box when not in use or as a permanent attachment (Model R 900) pivoted on top of the microscope objectives. The R 900 tonometer must be lifted off its pivot support if the photographic attachment or depth measuring device, which attach to the same pivot, are to be used. With a small bracket or metal mounting plate the tonometer can be attached to the Thorpe (Bausch & Lomb) and the Campbell (American Optical Corp.) of the United States or the Carl Zeiss and the Zeiss Jena of Germany. Gams of Lyons, France, and a few other manufacturers now produce competitive models (Fig. 7-4).

Currently the Goldmann is the most accurate tonometer available and presents large theoretic and practical advantages. Its use, however, is predicated on clear or essentially normal corneal tissue. Epithelial or stromal edema erroneously lower Goldmann readings, and scars make the readings very inaccurate. Weight applied to the eye and the resultant area of flattening or distortion are much less than with Schiøtz indentation. Actually the area of flattening with the Goldmann flat plastic face is essentially the size of the Schiøtz plunger (disregarding the foot-

---

*Ocular Instruments Inc., Redmond, Washington 98052.

*Manufactured by Haag-Streit, Berne, Switzerland.

Fig. 7-4. Goldmann Applanation Tonometer with biprism in contact with patient's right cornea; one ocular of the slit lamp is aligned for observation through the contact biprism.

plate), and the volume of intraocular contents displaced is about one-thirtieth of that caused by Schiøtz indentation. The distension characteristics or ocular rigidity of the globe are essentially of no concern in the minute disturbances effected by applanation. Similarly, intraocular pressure during tonometry is so nearly identical to the pressure (P_o) before the tonometer was applied that the instrument can be used on a cooperative patient at almost any time after intraocular surgery.

In actual testing, both patient and examiner are comfortably seated at a slit lamp. Topical anesthesia is induced as for Schiøtz measurement, avoiding tetracaine and cocaine, which cause some softening and staining of the epithelium. A thin film of fluorescein is obtained by touching the tip of a dry sterile fluorescein paper (Ful-Glo, Fluor-I-Strip) to the outer canthal conjunctiva of each eye. A theoretic equilibrium of 0.25% in tears should be achieved as evidenced by bright and solid yellow-green fluorescence. The small fixation light may be positioned

closely in front of the eye not being tested to keep both eyes directed steadily forward.

The cobalt blue light filter* is brought into the light beam and the slit diaphragm opened fully. The light arm is angulated to focus on the applanation prism in the region of the encircling black line near its tip, and at an angle of about 60 degrees to the line of observation. The voltage is turned to maximum and the low-power microscopic system is focused through the plastic prism so that its front face is clearly seen through the one (right or left) eyepiece as chosen. The pressure knob of the tonometer is turned to 1 gm. (10 mm. Hg), bringing the prism arm to its forward stop so that when corneal contact is made the prism will be exerting only light pressure. Room light is lowered.

The patient's eye and the applanation prism are watched from the side (or with the eye not sighting through the microscope) as the instrument is brought forward by the "joy stick" control until gentle contact is made be-

*Wratten Gelatin filter 47B.

tween the prism face and the corneal center. This is evidenced by an immediate bluish glow throughout the limbus. With the single eye aligned through the microscope, the examiner then sees two blue semicircles (actually encircling the flattened area of cornea), each bordered by an arc of green light and pulsing synchronously with the cardiac rate. Small vertical or horizontal adjustments may be needed to center the pattern.

If there is distortion of high anterior corneal astigmatism (about 4 diopters or more), the scale reading on the applanation prism should be rotated so that the minus cylinder axis coincides with the red mark. The semicircles should be of equal size and their width about one-tenth the diameter of the flattened surface contained within either one. If the semicircles are grossly widened, excessive tears are present or the prism was probably wet before contact and therefore must be withdrawn, dried, and reapplied (Fig. 7-5). If the semicircles are grossly narrowed, the tear film has dried excessively and the prism must then be withdrawn and the patient instructed to blink several times before recontacting the cornea (Fig. 7-6). If the semicircles are so broad as to extend beyond the illuminated field, there is excessive flattening and the slit lamp must be drawn back.

Readings in the presence of this ever-changing pattern should be taken at approximately the midpoint between systole and diastole, when the inner (concave) boundaries of each semicircle just meet in contact, or as they rhythmically glide past each other through excursions of equal distance (Fig. 7-7). Adjustment to the reading point or end point of properly located and sized semicircles is finalized by rotating the pressure knob back and forth. With applanation pressure exceeding intraocular pressure, the semicircles overlap excessively. With applanation pressure lower than intraocular pressure the semicircles are too small to intersect (Fig. 7-8).

At the actual end point there is a flattened disc area 3.06 mm. in diameter within the 7-mm. diameter of the prism face. Here the attractive power of the tears toward the prism is balanced by counterpressure of the elasticity or springiness of the cornea, and at this point the grams of force applied through the prism (indicated on the pressure knob) are directly convertible when multiplied by ten into millimeters of mercury, expressing intraocular pressure. With this instrument the average ocular tension of a seated adult is 14 to 17 mm. Hg.

After use, the tonometer should be carefully wiped dry and rotated to either side (or folded upward on the Bausch & Lomb model) if the slit lamp will then be used for other purposes. The pressure adjustment should also be verified every few weeks with the test weight or metal balance bar provided. This is attached to the main pivot above the pressure knob. With the test bar at its zero (center) position, the prism should move on rotating the pressure knob either plus or minus 0.1 gm. With the test bar decentered backward to its first black line (two position), the prism should move when the pressure knob is advanced to 2 gm. With the test bar decentered backward to its last black line (six position), the prism should move when the pressure knob is advanced to 6 gm.

A table-mounted, free standing Goldmann Haag-Streit tonometer (1080) is available with appropriate illumination and a single ocular but without a full slit lamp. This is particularly suitable for mass screening or use in large glaucoma clinics.

A hand-held model* of this equipment has been devised (1966) by J. Draeger particularly for use in the operating room under general anesthesia or in field survey conditions. Its greatest utility seems to be for children who cannot be examined in usual clinical settings but who require general anesthesia. A motorized image splitter is substituted for the Goldmann biprism. The instrument is rugged in construction and completely free of any relation to vertical or horizontal positioning of either the patient or the instrument.

*Hand-Applanation Tonometer, manufactured by J. D. Möller Optische Werke, Wedel-Hoist, Federal Republic of Germany.

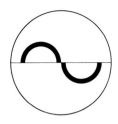

Fig. 7-5   Fig. 7-6   Fig. 7-7   Fig. 7-8

Fig. 7-5. Schematic representation of semicircles seen through contact applanation prism of Goldmann Tonometer showing semicircles that are too wide. This suggests excessive moistening of the prism or cornea. Prism must be withdrawn and dried.

Fig. 7-6. Schematic representation of semicircles seen through contact applanation prism of Goldmann Tonometer. Semicircles are too narrow, suggesting that the lacrimal fluid has dried out as during a prolonged measurement. The prism must be withdrawn so that the patient may blink a few times and the measurement then repeated.

Fig. 7-7. Schematic representation of correct end point seen through contact applanation prism of Goldmann Tonometer; semicircles are of appropriate width and their inner borders just touch. Cardiac pulsations transmitted through the globe cause rhythmic or pulsating movement of the semicircles over each other through small amplitude.

Fig. 7-8. Schematic representation of proper width semicircles seen through contact applanation prism of Goldmann Tonometer. Semicircles are slightly separated indicating applied pressure below that of the eye. The measuring drum must be turned to increase applanation pressure until end point is reached.

Weight is 700 gm. and an electric power supply is necessary.

The Perkins* hand-held Applanation Tonometer (1970) is a lightweight, simplified, battery handle, version of the Draeger instrument. An adjustable forehead button is rested on the patient's brow and then the handle brought toward the patient's cheek. As the contact prism is extended forward, a light source emerges at the appropriate angle. Monocular readings are made with a thumb controlled, knurled ring protruding slightly through the handle on the examiner's side. This is an excellent instrument unaffected by temperatures from 9° to 57 °C. Correlation with Goldmann readings is excellent (Fig. 7-9).

The Halberg hand applanation tonometer† was introduced in 1967 as a refinement of the Maklekoff (1885, later Filatov-Kalfe modification) or Posner-Inglima (1964) tonometers, offering simplicity, portability, and direct optical reading without a slit lamp. Like the Goldmann instrument, it requires topical

anesthesia and a clear, regular cornea. It is based on fixed force and variable applanation area created by a flat glass plate bearing a millimeter scale. Applanation is by a transparent, 5 gm. methyl methacrylate cylinder gravitationally applied (Fig. 7-10). One or two metal rings weighing 2.5 gm. may be added to the cylinder by simple twist release from the carrier portion of the instrument. The patient must be supine as for Schiøtz tonometry. The applanation area is directly seen through two convex lenses and the transparent acrylic cylinder; scale readings are seen simultaneously, but as a safeguard, sharp focus is limited to the midportion of the scale from 3.8 to 5.6 mm. This is the area of greatest reliability. The applanation diameter to the nearest 0.1 mm. is converted to mm. of Hg pressure by the Posner-Inglima table (Table 2). The foot plate has been reduced to 10 mm. in diameter and an optional light source made available. Readings show high correlation with Goldmann figures. The absence of moving parts further recommends this tonometer, but all users agree that at least 100 trial measurements are necessary before reliable readings can be derived.

For fixed force, hand applanation screen-

*Clement Clarke, London W1H ODH, England.
†Rynco Scientific Corporation, Floral Park, New York 11001.

ing a Glaucotest has been designed by Dr. J. Bruun-Jensen and produced by Heine in the Federal Republic of Germany. The instrument is read optically under 8× magnification and therefore necessitates a clear cornea free of pathology. Preselected test bodies of 1.8, 2.2, 2.6, or 3.0 gm. give gravitational applanation levels corresponding to 18, 22, 26, or 30 mm. Hg. A test streak mark of 3.06 mm. length is etched on the front surface of the flat transparent applanating plane. A reference ring within each of the four test weights is visualized as being of larger diameter than the reference streak mark (intraocular tension under the reference load), of smaller diameter than the reference streak mark (intraocular pressure higher than the reference load), or coinciding with the reference streak mark (intraocular pressure equal to the reference load). Cobalt filtered light is focused on the applanation plane, which is intensified with fluorescein. A battery handle provides current for illumination. For mass screening, the examiner selects the test body (test load) that he feels differentiates pathologic from nonpathologic intraocular pressure. Sterile disposable tips are supplied in boxes of ten.

Electronic measurement. The Mackay-Marg Electronic Recording Applanation Tonometer was introduced in 1959. Its operating head is a plunger, tipped by a fused quartz transducer 1.5 mm. in diameter that extends 5 mμ beyond a supporting silicone rubber annulus. Range of excursion is only a few micra but movements of less than one micron are detected. The supporting annulus essentially negates effects of (1) corneal resistance to deformation and (2) surface tension of tears. (These two opposite forces tend to cancel each other out with the Goldmann

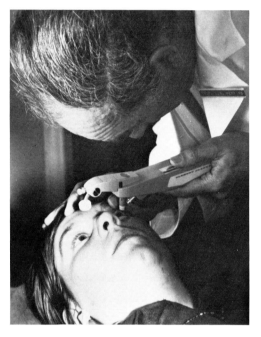

Fig. 7-9. Perkins Hand-held Applanation Tonometer in approach position to supine patient. Thumb of examiner's supporting hand rests on milled wheel to adjust the indicator semicircles. (Clement Clarke, Ltd., London, England.)

Fig. 7-10. Halberg Fixed-Force Variable-Area Hand Applanation Tonometer. Disposable flashlight (Concept) is attached for manual support and illumination. (Rynco Scientific Corp., Floral Park, New York 11001.)

Applanator.) The probe touches the cornea only for a few tenths of a second during which time a paper tracing of a few crests and troughs is created. The initial crest represents the total force of corneal resistance and intraocular pressure. With further applanation the corneal resistance acts only on the annulus and therefore a drop in the tracing to an *initial trough*, records intraocular pressure. Though topical anesthesia may be omit-

Table 2. Conversion table for the Halberg Hand Applanation Tonometer

Diameter (in mm.)	Intraocular pressure (in mm. Hg)		
	5 grams	7.5 grams	10 grams
3.5	42	59	80
3.6	40	56	75
3.7	38	53	72
3.8	36	50	68
3.9	34	47	65
4.0	32	44	62
4.1	30	42	59
4.2	28	40	56
4.3	26	38	53
4.4	25	36	50
4.5	24	34	47
4.6	23	32	44
4.7	22	30	42
4.8	21	29	40
4.9	20	27	38
5.0	19	26	36
5.1	18	25	34
5.2	17	23	32
5.3	16	21	30
5.4	15	20	29
5.5	14	19	27
5.6	13	18	26
5.7	12	17	24
5.8	11	16	23
5.9	10	15	22
6.0	9	14	21
6.1	8	13	20
6.2	7	12	19
6.3		11	18
6.4		10	17
6.5		9	16
6.6		8	15
6.7		7	14

Posner, A., and Inglima, R.: Principles of tonometry, New York, 1962.
For greatest accuracy, use only the readings between the dotted lines.

ted, it usually makes the procedure better tolerated and less affected by avoidance movements. The instrument requires frequent calibration. It may be used in any position and presents particular advantage and accuracy when corneal scars, irregularities, or edema render optical applanation inaccurate.

Pneumatic pressure balance tonometry. The Durham Applamatic Tonometer* is a nonrigid applanation instrument using a pressure balance system, developed by Maurice in 1951, between the flexible cornea and a thin (2 mil.), nonporous silastic membrane mounted over a small flat plate. This sensor tip is the operational end of a lightweight piston that floats on a thin layer of freon in a cylindrical handle. The tip is applied to the cornea in its terminal alignment, not by the examiner's hand, but by the gentle pressure of gas acting on the back end of the piston. During use, freon is delivered at a constant rate between the flexible membrane and the rigid plate. Unneeded gas escapes through several small (0.9 mm.) holes in the perimeter of the plate. As the sensor tip progressively presses against the cornea, the freon has greater difficulty passing between the plate and the membrane. This membrane moves only 5 to 6 mμ to cover the entire recording range of the instrument, which is 0 to 50 mm. Hg. When pressure under the membrane equals the intraocular pressure, the membrane flattens and a stylus tracing on heat sensitive paper levels off. Virtually instantaneous readings are made from the level midway between peaks and troughs of the superimposed cardiac pulse. A permanent strip chart is obtained. The sensor may be applied in any position, but readings on the supine patient tend—as with the Goldmann—to be 1 to 2 mm. higher than when taken on the same patient in the sitting position. Volume displacement by the Durham and the Goldmann instruments are very similar and derived corneal applanation pres-

*Manufactured by Block Engineering, Inc., Cambridge, Massachusetts, and distributed by Bausch and Lomb.

sures are quite comparable (Durham et al.: 1965).

Air blast applanation. Principles of air blast tonometry have been under study since the early 1960s but did not reach a production stage until 1972 when the American Optical Corporation's Non-contact Tonometer was marketed (Fig. 7-11). A collimated beam of light is directed to the corneal vertex and gauged by its reflection into a monitoring ocular at an angle of reflection equal to the angle of incidence. When so aligned, a single air blast of linearly increasing force is directed to the corneal site of incident light. Applanation progresses to a pre-elected (fixed) area at which time the corneally reflected light is received by a separately focused registering ocular. Time required for maximum reflection is converted to mm. Hg. Reading time is about 3 milliseconds, but don't leave the windows open. The standard deviations of readings with this instrument are about four times as large as those with the Goldmann, but are more reliable if several measurements are averaged and unusually high or low readings discarded (Stepanik, 1974). Cited advantages are reduced time for use, less discomfort to the

Fig. 7-11. Grolman Air Blast Tonometer as viewed from observer's side. (American Optical Corp., Scientific Instrument Division, Buffalo, New York 14215.)

patient, no need for a topical anesthetic, and little likelihood of transmitting mechanically-borne contaminates. Accuracy is not projected to exceed that of the Goldmann applanation system or any of its direct adaptations.

Summary of tonometer usage

Refinements of applanation tonometry in the last 25 years have established Hans Goldmann's applanator as *the* standard of accuracy for indirect measurement of intraocular pressure. This is predicated on a nonedematous, unscarred cornea of high catoptric quality. Necessarily combined use with almost any slit lamp, easily integrates Goldmann tonometry into office or clinic practice. The small, fixed applanation area of 3.06 mm. diameter causes little change (perhaps 0.5 mm.[3]) in intraocular volume. Readings are essentially unaffected by scleral or ocular rigidity, high ametropia, or endocrine disturbances. The small effects of surface tension in the tear film (minus) and corneal resistance to bending (plus) empirically have been found essentially to neutralize each other. Reading by vernier or aligning acuity increases the accuracy of endpoint determination. This procedure should now be the usual or conventional office practice wherever applicable. The single-hand operated Draeger or Perkins tonometers are of similar principles and accuracy: they can be used in any position, need no slit lamp, and are therefore well adapted and accurate for hospital rounds.

Indentation tonometers, classically exemplified by the familiar Schiøtz instrument, cause greater disturbance of intraocular volume and give significantly lower readings in high myopia or disturbances of ocular rigidity. Over all, about 20% of patients will be underestimated by Schiøtz tonometry. The instrument is unsuitable for scarred corneas or unusual corneal curvatures. Schiøtz tonometers—or with less precision, their simplified screening version by Berens and Tolman—may be used by understanding and instructed families for home follow-up of verified glaucoma patients under therapy.

With recognized limitations, this tonometer may also be used for screening or restive patients in home or institutional confinement. The 1948 calibration scale of J. S. Friedenwald,* as contrasted to the 1954-1955 scale, retains an added margin of protection for the patient because readings in the clinically important range are 3 to 6 mm. Hg higher. These are closer to comparable Goldmann applanation values.

The Mackay-Marg Electronic Tonometer is soundly and elegantly designed with a transducer probe only 1.5 mm. in diameter as a *fixed area* applanator. Because the applanation diameter is about half that of the Goldmann and optical systems are *not* involved in reading, it is particularly indicated and accurate in the presence of corneal edema, scars, or irregularities. This is a compact and portable (30 lbs.) unit with the advantages of reading in only a few tenths of a second and a permanent record by hot stylus strip recorder. Its cost is about four times that of the Goldmann and it offers no greater precision for office use with clear corneas. Calibration and standardization must be done more frequently than with the Goldmann. The Durham applamatic tonometer, though limited by a larger fixed applanation area, is nonoptical and delivers a permanent tracing on heat sensitive paper strip. It also correlates well with Goldmann readings on clear corneas but, like the 5-years older Mackay-Marg, has unique applicability in cloudy, edematous, or scarred corneas. Both instruments can be used in any position but neither affords comparable precision if applied over the bulbar conjuctiva and sclera.

Wide acceptance and utilization of the Goldmann has also stimulated in the past decade interest in the simplified (no moving parts), fixed force, hand-held applanation tonometers (Posner-Inglima Tonomat, Halberg variable weight, hand applanation tonometer). These offer high accuracy, low

---

*Committee on Standardization of Tonometers, American Academy of Ophthalmologists and Otolaryngologists, Rochester, Minnesota 55901.

cost ($135 to $200), gravitational operation, and are pocket-sized. They require clear corneas, topical anesthetics, and supine patients. With appropriate examiner practice their readings correlate well with the Goldmann. The Halberg can be used much more rapidly by virtue of direct readings rather than dye transfer prints. The Halberg is splendid for rapid hospital or nursing home rounds, periodic health examinations, and screening by general practitioners or technicians.

Tonography: indentation and applanation

Massage or pressure against the eyes has been recognized as reducing ocular tension since the work of Donders and of Pagenstecher in the 1870s. Similarly, Schiøtz and Priestly Smith in the early years of this century noted that holding a tonometer on the globe or repeatedly measuring ocular tension would lower these values, apparently by expressing some of the intraocular fluids. Quantitation of this "rate of ocular drainage" in terms of duration of application of the tonometer was begun by Gelder (1911) and Schoenberg (1912). This was improved somewhat by Kronfeld and his colleagues (1934) using a 2-minute application period. In the late 1940s two diagnostic aids, the electronic tonometer by Mueller and the practical understanding of gonioscopy evolved by Troncoso, laid the groundwork for modern, recorded tonography against a constant weight applied to the globe. In 1950 Moses and Bruno, as well as Morton Grant, presented mathematic foundations and prototype instruments for recording the "rate of outflow" over a standardized 4-minute period.

Usual tonography of the 1950s and 1960s is an extension in time of Schiøtz indentation tonometry and therefore incorporates the problems of indentation tonometry such as (1) ocular rigidity, (2) problems of clogging versus corneal attraction in the space between the plunger and footplate cylinder, (3) variations introduced by atypical or irregular corneal curvatures, and (4) defects of instrument manufacture or maintenance. In addition, the electronic tonometer and its recording equipment are subject to line voltage variations, influence of nearby metal masses or electric fields from other sources, drifts in electronic circuitry, and variations in function before complete warm-up. More than a thousand models of strip recorders are available for adaptation to electronic tonometers, though generally the narrow types are superseding the wide because of economy achieved at the expense of vertically compressing the tracing and making the reading of smaller variations difficult. Newer instruments contain well-matched recorders and often have built-in line voltage stabilizers. In addition to continuous refinements by V. Mueller[*] nuvistor circuitry and miniaturization, other quality instruments are available: Berkeley Bio-Engineering Inc.[†] transistorized circuits, low center of gravity plunger head, inkless recording, second scale for ophthalmodynamometry, solid state electronics, snap-on wristwatch type, digital read-out unit giving time of trace in seconds and continuous display of intraocular pressure in mm. Hg, Schwarzer Corporation's[‡] table-model and console stands, and Takata Ophthalmic Instrument Company's[§] small tonometer with built-in narrow strip recorder.

In use, the patient must recline on a suitably padded cot, stretcher, or tilt-back lounge chair, which must be relaxing and comfortable. A fairly large, and preferably luminous, ceiling fixation device should be centered above the patient's eyes. Drews recommends a decorator's handsome, four-bulb, frosted glass ceiling fixture about 12 to 24 in. square with an opaque knob in its center. The technician should be supplied with a comfortable stool with a backrest and should have some structure or available edge of the cot where she can steady her forearms. A foot switch for the recorder is highly desirable to reduce distracting move-

[*]V. Mueller, Chicago, Illinois 60648.
[†]San Leandro, California 94577.
[‡]Germany and 46 Salmi Road, Framingham, Massachusetts 01701.
[§]Tokyo, Japan.

ments around the patient. All disturbances of buzzers, telephones, intercoms, and incidental traffic must be excluded from the area during tonography. The recorder and tonometer dial must be positioned to be seen by the technician with no more than eye movement, because head movements are distracting to the patient.

The tonometer calibration should be checked before each run and before the patient is brought into the room, in accordance with the manufacturer's instructions. Gentle and reassuring explanation should be given as the patient is positioned. The patient's face must be parallel to the ceiling and must be maintained in this position without blinking or ocular movement for the 4 minutes of the test. Both local and vocal anesthesia should be administered as for Schiøtz tonometry. Tear evaporation from the open, fixing eye may create an unpleasant problem of drying and visual obscuration, which may be reduced if the patient shifts gaze, but only within the fixation target. Grant prefers to reduce tear evaporation by fixing a thin sheet of clear plastic Saran Wrap over this eye.

After achieving good patient understanding and relaxation, the tonometer must be lowered very slowly and gently onto the anesthetized right cornea, avoiding any mechanical bang or impact touch. The heel of the technician's hand should rest on the patient's forehead. Conversation cannot be allowed during the tracing, though the technician may have to remind or reassure the patient softly during the procedure. At the conclusion of tracing, the tonometer is gently lifted away, cleaned, and dried. A little movement, a compliment to the patient, and a few more drops of anesthetic in the left eye will prepare for the second tracing. The technician should not comment on the quality or the implication of the tracing, both of which the physician must interpret to the patient. As a single laboratory test, this is only one component in the study of the disease.

The finished tonogram must bear (1) calibration marks, (2) patient's name, (3) date,

(4) hour, (5) eye, (6) weight used, (7) technician's name, and (8) instrument used. The tracing itself is a complex of superimposed variables including the falling slope of intraocular pressure induced by the tonometer, the clearly visible cardiac pulse, the Traube-Hering slow undulations in systemic blood pressure, and the respiratory pattern. To plot the reading, a smooth line is drawn through the center of the tracing, averaging out the extraneous variations. Gross artifacts should be excluded, as should abrupt changes in slope at either the beginning or the end of the tracing. The averaging line is almost always a gentle curve and practically never a straight line. Once this has been constructed, or merely located visually, the scale readings (R) at the beginning and end of the 4-minute run can be read. In relation to the weight used, it is then possible to calculate the initial or opening intraocular pressure (P_0), which is assumed to have been present before the tonometer was applied, by use of the Friedenwald nomogram* based on the 1955 Friedenwald tonometer table. This should be essentially the same as applanation tension recorded before tonography. The difference between initial and final scale readings is then calculated and this figure ($\triangle R$) located in the row across the top of the table for the appropriate weight employed. The number in the column below this ($\triangle R$) difference, which lies in the row across from the initial scale reading (R), is the facility of outflow (C).

For the clinician these two values, P_0 and C, are the most important facts to be derived from tonography. Corrections for the influence of ocular rigidity on P_0 and C are not clinically significant. Similarly, other numerical values derived by manipulation of P_0 and C have statistical interest and value but do not merit the mathematic labors of derivation for individual patient care.

C values above 0.18 are generally normal,

---

*The Tonography Table of Moses and Becker based on the eye of average ocular rigidity and normal radius (7.8 mm.) of anterior corneal curvature may also be used to derive P_0 and C. Am. J. Ophthalmol. 45:196, 1958.

those between 0.13 to 0.18 are borderline, and those below 0.13 are abnormally low.

A crude or fixed pressure form of tonography is the bilateral Bulbar Compressor Test* of Berens and Tolman (1959). Applanation tension is measured in each eye and then a pressure of 50 gm. is applied simultaneously to each eye through the concave base of two spring-loaded compressors placed 7 mm. proximal to each limbus and below the lateral rectus borders. The examiner maintains these compressors in radial position for 2 minutes, then removes them and immediately repeats the applanation readings. Simultaneous testing theoretically avoids the possibility of pressure on one eye unduly affecting the other. Results should be expressed as the change in ocular tension. Normal values are not well documented, but generally normal eyes may be expected to show a greater drop than those with glaucoma or reduced facility of aqueous outflow.

Applanation tonography

Recording applanation tonometers usable in supine as well as the sitting position have been acceptably validated in the 1970s. Among these, the Durham Applamatic Tonometer (Bausch and Lomb) has been particularly studied by Langham and others. The Mackay-Marg Electronic Tonometer is adaptable for tonography, but has been less used by medical investigators of disease and apparently requires calibration at intervals considerably more frequent than a year. The Durham instrument, when handled with care, holds accuracy for periods much longer than a year without recalibration. Langham et al. have validated the 2-minute pneumotonographic techniques using a 10 gm. weight with this instrument. This establishes modified and possibly more precise values for tonographic coefficients that are free of previous indentation artifacts. A compact unit suitable for office use is available commercially as the Applanation Pneumatonograph.†

---

*Matalene Surgical Instruments Co., New York, New York 10017.
†Alcon Laboratories, Inc., Fort Worth, Texas 76101.

By simple movement of a switch this can be used for basic tonometry or for tonography timed at either 2- or 4-minute runs.

Provocative tests

Provoke: (from Latin) to irritate; to offend

"Don't challenge and thus gamble with the vitality of the patient by quickly subjecting him to more tests and treatments than he can tolerate with reasonable safety."

DAVID SEEGAL, 1964

Provocative tests—such as the Marlow prolonged occlusion technique for heterophoria, intravenous curare in suspected myasthenia gravis, digital compression of the carotid artery to evoke amaurosis fugax, or the mydriatic examination in narrow-angle glaucoma—are generally secondary procedures and should be avoided if possible. Each of these examples has been followed at times by near catastrophic results. Resort to such methods to establish a diagnosis generally suggests inadequate development of the state of the art or the state of the examiner. More widespread use of modern applanation tonometry, gonioscopy, and tonography has lessened the need for provocative testing in individual patients, though such procedures may have both predictive and statistical value.

The possibly intermittent character of open-angle glaucoma (elevated P_0 or depressed C values) in its early stages may at times yield negative provocative procedures as well as standard tests. In such patients, the longitudinal studies and follow-up observations of the regularly attending ophthalmologist may be of greater value than the one-time or "cross sectional" view of the consultant, even though the latter has the virtues of *freshness* and possibly unencumbering *set* from previous experience with the particular patient.

Provocative tests are subdivided in correspondence with the major types of glaucoma into those applicable to open-angle glaucoma and those applicable to narrow-angle glaucoma. Anatomically narrow iridocorneal angles, however, can be present incidentally in an eye with the underlying fault of open-angle glaucoma, and thereby both major forms of the disease may be present at the same time.

When anatomically narrow angles cause glaucoma (in the absence of open-angle defect) it is by the mechanism of angle closure or forward displacement of the peripheral iris blocking access of aqueous flow into the trabecular drainage meshwork. This may be independent of or secondary to a pupillary block, wherein the iris sphincter adheres to the anterior lens surface physiologically (such as with increased convexity of the lens surface and rigidity of the iris), pharmacologically (such as with tight sphincter contraction by strong miotic medications), or anatomically (such as following inflammatory adhesions of iritis). The symptoms of pain, blurred vision, and tearing, as well as the signs of deep conjunctival injection and increased ocular tension, initially tend to be intermittent and frequently mild until a major angle closure occurs with subsequently intense pain, nausea, and vomiting. Gonioscopic inspection with a contact lens identifies the anatomic proximity of the iris to the corneal endothelium and should define the likelihood of acute glaucoma being induced. In some patients, either during or between angle-closure episodes, the acute iridocorneal angulation of 10 degrees or less is so apparent (closed, Shaffer grade 0; extreme narrow angle, Shaffer grade 1) as to leave no doubt in the examiner's mind concerning the induction mechanisms. In other patients, the reverse end of the scale (wide open angle, Shaffer grade 4) is so obvious that closure is impossible. Between these extremes lie the moderately narrowed configurations with angles of approximately 20 to 40 degrees (Shaffer grades 2 and 3) where the examiner might wish to quantitate better the closure potential. Basically two provocative tests are suitable under these conditions.

The *dark room test* is the most conservative provocative procedure. Initial applanation measurements are made with or without tonograms, as desired, and then the patient is placed in a totally dark room. Both eyes are covered lightly with patches or a bandage. The test cannot be done on one eye at a time, as is done in mydriatic tests. After 60 minutes, the dressings are removed and very prompt applanation readings are made again, but with the added precaution that lighting is kept very dim and directed away from the patient. An increase of pressure exceeding 5 mm. Hg should be considered positive. Generally the degree of dilation by this technique is less than with topical drugs, and it is progressively less in advancing years as iris rigidity increases and physiologic miosis develops.

Mydriatic testing generally produces larger pupils, more positive results than does dark room testing, and greater likelihood of induced glaucoma necessitating surgical relief. Because of this danger, only one eye should be tested at any examination. Long-acting drugs such as atropine, difficultly reversible drugs such as 10% Neo-Synephrine, or rapid and potent drugs such as 1% cyclopentolate (Cyclogyl) should be avoided. Shorter acting and weaker mydriatics such as 3% eucatropine hydrochloride (Euphthalmine), 0.5% tropicamide (Mydriacyl), or 1% hydroxyamphetamine Paredrine) are preferable. The pupil should be brought to a midposition of dilation (diameter of 5 to 7 mm.) thus avoiding the tendency for the iris to fall back on the receding lens surface as occurs in extreme dilation. Ambient light is not important, but the pupillary diameter should always be recorded before and after the dilation period. Results may be considered positive when ocular tension increases by more than 8 mm. Hg, when there is distinct flattening of the tonogram, and when gonioscopy shows the angle to be closed. Following this test it is necessary to instill a weak miotic such as 0.5% or 1% pilocarpine and have the patient remain in the office long enough to see that the dilation has been reversed. This may require 30 to 45 minutes. Strong miotics are contraindicated because of their ability to cause pupillary block and subsequent angle-closure glaucoma.

In the presence of distinctly wide or open

angles, or where a concomitant open-angle defect is suspected in the presence of anatomically narrowed angles, two provocative procedures are again available.

The water provocative or hemodilution test, as all of these procedures, requires tonometry and preferably tonography before the test. Manifestly, if the tonography is abnormal there can be no additional information obtained by hemodilution, and the test is not indicated. The patient should be off all medication that may affect pressure and should be restricted from all food and liquid for at least 4 hours before the test. The test is often thus best scheduled for an early morning office appointment. Fourteen milliliters per kilogram of body weight, or approximately a quart, of water is then drunk as rapidly as comfortable. Practically all beverages are hypertonic to water; therefore, they will have a lesser effect and should not be used. Repeat tonometry is done 15 and 30 minutes after ingestion of the water or until the pressure starts to fall. A rise of at least 8 mm. Hg in ocular tension should be interpreted as positive. The effects are bilateral. Of the provocative procedures, this is the least apt to be followed by complications. To obtain mathematical indices such as P_0/C after water drinking, it is, of course, necessary to do repeat tonography.

Steroid testing may not only evoke positive pressure increments in a given patient, but such response in apparently nonglaucomatous members of a family may yield statistics on predisposition and the three known phenotypic patterns for inheritance of steroid responsiveness. This seems to be a recessive trait. Though various topical corticosteroids have been employed, most testing has been done with 0.1% betamethasone and 0.1% dexamethasone, 1 drop in each eye three or four times a day. Tensions are checked weekly and drops may be continued until a significant increase is noted or for a maximum of 6 weeks. Modifications of this routine for more frequent instillations on a short-term basis may prove to yield similar responses. Steroids administered systemically generally do not have this capacity to elevate intraocular pressure. Though topical steroids are also known to "provoke" subclinical or latent herpes simplex, this has appeared to be of little clinical significance thus far. There is a further potential for topical steroids to cause lens opacities, which the physician must always weigh in the extended use of these drugs.

Diurnal variations

Glaucomatous elevation of pressure may be intermittent but may also vary with the time of day and the cycle of ocular rest or reduced mobility during sleep in comparison to the massaging action of waking hours. Diurnal fluctuations are more marked in eyes with increased tension or impaired outflow facility than those with normal facility. Careful measurement by the same instrument and same examiner every 2 or 3 hours around the clock may reveal significant diurnal rises that would be missed during routine office hours only. The patient is commonly hospitalized for such studies, but he is reassured and less disturbed if this can be done in a self-care or convalescent unit. In some medical centers, a type of "Medical Inn" of motel design serves well for such studies.

Normal diurnal fluctuations are usually within 2 to 4 mm. Hg, but in open-angle (chronic simple) glaucoma they may reach 15 to 20 mm. Hg. Commonly the greatest rise in pressure is in the early morning hours of 4 to 7 A.M., but there may be reverse cycles with highest pressure in the late afternoon. Differences between the two eyes particularly raise suspicion of the eye with the greater increase.

Ballistic tonometry or viscoelastometry

Since the late 1950s several refinements of measurement (vibration tonometry: Hargens, Keiper, Sarin, 1965; viscoelastometry: Hargens, Keiper, G. Spaeth, 1962) have been designed to extremely minute disturbances of the globe and self-recorded information (signatures drawn automatically on an oscilloscope with X and Y axes representing strain and stress) of deformation and reformation or viscous and elastic moduli. Permanent records are obtained on Polaroid camera film. Such equipment yields a new dimension in study of both tissue characteristics and pressure factors within the globe, but it is expensive and cumbersome as yet. These new concepts, however, have far more potential than did earlier attempts in the modification of indentation techniques (fixed indentation: Maurice, 1958; microplunger movements: Mackey-Marg, 1960) or use of the less sensitive—and less consistent—scleral portions of the globe (Wolfe, 1948). At present, however, such equipment in practical or production models is not available.

GONIOSCOPY

Gonioscopy (Greek *gonia*, angle, and Greek *skopein*, to examine) is a contact lens technique of visualizing the anterior chamber recess or filtration angle, which is hidden to direct inspection by the overhanging opaque scleral limbus and obscured to view from the opposite limbus by internal corneal reflections and often by forward bulging of the peripheral-most or "last roll" of the iris.

Gonioscopic visualization of the iridocorneal or filtration angles has led to probably the most fundamental advance of this generation in understanding and diagnosing causative mechanisms in glaucoma. This has also produced far more rational and effective therapy. Basically this is the identification of the anatomically narrow angle mechanism and its precipitating role in both acute and progressive angle closure. Gonioscopy thus affords direct and immediate differentiation of such pathology from chronic simple or open-angle glaucoma. Unfortunately the presence of narrowed angles or the catastrophe of angle closure does not exclude coexistence of open-angle mechanisms or "mixed glaucoma." On the other hand, a wide open and accessible angle does not rule out likelihood of angle closure episodes. It is therefore important to examine gonioscopically all glaucoma patients and those with suspect episodes of pain, blurring, or congestion. Progressive thickening

of the lens throughout life also has a narrowing effect, both on the anterior chamber and on the angle itself. A progressive or "creeping" angle closure may occur; this calls for repeated gonioscopy in open-angle glaucoma patients at intervals of a year or so.

Gonioscopy is also essential in the location of small, radiolucent foreign bodies whose concealment in an angle recess may cause localized corneal edema. Similarly, it is vital in the study of peripheral iris or angle recess tumors to determine their invasion into the angle and the possibility of excision by methods less than removal of the eye.

Modern practical gonioscopy has been made possible by the contact lens designs and procedure introduced by Troncoso for "direct" visualization of the angle (1925). Technical evolutions were spearheaded by Salzmann (1914-1915) and by Koeppe (1919-1920), primarily in the area of circular or 360-degree (direct) goniolenses for use with the recumbent patient. Koeppe also developed early contact lenses for use at the slit lamp with the patient seated, and Goldmann in the mid-1930s presented the first of his mirrored or "indirect" contact lenses for slit lamp use. These became the prototypes for more recent refinements such as the Goldmann three-mirror lens, which is now one of the most widely used models. In the mid-1930s, Barkan also began a series of handled and truncated lenses to facilitate surgical introduction of a knife for goniotomy under visual control.

Lens designs

Goniolenses are divided into those for examination with the slit lamp or gonioscope, and those for surgical use with the operating loupe, microscope, or other mechanically mounted gonioscope (Troncoso, Heine, Haag-Streit, Barkan floor stand).

Gonioscopy is one of the most fundamental or pivotal examinations in both diagnosis and control of glaucoma. It should be part of every initial work-up and repeated in controlled patients about once each year.

Techniques of use are modified according to the design of the retention mechanism for the lens:

1. Smooth, nonflanged base for retention with fingers and capillarity. The Zeiss four-mirror lens, the Barkan surgical lenses, the Thorpe four-mirror gonio-lens, the Worst Prismatic lens, the

Fig. 7-12. Koeppe Flange Retention Direct Goniolens for 360° visualization of filtration angle with focal light and magnification. Basic magnification by this lens is 1.5×.

Worst Lovac six-mirror gonioscope lens, the von Beuningen goniopyramid (Zeiss-Jena), the Haag-Streit Goldmann three-mirror lens, and its Franklin three-mirror adaption are available in this type.

2. Flanged or scleral haptic base for retention between the lids. Early models of the Goldmann three-mirror lens (and the earlier single-mirror version), the Koeppe (Fig. 7-12), the Troncoso, the Worst Lo-Vac spherical modification of the Barkan, the Franklin direct, the Richardson, and the four-sided Allen-Thorpe are of this type and therefore contribute to their own self-retention. A silicone rubber (as in the Franklin direct lens) or similar plastic surface to the flange reduces the likelihood of corneal abrasions.

3. Vacuum retention lenses. These lenses (Lo-Vac) of J. G. F. Worst are small, light lenses of original design (direct goniolens with tilted flat anterior sur-

Swan-Jacob
gonioprism

Fig. 7-13. Swan-Jacob direct gonioprism with magnifying convex surface. (Ocular Instruments, Inc., Redmond, Washington 98052.)

face allowing nearly a 180-degree view of the angle; six-mirror indirect gonio-lens; double-focus lens for gonioscopy with direct or indirect ophthalmoscope) or modifications of classical designs (Barkan and Koeppe), each fitted with connections for plastic tubing through which a small amount of vacuum is generated after the lens is placed on the cornea.

4. Hand-held lenses. This includes the Cardona goniofocalizing lenses, some of the Barkan lenses, the S.C. Becker fluid bridge gonioprism with two stand-off orbital rim supports, the Thorpe surgical lens, the Unger holding fork for the Zeiss four-mirror lens and the Swan or revised Swan-Jacob direct surgical examining lens (Fig. 7-13). The Cardona fiber-optic goniolens permits one-handed control of the lens and its direct illuminating system; a wide direct image field of 30° to 35° is afforded.

5. Headband-mounted lens on patient as designed by S. C. Becker (fluid bridge or noncontact indirect lens for totally undistorted viewing).

Fig. 7-14. Goldmann three-mirror contact lens in place with the aid of topical anesthetic. Small semicircular mirror shown in upper position is angulated for inspection of the filtration angle.

Design principles should minimize distortion of the cornea and *relationships of the angle*. Thus the corneal contact surface is preferably small and the angulation of the mirror extends close to the center of the pupil. These principles underlie the Becker stand-off or bridge gonioprism, which may be stabilized as much as 3 mm. above the cornea by two adjustable orbital supports. The interval is filled with Gonio-Gel. Exceptionally high (25 mm.) reflecting surfaces permit inspection of very narrow chamber angles without anatomically disturbing the anterior segment. This is the reverse of the modified direct Koeppe lens with a dimple in its crown for manipulation and compression by an applicator inserted into the recess. Corneal contact diameters vary from 9 to 14 mm. and the radii of curvature similarly vary between 7.16 and 8.15 mm.

Various diameters are available in several lens designs for use in children or those with small eyes: Koeppe 17, 19, and 21 mm. outside-flange diameter; Cardona small, medium, and large; Goldmann three-mirror, small and large; Worst spherical goniotomy lens, small and large.

In use, the adult must have a topical anesthetic such as Ophthaine or Ophthetic instilled. Infants and small children require light general anesthetic under proper preparation and with appropriate resuscitation safeguards immediately available. A small amount of 2% to 6% methylcellulose solution is placed in the concavity of the corneal surface of the lens both to complete the lens-corneal contact and to reduce possible edge trauma. When the sitting position is used for slit lamp gonioscopy, the patient is first positioned on the chinrest and the

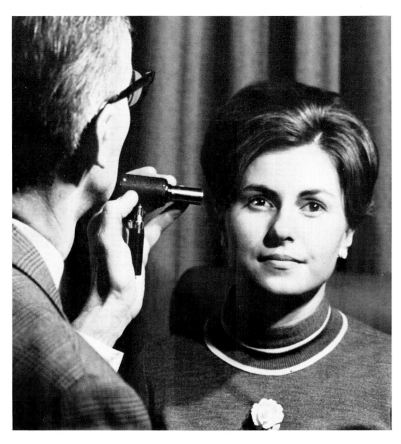

Fig. 7-15. Barkan hand-held illuminator used for external inspection or gonioillumination. Zeiss quick focusing hand lamp is similarly useful.

slit lamp turned on. With the lens held be-tween the thumb and forefinger of one hand, the thumb of the opposite hand is used to draw down the lower lid while the patient looks upward. The lower edge of the gonio-lens is then inserted against the center of the lower lid border, and the hand is moved to draw the upper lid away from the globe. At this time, the goniolens is rotated upward, bringing its concave surface against the pa-tient's cornea. At the same time, the upper lid is released to drop against the upper sur-face of the lens. The patient is initially asked to maintain the primary position of gaze and not to squeeze his lids (Fig. 7-14).

Illumination and technique

Light is no problem with indirect lenses used at the slit lamp, but for direct lenses used with a supine patient a small focal light is needed such as the Barkan illuminator (Fig. 7-15), the Zeiss Focusing Hand Lamp, or those built into the Troncoso, Heine, and Haag-Streit binocular gonioscopes. The latter three hand-held instruments afford good stereoscopic viewing at 6.5× to 16× and suitable coincidence illumination; the combinations however are heavy, cumber-some, and cannot be easily used at surgery. More recently, fiber-optic bundles built into goniolenses, such as the Worst prismatic or the Cordona design, afford direct illumi-nation and control handles in the same struc-ture. The head-mounted Beckerscope, orig-inally designed for ocular surgery, gives a magnification of 9 to 10×, and when fitted with dual fiber optic illumination provides excellent illumination for shadowless direct gonioscopy. For slit lamp gonioscopy, the light and line of observation are brought to coincidence first on the reflecting surface positioned at the upper pole to study the lower angle. It is generally necessary to tilt the lens at various points of examination to visualize the angle fully. Initial contact should be quite light against the eye, to avoid unknowingly manipulating open an angle that has been physiologically closed. The entire circumference of the angle is then inspected by rotating the goniolens and the

illuminating and observation systems or with multiple mirrors by moving the light and line of observation to successive mirrors.

Indirect slit lamp gonioscopy of the upper angle is at times slightly more difficult than the lower, and focusing into the medial and lateral areas is the most difficult because it affords the least latitude in aligning the light and observational axes. Sclerotic scatter (p. 90) may be used in the horizontal recesses if it seems impossible to obtain illumination and visualization in good coordination. The Leydecker (1969) goniolens directs light into the angle by incorporated fiber optics and has the added benefit of not requiring contact fluid between the lens and the cornea. This is an advantage at surgery as well as at ex-amination in that one additional step is de-leted from the technique.

Diffuse or broad-beam illumination should first be used in identification of the land-marks of the angle and major pathologic alterations. The beam should then be nar-rowed to a fine slit to demonstrate in optic section the precise curvature of the iris sur-face into the angle.

Landmarks

The landmarks should be sought serially from anterior (corneal) to posterior (iridic). The surgeon potentially operating in the angle must appreciate the actual size of angle structures. Schlemm's canal varies between 0.2 and 0.3 mm. in diameter. The width from Schwalbe's line to the scleral spur is 0.6 to 0.7 mm. and from Schwalbe's line to the depth of the normal angle is 0.7 to 0.8 mm. The landmarks include:

Schwalbe's line. Schwalbe's line (anterior border ring) or termination of Descemet's membrane appears as a whitish line, often projecting slightly into the anterior cham-ber.

Trabecular meshwork. The trabecular meshwork extends from its anterior limits at Schwalbe's line (corneoscleral portion) to the blending of its posterior (uveal) portion with the anterior iris surface.

Schlemm's canal. Found beneath the junction of the middle and posterior thirds of the trabecular meshwork, Schlemm's canal sometimes appears as a faint gray line or a blood-filled line deep to the trabeculum.

Scleral spur. The scleral spur is the most anterior projection of the sclera and often appears through the trabeculum as a gray-white line of varying width at the outer end of the angle recess.

Ciliary body band. The ciliary body band is a stripe created by the anterior portion of the ciliary body when it is within gonioscopic view. It usually appears to extend from the root of the iris to the scleral spur, but in some eyes it is completely veiled by the overlying posterior trabecular meshwork. In darkly pigmented individuals the band appears to be dark gray, and in light individuals it may be unpigmented. In angle recession, the ciliary muscle is torn from the scleral spur, and therefore exposed scleral whiteness may be seen in this area. The narrower the angle, or the farther forward the iris is attached, the narrower or less visible will be the ciliary body band.

Iris processes (pectinate fibers). The iris processes bridge the angle recess from the anterior iris surface to the trabeculum, usually in the scleral spur area. Some processes, however, may run as far forward as Schwalbe's line. The processes are pigmented and more conspicuous with brown irides; with blue irides they appear light gray and are difficult to identify.

Trabecular pigment band. The trabecular pigment band often appears in the proximal meshwork just anterior to the scleral spur. This results from uveal pigment being carried through the trabeculum with the aqueous flow. It is seen more commonly (1) in the inferior trabeculum, (2) in darkly pigmented eyes, (3) in advancing years, (4) in the presence of a Krukenberg spindle, (5) in the diabetic patient, (6) in eyes with anterior melanomas, (7) following uveitis, and (8) in pigmentary glaucoma. The width and intensity of this pigment band is graded from 1 through 4, and in the most advanced grade it fills about half or more of the trabecular width. Where iris processes are numerous, they may obscure trabecular pigment and require gonioscopy under transillumination.

Adhesions (synechiae). Adhesions occur between the iris surface and trabeculum or farther anteriorly. They may vary widely in appearance from small and tent-like types from localized injury, through columnar or broad adhesions of previous narrow-angle glaucoma attacks, to essentially circumferential apposition, or extensive strands and broad processes arching forward from the anterior iris surface to Schwalbe's line, as in the congenital anomaly of Axenfeld (1920).

Blood vessels. Vascular patterns vary widely in the angle. The normal radial iris vessels appear as irregularly corkscrew structures in the peripheral iris, particularly if pigmentation is light. Anomalous knuckles or hairpin loops of normal vessels may emerge through the iris or ciliary body. Pathologic or new vessels tend to be on the surface of the iris or trabeculum at indiscrimate angulations and with some fibrous proliferation about them.

Grading of iridocorneal angle

Accurate observation should be made of the openness or depth of the anterior chamber angle or iridocorneal angle. This is graded from 0 through 4. Unfortunately, contradictory systems exist for numerical designation of the width of the angle. The classification sometimes known as the Shaffer System* (Table 3) is in wide use and logically considers the zero angle to be the closed angle.

In quantitating the width of the iridocorneal angle and to avoid distortion of trabecular details by oblique inspection, the observer's line of view should be as nearly parallel as possible to the surface of the iris. In narrow-angled eyes (grades 1 and 2), however, the necessarily oblique view precludes critical evaluation of structures beneath the

*Adopted by the United States Public Health Service Committee on Glaucoma and by the Symposium on Primary Glaucoma of the American Academy of Ophthalmology and Otolaryngology.

Table 3. Shaffer system

Numerical grade	Terminology	Description
0	Closed	Anterior iris surface is in contact with peripheral corneal endothelium and trabeculum, or it is sufficiently displaced forward so as to preclude visualization of any anatomic details of the trabecular area. The lens is well anterior to the ciliary body ring. The central, endothelial iris surface is snug against a major area of the anterior capsule.
1	Extremely narrow	The iridocorneal angle is reduced to approximately 10 degrees, or "slit-like" appearance. It will close with slight iris edema or additional bombé, such as from physiologic pupillary block. Closure is probably inevitable in time. The lens is anterior to the ciliary body ring and a large area of endothelial iris surface is in contact with the anterior capsule.
2	Moderately narrow angle	The iridocorneal angle is approximately 20 degrees. The iris surface appears to be modestly convex but anterior trabecular details can usually be visualized without excessive tilting and manipulation of the goniolens, though these maneuvers may be necessary to inspect the narrowed posterior depths of the angle. The lens is slightly anterior to the ciliary body ring, and there is moderately broad contact between the endothelial iris surface centrally and the anterior capsule. Closure is certainly possible, and the earlier in life such angles are seen, the greater the likelihood of angle closure in later life. Such angles are more commonly found in later years of life and with hyperopia.
3	Open angle	The iridocorneal angle is approximately 30 degrees and there is only a little convexity of the iris surface. Anterior trabecular details are easily apparent, and posterior trabecular details can be seen with only modest tilting or angulation of the goniolens. The lens is approximately on a level with the ciliary body ring. Closure is most unlikely or impossible. This angle configuration is more likely in myopia than in hyperopia.
4	Wide open angle	The iridocorneal angle is approximately 45 degrees. All details of the trabecular area and recess are visualized with ease. The iris extends from its attachment at the inner anterior border of the ciliary body and generally appears flat. The lens is on a level with or slightly posterior to the ciliary body ring, and there is minimal contact between the endothelial iris surface centrally and the anterior lens capsule. Physiologic pupillary block and angle closure are both essentially impossible. This type of angle is commonly seen in youth, myopia, and aphakia.

trabeculum and gives a foreshortened illusion of the extent of the meshwork.

The normal corneal epithelium is very tolerant to both rotation and angulation of smooth, concave-based goniolenses. However, small grey patches, wrinkles, or breaks in the epithelium with such examinations suggest pathology as poor binding of epithelium to Bowman's membrane or recurrent corneal erosion.

Recording angle characteristics

Just as inflammatory adhesions may be limited to specific areas of the angle, so may the anatomic characteristics differ in various portions. At times the entire 360 degrees will be fully open grade 3 or 4, and in the presence of certain catastrophies the angle may be 0 throughout. The ophthalmologist should note configuration of the angle by quadrants or positions of clock hours. More

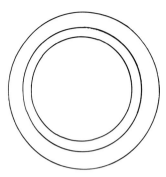

Fig. 7-16. Goniodiagram for recording details of the anterior chamber angle. Outer circle represents Schwalbe's line with trabecular meshwork extending to the middle circle, which represents the scleral spur. The angle recess is represented by the space extending to the inner circle, which indicates the iris root or iris insertion. The position and height of synechiae are recorded by drawing in radial lines to their anterior limit. The grade of angle width, 0 through 4, is noted by placing the appropriate number in each quadrant or clock position adjacent to the outer circle.

detail may be displayed graphically and in fewer words by use of a schematic set of three concentric circles in which the outermost represents Schwalbe's line, the middle represents the scleral spur, and the innermost represents the angle recess (Fig. 7-16). For the more compulsive gonioscopist a recording of angle width at selected hours may be derived from a goniometric reference grid inserted into one of the slit lamp oculars. For permanent records, a photographic slit lamp may be used and a corrected overlay graticule is available to read the angle width from a print enlarged ten times (Clark and Lowe, 1974).

Fluorescein photography

Fluorescein angiography of the optic nerve head offers prognostic assessment of disc susceptibility to glaucomatous pressure. The role of ciliary arterial supply, postlaminar vessels, prelaminar vessels, and peripapillary choroidal vessels can be estimated; vascular compromises may predispose the disc to ischemic atrophy even though central retinal artery circulation is excellent.

REFERENCES

Becker, S. C.: Clinical gonioscopy, St. Louis, 1972, The C. V. Mosby Co.

Becker, S. C.: Unrecognized errors induced by present day gonioprisms and a proposal for their elimination, Arch. Ophthalmol. 82:160-168, Aug., 1969.

Clark, B. A., and Lowe, R. F.: Slit lamp measurement of anterior chamber geometry, Ophthalmologica 168:58-74, 1974.

Draeger, J.: Principle and clinical application of a portable applanation tonometer, Invest. Ophthalmol. 6:132-134, 1967.

Dunn, J. S., and Brubaker, R. F.: Perkins applanation tonometer, Arch. Ophthalmol. 89:149-151, Feb., 1973.

Durham, D. G., Bigliano, R. P., and Mashino, J. A.: Pneumatic applanation tonometer, Trans. Am. Acad. Ophthalmol. and Otolaryngol. 69:1029-1047, Nov.-Dec., 1965.

Forbes, M.: Gonioscopy with corneal indentation for distinguishing between appositional closure and synechial closure, Arch. Ophthalmol. 76:488-492, 1966.

Friedenwald, J. S.: Tonometer (Schiøtz) Calibration Trans. Am. Acad. Ophthalmol. and Otolaryngol. 61:108-123, Jan.-Feb., 1957.

Grant, W. M.: Tonographic method for measuring facility and rate of aqueous flow in human eyes, Arch. Ophthalmol. 44:204-214, 1950.

Halberg, G. P.: Hand applanation tonometer, Trans. Am. Acad. Ophthalmol. Otolaryngol. 72:112-114, 1968.

Kaiden, J. S., Zimmerman, T. J., and Worthen, D. M.: Evaluation of the (Heine-Propper) Glauco Test Screening Tonometer, Arch. Ophthalmol. 92:195-197, Sept., 1974.

Keiper, D. A., Sarin, L. K., Leopold, I. H., and Chevrette, L.: The vibration tonometer, Am. J. Ophthalmol. 59:1007-1012, June, 1965.

Krakau, C. E. T.: A vibration tonometer, Ophthalmol. Research 1:129-139, 1970.

Maurice, D. M.: An applanation tonometer of new principles, Br. J. Ophthalmol. 35:178-182, 1951.

McMillan, F., and Forster, R. K.: Comparison of Mackay-Marg, Goldmann, and Perkins tonometers in abnormal corneas, Arch. Ophthalmol. 93:420-424, June, 1975.

Moses, R. A., and Becker, B.: Clinical tonography: The scleral rigidity correction, Am. J. Ophthalmol. 45:196-208, 1958.

Moses, R. A., and Bruno, M.: Rate of outflow of fluid from the eye under increased pressure, Am. J. Ophthalmol. 33:389-397, 1950.

Nesterov, A. P., and Vurgaft, M. R.: Calibration tables for the Filatov Kalfa elastotonometer, Vest. Oftalmol. 2:20-25, 1972.

Quigley, H. A., and Langham, M. E.: Comparative intraocular pressure measurements with the pneumatonograph and Goldmann tonometer, Am. J. Ophthalmol. 80:266-273, 1975.

Schwartz, B., Henkind, P., Hayreh, S. S., Kronfeld,

P. C., Spaeth, G. L., Hitchings, R. A., Sivalingam, E., and Drance, S. M.: The optic disc in glaucoma, a symposium, Tr. Am. Acad. Ophthalmol. and Otolaryngol. **81:**192-238, Mar.-April, 1976.

Shaffer, R. N., Ridgway, W. L., Brown, R., Kramer, S. G.: Diagrams to record changes in glaucomatous discs, Am. J. Ophthalmol. **80:**460-464, Sept., 1975.

Stepanik, J.: The AO noncontact tonometer: Clinical measurement in normotensive eyes, Graefes Arch. Ophthalmol. **190:**47-49, 1974.

van Herrick, W., Shaffer, R. N., and Schwartz, A.: Estimation of width of angle of anterior chamber, Am. J. Ophthalmol. **68:**626-629, 1969.

Weisman, H.: Anesthesia and glaucoma, Ann. Ophthalmol. **3:**1129-1131, 1971.

Worst, J. G. F.: Goniotomy lens with internal fiber illumination, Am. J. Ophthalmol. **65:**251-254, Feb., 1968.

CHAPTER 8

The uvea and its inflammations

Differentiating the red eye of intraocular inflammation from the generally less serious external infections of conjunctivitis and the major problem of congestive, acute, or subacute glaucoma presents an immediate and pressing problem. Probably the most pivotal sign is the pupil: this usually is normal in external infections, tends to be smaller and somewhat irregular in uveitis, or larger and somewhat vertically ovalized in acute or angle-closure glaucoma. Thus a normal-size and reactive pupil tends to rule out acute or severe intraocular disturbances in the presence of a red eye. Secretions also furnish some guide: external infections produce tenacious or purulent secretions with matting or adherence of the lids on awakening; both uveitis and glaucoma produce excessive secretions, but these are clear, watery tears. Pain is generally mild in posterior uveitis and conjunctivitis, moderate in anterior uveitis, and severe in acute glaucoma. Severe uveitis in childhood, however, may be deceptively devoid of discomfort.

Color of the irides should be noted and any unusual characteristics, such as heterochromia or sector differences, verified as to whether they are congenital or acquired. Anticipated testimony from parents and siblings often is noncontributory, but a search for previous close-up photographs such as Polaroid color prints, may document the time of onset. Segmental darkening or appearance of one or more dark spots in the iris—later than the freckles of puberty—suggests the localized and low malignancy iris melanoma. Lightening of one iris with faint inflammatory signs and few keratic precipitates (K.P.) suggest indolent heterochromic uveitis of Fuchs. Diffuse and uniform darkening throughout one iris in the adult patient suggests the vi-

cious ring melanoma with pain of secondary glaucoma. Unilateral, acquired extra pupils and eccentric movement of the true pupil of the young adult patient suggests essential iris atrophy and difficult secondary glaucoma.

Diagnosis in any illness is best made on the basis of specific cause. Often, however, in uveitis no specific cause, either local or general, is identified even after extensive search. In studying disease manifestations and in considering prognosis, it is important to make at least a morphologic description and classification of the ocular process. Uveitis may appear only as a local inflammation. In such cases always suspect an occult foreign body, even with a negative history. X-ray scout films should usually be made unless the morphology is classically distinct (e.g. candle wax drippings of sarcoid, budding daughter lesions of posterior polar toxoplasmosis, or punched-out configuration of presumed histoplasmosis). Search for a wound track. Small linear corneal scars and telltale iris holes will remain forever, but external evidence of perforation in the bulbar conjunctiva and sclera will usually be obscured. The frequency of perforating foreign bodies decreases linearly from the anterior to posterior poles, but the weight of such retained foreign bodies increases linearly with the depth of perforation. In a small percentage of cases, uveitis seems to be the ocular manifestation of systemic diseases, such as Boeck's sarcoidosis, toxoplasmosis, Weil's disease, Behçet's disease, Still's disease, Marie-Strumpel's disease, leprosy, or presumed histoplasmosis. Rarely, uveitis is a component of a distinct uveomeningeal infection, as in torulosis or cryptococcosis, or the etiologically less defined syndromes such as Vogt-Koyanagi and Harada's uveomeningitis. The latter has a

162

significant fatality rate. The following interim classification provides valuable working data:

Classification of uveitis

A. Anatomic area of inflammation

1. Anterior uveitis or iritis: swelling and inflammatory signs confined primarily to the iris and circumcorneal area. White cells and increased protein density in the aqueous may lead to secondary glaucoma. Recurrent acute glaucomatocyclitic crises in the young adult, however, may have only mild inflammatory signs.

2. Iridocyclitis: inflammatory disturbances involving both the iris and ciliary body (This is more frequent than iritis alone, generally produces uncomfortable disturbances of accommodation, and causes ocular hypotony because of impaired aqueous secretion.)

3. Posterior uveitis (chorioretinitis): appears in many forms and should be specified as to whether the retina or the choroid is primarily inflamed (Disturbances in the retina as in acute toxoplasmosis commonly produce marked cellular debris and haze in the vitreous, whereas those largely confined to the deeper layers, as in histoplasmosis, may be associated with a clear vitreous.)

   a. Macular or posterior polar involvement: an almost exclusive localization

   b. The pars plana (pars planitis): may be principal site of involvement

   c. Peripheral or disseminated involvement: primary localization of pathology

   d. Diffuse

B. Stage of activity

1. Acute: sudden onset of findings in a previously clear and quiet eye

2. Subacute: modest or mild onset without sudden, disabling symptoms

3. Chronic: persistent inflammation, though subject to variations in severity

4. Recurrent: intermittent inflammation with complete clearing and quieting between episodes

C. Degree of severity

1. Mild: slight discomfort, little lid edema, minimal disturbance of vision, and almost no disturbance of pupillary reaction

2. Moderate: discomfort requiring medication and particularly troublesome at night, mild lid edema, significantly depressed vision, small and irregular pupil (if involvement is anterior)

3. Severe: pain not completely controlled by simple or oral medications, marked lid edema, poor vision, pupil small and caught by inflammatory adhesions to the lens capsule (if involvement is anterior)

D. Type of inflammation (this may vary from time to time)

1. Nongranulomatous: usually diffuse edema without lumpy infiltration of uvea; small gray or slightly pigmented inflammatory deposits on corneal endothelium

2. Granulomatous: chronic inflammatory signs with localized thickening of the uveal tissue; fatty or lardaceous deposits on the corneal endothelium (as in sarcoidosis or sympathetic ophthalmia)

3. Acute choroidal effusion; this idiopathic collection of fluid within the choroid may be associated with mild meningeal signs, often appears bilaterally, and may pose a differential from serous retinal detachment with or without peripheral holes. The major key in diagnosis is bright transillumination through the sclera.

Such notations produce an orderly ocular base on which to seek associated systemic disturbances and to obtain special tests. The patient with nongranulomatous and nonsuppurative uveitis should be questioned about five symptoms to identify causally-related inflammations:

1. Joint pain (rheumatoid arthritis, Still's disease, Marie-Strumpel's disease)

2. Abdominal cramps or diarrhea for more than two days (Crohn's regional enteritis, ulcerative colitis)

3. Allergies and sensitivities

4. Mouth ulcers or aphthous stomatitis (Reiter's syndrome)

5. Dysuria or penile or vaginal pain (Behçet's relapsing disease)

Previously many clinicians felt that a diagnosis of uveitis was automatically an indication for a "uveitis survey" or "uveitis work-up." This has often been time consuming, uncomfortable for the patient, and fruitlessly expensive. Instead of widely scattered and frenetic activities, from general physical examinations through exotic serologic tests for leptospirosis (which can cause uveitis), the examiner should (1) recheck his questions concerning previous medical history for any inflammatory disease associated with uveal inflammation (such as histoplasmosis, tuberculosis, toxoplasmosis, sarcoidosis, rheumatoid arthritis in children, or syphilis), (2) inquire into any active focal infection that may be troubling the patient (periapical dental inflammation, sinusitis, prostatitis, or tonsillitis), and (3) order such x-ray films or laboratory tests as may be related to the type of uveitis or suspect areas of medical disturbance. Thus an active granulomatous process particularly involving the retina at the posterior pole suggests skin sensitivity tests and agglutination tests for toxoplasmosis. The appearance of so-called candle wax drippings about vessels in the posterior pole particularly indicates study of the long bones and serum albumin–globulin ration for sarcoidosis. Chronic dental sepsis in the presence of acute serous anterior uveitis suggests dental x-ray films for periapical abscesses.

Skin tests for sensitivity to tuberculoprotein, histoplasmin, or toxoplasmin are significant to indicate a previous exposure to the organisms of these diseases. On the other hand, skin testing for sensitivity to *Streptococcus* is a remote and almost desperate last-ditch search for an unlikely cause after more logical efforts have failed.

In examining the eye with uveitis, the slit lamp is the principal tool. This is necessary to determine the character of inflammatory precipitates on the corneal endothelium and to evaluate changes in the iris architecture. A fine or small beam is necessary to quantitate the flare or Tyndall effect of increased protein in the anterior chamber. This should be graded 1 to 4, and at the same time effort should be made to quantitate cells that may be floating in the anterior chamber or fixed there if the chamber appears "frozen."

In posterior uveitis, the intense light of an indirect ophthalmoscope is often obligatory to see through a hazy vitreous. It is also necessary, along with scleral depression, to visualize the pars plana and to identify the inflammatory foci often called "snowballs," which tend to be chronic in this area.

Slit lamp examination of cellular precipitates (KP) on the corneal endothelium gives a fair guide to the type of inflammation. Polymorphonuclear leukocytes tend to form a very thin cellular layer and may resemble tiny drops before larger volumes of cells gravitate to the inferior chamber angle as hypopyon. Lymphocytes tend to form compact and globular aggregations that are tightly localized. The cells of chronic active uveitis, which are often monocytes, tend to form keratic precipitates that are large, greasy, or mutton-fat in character; these are commonly found in granulomatous inflammations classically related to sarcoidosis, sympathetic ophthalmitis, and possibly tuberculosis.

In very low-grade inflammation such as heterochromic iridocyclitis, the KPs tend to be small, round, and whitish. Precipitates of fibrin in acute and severe uveitis may overlay or obscure the character of the inflammatory cell precipitates and also create extremely turbid or even "frozen" aqueous with the loss of all thermal convexion currents in the anterior chamber. Such dense or plastic exudates generally respond quickly to appropriate treatment, whereas the very low-grade and minor inflammatory reactions may drag on for months and even years, with poor response to anti-inflammatory management.

As the uveitis subsides, KPs tend to thin and the edges become crenated, forming somewhat stellate configurations. Pigmentary deposits, either uveal or fibrinous in origin, are usually the slowest in resolving and may persist weeks after other characteristics of the inflammatory deposits clear.

Roentgenographic examination is also important in diagnostic support of several causative mechanisms. The most obvious is x-ray films of the eye for possible retained foreign bodies. Skull x-ray films may reveal several important corollaries such as medium-sized cortical calcifications in congenital toxoplasmosis or finer calcific deposits deeper and near the ventricular system in cytomegalic inclusion disease. The same skull x-ray films will give an indication of inflammatory clouding of the paranasal sinuses, which may merit treatment in its own right. Chest x-ray films are important in parenchymal shadows of tuberculosis or hilar and mediastinal shadows of histoplasmosis. The fingers and long bones may show osteolytic or punched-out areas in the presence of sarcoidosis, and dental x-ray films are necessary to reveal the common periapical infection that may be a quiet nidus of intermittent bacteremia.

Paracentesis of the anterior chamber (keratocentesis) is at times critically differential for determining the type of cellular response, or less often recovering specific pathogens. This should be done under sterile access and with the patient supine on a firm examining table. Rarely the critically ill patient such as one with Harada's disease will be better served by keratocentesis in bed. A short, sharp needle of 25 to 30 gauge and about ⅜ inch long should be used on a tuberculin or similar syringe.* External infection (blepharitis, conjunctivitis, dacryocystitis) contraindicate the procedure. Topical anesthesia, a speculum, good light, and loupe magnification are needed. Slightly opened, toothed forceps in the nonpreferred hand should be pressed firmly against the limbal conjunctiva just below three o'clock in the left eye or nine o'clock in the right eye. Tight closure will then engage both the bulbar conjunctiva—which alone is inadequate for fixation— and episcleral tissue. The site for entry just proximal to the limbus is touched with a sterile cotton applicator moistened with tincture of iodine. After allowing a moment for drying, the bulbar conjunctiva is picked up with

*Alternatively, a prepackaged, disposable, 32-gauge, Thomas Micro Paracentesis needle, 2 mm. long, may be used. This is bonded to a 0.4 cc. pipette (Edw. Weck & Co. Inc., Long Island City, New York 11101).

the needle tip about 2 mm. from the limbus. The needle is then advanced subconjunctivally and positioned for a controlled thrust through the limbus in a plane parallel to the iris. As soon as the tip is visualized in the chamber, advancement stops and about 0.1 cc. of aqueous should be aspirated. This is followed by temporary, forward displacement of the lens–iris diaphragm. Quick withdrawal of the needle minimizes subsequent leakage. The specimen should be handcarried to the laboratory at once or entrusted only to a close associate intimately familiar with plans for smear, culture, staining, or phase contrast examination.

The diagnostician in uveitis neither throws up his hands in therapeutic nihilism nor spins the prayer wheel of countless laboratory tests and special procedures. He must follow the indications of a penetrating medical history and the leads furnished by the characteristics of the patient and the eye toward a sensible plan of well-oriented studies.

REFERENCES

Gamble, C. M.: Pathogenesis of recurrent uveitis, Arch. Ophthalmol. **84:**331, 1970.

Sawelson, H., Goldberg, R. E., Annesley, W. H., and Tomer, T. L.: Presumed ocular histoplasmosis syndrome: the fellow eye, Arch. Ophthalmol. **94**(2):221, Feb., 1976.

The lens and its disturbances

The lens is a small, biconvex, and normally transparent focusing component of the optic system of the eye. It is encased in a clear and highly elastic capsule, which in turn is supported by zonular fibers encircling the 360 degrees of its equator and attaching to the ciliary body, generally between the ciliary processes or into the pars plana and ora serrata. The lens normally goes through marked variations in its curvature, softness or moldability, zones of optic discontinuity, and even clarity during the normal lifetime. At birth it tends to be nearly spherical and contributes to the shallow anterior chamber of infancy. In the first years of life there is apparent flattening that may be related to increased tension of the zonule and the elastic capsule. Throughout life, new cortical layers of lens fibers continue to be laid down at the periphery or subcapsular portions of the lens. With age, this causes increasing lens thickness, consequent shallowing of the anterior chamber, and, with the swelling that may lead to senile cataractous changes, some "myopic shift" in total refraction.

ZONES OF DISCONTINUITY

Zones of optic discontinuity may be visualized within the lens by thin beam slit lamp examination. These are variable in relation to (1) age; (2) medical, nutritional, or endocrine disturbances that may be experienced; and (3) individual characteristics of the particular patient under study.

In a high light intensity, narrow slit beam (the "cut" of an optic section in direct or focal illumination), the anterior capsule appears as a distinctly bright or relucent surface layer. The posterior capsule is anatomically thinner as well as somewhat obscured by diffraction of light passing through the lens and is therefore less clearly visible. The capsule generally increases in thickness until about age 50.

Beneath the capsule is a less relucent, concentric layer, the cortex, composed of young and superficial fibers. Deep to the cortex, various nuclear zones of optic discontinuity can be identified; these have often been given conflicting names by different observers. The most central and normally the most clear is the embryonic nucleus. A fetal nucleus, commonly seen as areas of slightly greater relucency immediately anterior and posterior to the embryonic nucleus, can usually be identified. Often suture lines, appearing in Y shape anteriorly and in Λ shape posteriorly, can be seen in this area or extending to the next most superficial nuclear layer, usually called the infantile nucleus. Superficial to this can be seen various lines of discontinuity representing the adult nucleus, which forms after puberty until about the age of 30.

More complex second- and third-order bifurcations of the simple, deep, tripartite suture lines can often be seen extending normally through the adult nuclear layers. Following contusion trauma or early transcapsular fluid imbibition, these may be accentuated or "feathered." In mild injuries this may be reversible by absorption of such fluid, but in more severe trauma (capsular tears, subluxations, intralenticular foreign bodies, angle recession) or with the quiet inroads of maturity this may proceed to major cataractous opacification.

Notation of total lens thickness as well as thickness of nuclear and cortical components may furnish vital information concerning impending cataractous changes. This is particularly valuable when comparison can be made with an uninvolved fellow eye. In the juvenile or adolescent lens, interruptions in growth, such as are caused by contusion damage, may be followed in a matter of weeks or a few months by distinct lens thinning. Subsequent thickening seen in the zones of discontinuity is associated with loss of transparency and increased total thickness. In advanced age, the nuclear zone increases excessively and apparently at the expense of cortical thickness. Growth inhibitions in late life primarily affect the thin cortical layers rather than the nuclear zone. Thus an apparently thin nuclear zone in advanced life probably reflects metabolic impairment or contusion injury many years previously. Lenses that remain clear in the presence of other disturbances such as Coats' disease, retinal detachments, or early-onset diabetes tend to be thicker than lenses in the healthy individual.

POSITION OF THE LENS

Position should be the first element noted in diagnostic examination of the lens. Ordinarily the lens supplies physical support to the iris through its posterior surface. When not uniformly supported in this frontal plane, the lens may be partially dislocated (*subluxated*) or completely freed of its zonular attachments (*luxated*) and moved through the pupillary area (*anterior*) or into the vitreous (*posterior*). Vertical and horizontal directions may also be indicated.

Tremulousness of the iris or iridodonesis suggests posterior subluxation. This may usually be detected with sharp focal light and direct observation while the patient shifts his gaze back and forth between such easily available targets as the right and left ears of the examiner. Infrequently this is noted only with the aid of slit lamp magnification, which may also confirm the positional disturbance of the lens through its own phakodonesis. Sometimes minimal posterior subluxation is only detected when the patient is supine, as for indentation tonometry. The examiner should take advantage of the patient's horizontal position to watch for slight iridodonesis, which would warn of a discontinuous anterior hyaloid face, or possibly vitreous prolapse about the lens equator. Either of these

signs increases the likelihood of vitreous loss at subsequent lens extraction. If the lens is not seen through the pupil at all, it may be luxated posteriorly or remain hinged below. The posterior subluxation in Marfan's disease is nearly always upward, so that the lower lens equator encroaches on the pupil. Aside from visual distortions, these posterior positions create no acute distress to the patient.

Anterior subluxation is usually marked by lodgment of the lens partially through the iris sphincter with consequent ovalization of the pupil and impaired reactions. With complete positioning of the lens in the anterior chamber (anterior luxation) the iris is behind the lens, but the pupil is again commonly irregular and impaired in its reaction. Lenses encroaching on the anterior chamber commonly evoke a painful secondary glaucoma and require emergency measures to reduce intraocular pressure preparatory to surgical removal of the lens.

Posterior subluxation may not only give intermittent distortion of vision, but may harass the examiner's attempt at direct or indirect ophthalmoscopy. Fundus visualization may be aided by having the patient lie down or by positioning the head in relationship to the point of remaining zonular "hinge" or attachment. This may let the lens drift out of the pupillary axis and facilitate aphakic ophthalmoscopy.

PATHOLOGIC ALTERATIONS IN THE LENS

In general the lens has only one major response to any type of insult or injury and that is loss of clarity or the development of opacity. Any opacity occurring within the normally clear lens may be technically called a cataract. A few small, punctate, or eccentric opacities, however, are so commonly uncovered on detailed search of the lens that they may almost be considered normal variations. Indeed, the word "cataract" should not be invoked for small opacities of no visual significance, particularly when they present no symmetric pattern or configuration (such as lamellar separation, subcapsular vacuoles, posterior cupuliform, or the snowflake cataract of diabetes) indicative of progression.

Congenital defects

Many morphologic variations of lens opacities seen in early life may be identified (zonular or lamellar, anterior polar, stellate, centralis pulverulenta). Most of these represent autosomal dominant genetic traits. The anterior capsule often shows small, stellate aggregates of iris pigment (congenital and stationary lens stars), which may at times be connected to the iris collarette by strands of persistent pupillary membrane having the same color as the iris. At times the lens equator will be notched and its suspensory ligaments missing at that point in association with congenital colobomas of the iris or the retina and choroid. Rarely the lens configuration will be quite small and round though completely clear (spherophakia). This infrequent morphologic variation presents a constant threat of inducing pupillary block glaucoma by wedging of the lens within the iris sphincter.

Cataract formation other than congenital

Noncongenital cataract formation is one of the most common problems among all the disturbances of the eye. It may be apparently primary, senile, or without cause. At other times it follows injuries such as mechanical contusions, foreign body wounds, electric shock, chemical burns of the anterior segment, x-ray or beta ray exposure, and so forth. It may also be associated with other general medical disturbances such as diabetes, tetany, galactosemia, or myotonic dystrophy or with dermatologic conditions such as atopic dermatitis.

Follow-up statistical incidence data from World War II personnel exposed to microwave irradiation suggest in the mid 1970s that earlier implications of cataractogenesis by microwaves can no longer be supported.

The stages of cataractous opacification should be described as incipient, then immature, mature, and hypermature. The many morphologic variations occurring in each stage should be recorded either in descriptive terms or by external photography.

Vision undergoes progressive embarrassment as opacity increases. It is most important, however, to identify the stage of incipient intumescence or approaching hypermaturity because this is associated with increasing lens convexity and thickness. Such changes may shallow the anterior chamber and filtration angle leading to lens-induced glaucoma from mechanical swelling of the lens (phakomorphic glaucoma).

A mature cataract is one that has developed complete opacification throughout. Generally this indicates surgical removal of the lens —particularly if the anterior chamber is shallow—regardless of the clarity of vision in the other eye. This is because of the threat of acute, secondary glaucoma.

Foreign bodies

Small foreign bodies that penetrate only the anterior and not the posterior capsule of the lens may be tolerated without major cataract formation. This is particularly true if the anterior capsular laceration is so small that the capsule edges tend to fall back onto the lens cortex or into near apposition. The foreign body, of course, must be of an inert material such as glass, aluminum, or stainless steel. Ferrous or copper foreign bodies cause destructive chemical reaction and must be removed except when they are of minute size.

In the presence of an unexplained unilateral cataract it is always essential to make careful slit lamp search for a perforating linear scar through the cornea or a small hole in the iris. Bone-free x-ray studies made with small squares of dental film firmly pressed into the inner canthal area may confirm even low-density material such as glass fragments. When these are negative, then PA Waters views and oblique lateral views should be taken as scout films.

Reexamination of patients with cataracts

Patients with cataracts generally must be reexamined more often than patients without active pathology. Early (incipient or immature) cataracts cause changes in refraction particularly marked by increasing myopia at an age when refraction should either be stable or show increasing hyperopia. Nearly mature lenses, with their threat of maturity and intumescence, also call for frequent examination. In the absence of pain or marked subjective symptoms, cataract patients should probably be reexamined about three times a year. It must also be remembered that senile cataracts occur at a time in life when the incidence of chronic simple glaucoma is increasing. Therefore such cataract patients should be carefully examined for chronic simple or open-angle glaucoma as well as for the state of lens opacification and swelling.

With the diagnosis of cataract—the most common pathologic alteration encountered in the lens—a morphologic description of the opacities and the areas of involvement should always be noted. An investigation for both local and systemic causes should always be undertaken. One of the most valuable of all diagnostic tools, the subsequent examination, should be scheduled at appropriate intervals of 6 months or less, depending upon the suggestion of progressiveness. Remember, too, that scattered or even localized opacities such as relatively dense nuclear sclerosis generally cause visual distortion that may be ameliorated by spectacle correction. It is important, therefore, to repeat the refractive examination at more frequent intervals than in the noncataractous eye. This may be the greatest contribution made to the patient's visual life.

A record of myopic shift is a documentation of cataract progression and intumescence. This may occur in the diabetic patient (more commonly the young than the old, and more commonly the undiagnosed than the diagnosed) or in the presence of usual senile cataracts. Diabetes and pathology of the lens should be particularly suspected in the adult requiring significant change in spectacle prescription, such as two or three times a year.

Lens-induced inflammation and glaucoma

Phacogenic disturbances, other than the painless progressive loss of vision associated with senile cataract, are divided into *inflammatory* and *glaucomatous* types. Probably the most common of these are the *phacomorphic glaucomas* in which a swollen or intumescent lens pushes forward against the iris obstructing aqueous outflow, either by pupillary block (iris sphincter tightly against the convex anterior lens surface) or by angle closure (iris root pushed forward and precluding aqueous access to the filtration angle). This causes an acutely painful congestion, usually uniocular, which may evoke nausea and vomiting. *Phacolytic* or *phacotoxic* uveitis is a chronic nongranulomatous, monocular or binocular uveitis initiated by minor trauma to the anterior capsule or pressure from liquefaction swelling within the lens causing lens protein diffusion into the aqueous. *Phacoanaphylactic enophthalmitis* (or *uveitis*) is a severe granulomatous iridocyclitis with mutton fat KP. This is usually initiated by lens fragmentation following lacerations of the capsule and cortex, or following extracapsular extraction. This may involve the second eye. In each of these three types of phacogenic reactions both the inflammation and glaucomatous elevation of pressure must be controlled and then the lens removed surgically as an urgent procedure.

The vitreous and its disturbances

The vitreous body has become of increasing diagnostic importance with improvement in understanding of retinal detachment mechanisms. Refinements in ophthalmoscopy and slit lamp examination of the vitreoretinal interface have also added new clinical significance to examination of the vitreous.

STRUCTURE OF THE VITREOUS

The normal vitreous body is a semisolid, jelly-like mass enveloped within a boundary condensation or "hyaloid surface" variously identified by the anatomic position of its components. Thus the *posterior hyaloid* is generally considered to be the portion in intimate relationship with the internal limiting membrane of the retina from the ora serrata to its generally discrete encirclement of the optic disc. The *base of the vitreous* is a ring varying between 2 and 3 mm. in width and characterized by firm adherence to the ciliary epithelium, with subordinate strands attached to the ciliary processes and some of the zonular fibers.

The *anterior hyaloid* extends forward from the pars plana and almost immediately begins to curve backward, forming a concavity in the phakic eye known as the patellar fossa. A faint and inconstant ring 8 to 9 mm. in diameter, the hyaloideocapsular ligament of Wieger, occurs about the center of this concavity. In youth this constitutes a relatively firm attachment between the posterior capsule and the anterior hyaloid. It is generally difficult or impossible to identify even under optimal conditions of slit lamp examination.

The anterior hyaloid in the aphakic eye generally loses its concavity (patellar fossa) and may variously appear to be flat, convex through the pupil, discontinuous, mushrooming into the anterior chamber, or marked only by irregular fimbria floating forward.

In early life there may be seen a canal of Cloquet of optically less dense or primary vitreous several millimeters in diameter immediately behind the posterior lens capsule. This funnels into a narrower tubular diameter and sags loosely across the main mass of the vitreous to dilate again into the prepapillary space of Martegiani.

Actually the vitreous represents the simplest type of connective tissue and is the largest single speciment of intercellular material that can be found in the body. The vitreous does possess greater relucency than the aqueous when examined in a concentrated light beam. Optically identifiable micellae and fibrillar lines tending to criss-cross irregularly are sometimes called "pseudostructures," but they give objective evidence of the physical consistency of the vitreous. When normal gel consistency is preserved, such micellae and vitreous landmarks swirl gently within the vitreous in response to movement of the globe. When the vitreous has undergone liquefaction, these components drift without restraint and fall freely in response to gravity.

If the vitreous space appears optically empty or the space is only crossed by membranous strands, serious congenital defects in the retina, choroid, and facial architecture should be sought.

PRELIMINARY INSPECTION

Preliminary inspection of the vitreous can be accomplished with either the ophthalmoscope (pp. 192-193) or the slit lamp. Dilation of the pupil greatly increases the available angle of observation and detection of details away from the visual axis. The high-voltage direct ophthalmoscope, when used in the preliminary position a foot or two from the pupil, immediately reveals the shadows of any vitreous opacities in the line of illumination. The movement of such shadows with or against the direction of rotation of the globe indicates whether the opacities are respectively anterior or posterior to the center of rotation, which is generally 13 to 14 mm. behind the apex of the cornea. The freedom or constraint of movement within the vitreous also indicates whether the vitreous is normal and gel-like or abnormal and liquefied or replaced. With a high plus lens in the ophthalmoscope it is possible to study the size, approximate character, and distribution of many opacities.

The focal beam of the slit lamp also offers a sometimes neglected preliminary view of the vitreous with the unaided eye. Such an initial maneuver establishes the clarity of the media and the presence or absence of gross disturbances. The red color of fresh blood in the vitreous is best identified by this macroscopic technique. Membranous and trabecular formations can also be oriented promptly. With either direct view or use of the biomicroscope, only about the anterior third of the vitreous is accessible to examination.

The indirect ophthalmoscope immediately combines the advantages of high illumination, broad field, and stereopsis. This assists in overcoming impediments of partial opacities in the cornea, lens, and vitreous. The colloquial phrase "to burn through" vitreous haze aptly applies to the advantages of illumination and binocularity in visualizing retinal details through blood, inflammatory cells, or other debris in the vitreous.

DETAILED EXAMINATION

Detailed examination of the vitreous is best done with slit lamp biomicroscope and diagnostic contact lens to overcome the strong power of the corneal curvature. The preset Hruby −55D lens mounted on a slit lamp gave pioneering access through the central vitreous and its most posterior portions, including its attachment at the disc and overlying the macula. Because the Hruby lens is not in direct contact with the cornea, how-

ever, it affords poor accessibility anterior to the equator and into the peripheral portions of vitreous and retina. It does afford detection of posterior and large detachments of the vitreous.

Contact lenses for vitreous and fundus examination increase the range and angulation of accessibility. The Goldmann fundus lens has a 12-mm. diameter optic surface and will afford inspection of a 30-degree field well into the equator. Similarly the Schirmer-Marie wide-angle lens, the Krieger fundus lens, and the Worst Lo-Vac fundus contact lens afford considerably larger areas for examination than can be reached with the old Hruby lens, or its hand-held Hruby-Friedman successor which are not in contact with the cornea.

More peripheral access to vitreous and fundus with contact lens examination is afforded by a nonflanged Goldmann (Fig. 10-1) three-mirror contact lens. Through its flat front surface, visualization to the posterior pole is easy; by shifting the lines of illumination and observation, three separate steps or angulations of inspection are available. The smallest and semicircular mirror presents the most angulation and therefore gives visualization not only of the anterior chamber angle but also of the pars plana and ora serrata. Inspection of the vitreous base attachment here is under greater magnification than can be achieved with indirect ophthalmoscopy. The intermediate width mirror affords visualization from the ora serrata to the equator, and the widest mirror (most closely angulated to the line of inspection) generally bridges the area between the equator and the field of direct observation through the flat front surface. Practice is required in rapidly shifting from one mirror to another, but this technique affords precise information about vitreous attachments to the retina, and specifically their relation to retinal breaks or suspect traction sites. The examiner, however, must adapt to interpretation of inverted images.

Scleral depression as an adjunct to examination with the intermediate width mirror sometimes facilitates visualization of the pars plana, ciliary processes, and zonular inser-

Fig. 10-1. Diagrammatic representation of approximate intraocular areas visualized with aid of Goldmann three-mirror contact lens. *1,* Thirty-degree area of posterior pole seen directly through center of lens face without use of mirror. *2,* Area between posterior pole and equator seen through the wide mirror, which is most nearly parallel to the line of inspection. *3,* Area from equator to near the ora serrata seen through the medium width and medium angulated mirror. *4,* Area including anterior chamber filtration angle, posterior chamber, vitreous base, and pars plana seen through the smallest or semicircular mirror.

tions particularly in the hyperopic, phakic eye. The George Eisner funnel is available as a carrier cone into which the Goldmann three-mirror lens may be placed. The funnel is held between the examiner's thumb and middle finger while the index finger is applied to the near or widemouth end of the funnel, at a point corresponding to the region to be indented. A small spur affixed to the funnel transmits the indentation pressure to the sclera.

The unique Lo-Vac Peripheral Fundus Contactlens gives unmirrored or direct (not indirect, as in the Goldmann) view of the region between the equator and the ora. Scleral depression is needed in the farthest periph-

ery, and the lens must be rotated around its axis to reach each quadrant. Though the Lo-Vac series of contact lenses from Holland is of progressive design, actually the question of the lens adhering to the globe presents little need of even finger assistance in most cases. This is because of good corneal curve design and the aid of capillarity.

Posterior detachment of the vitreous may be circumscribed in area, but more commonly the inexperienced examiner is circumscribed in his visualization. Occasionally a large area of posterior cavitation will be mistaken for detachment if the examiner is unable to follow the vitreous boundary. The most resistant sites to vitreous detachment tend to be the base and the optic nerve. Frequently, however, the posterior detachment is well evidenced by a boundary ring configuration (disinsertion from the optic disc) in the posterior hyaloid as it floats in front of the disc.

Though complete detachments may occur in young and nonmyopic individuals without cavitation and disorganization of the vitreous, this type of pathologic change is commonly associated with vitreous collapse and occurs more often in the elderly and the myopic. Funnel-shaped detachment, seen from time to time in old or unsuccessfully treated retinal detachments, is unusual as a type of vitreous detachment. On the other hand, massive vitreous retraction following vitreous hemorrhage, inflammatory complications, fibrosis, and membrane formation is an unfortunately frequent late-stage problem associated with fixed and star folds in the detached retina.

Vitreous opacities may be hemorrhagic, inflammatory (exudative), pigmentary, asteroid, or crystalline (synchysis scintillans). They rarely may be larval invasions, neoplastic cells, or foreign bodies. All complaints of recent or increasing opacities that impose themselves on the patient's awareness *are* significant. The complaint of suddenly-appearing dark spots of floaters in the visual field must be investigated, with particular attention to the peripheral retina and hole formation. These symptoms of opacities are

Fig. 10-2. Bronson-Turner Ophthalmic Ultrasound equipment that provides B-scan display on face of cathode tube. Top right, hand control adjusts decibel level in steps of 10 decibels from 80 to 40. Lower knob on right adjusts depth of scan from midglobe to deep orbit. Hand-held scanner, right front, is coupled into lower side of control panel. Scanning heads are not interchangeable and each must be calibrated specifically to its unit. Polaroid camera at left is detachable.

more suggestive of serious retinal traction or tugging when accompanied by flashes of light, lightning streaks, or "sparklers." The early identification of a retinal break or hole may afford an opportunity for relatively simple measures such as cryotherapy and thus avoid more complex surgery that would be needed for a major retinal detachment.

Opacities incidentally discovered during ophthalmoscopy and appearing as small spheres suspended in semifluid vitreous are usually unilateral and without serious significance. They are commonly found in the mature age group and are designated "asteroid bodies." At times their quantity and density will surprise the examiner who anticipates visual handicap from them. Patients with asteroid hyalitis should be studied for diabetes mellitus.

ULTRASONIC EXAMINATION OF THE VITREOUS

Since the early 1960s ophthalmic ultrasound has made available specific information based on acoustic densities within the vitreous. In health, the vitreous is acoustically homogeneous and free of echoes. Since the late 1960s quantitative ultrasonography, both A-scan and B-scan, has greatly increased the range of available and significant information. Near surface accessibility makes ultrasonic examination relatively free of intervening disturbances and artifacts such as reverberation echoes. Relatively low levels of sonic energy are needed in comparison to those for retrobulbar examination, and of course, occlusion of the pupil or opacities of the cornea or lens, make ultrasound the major diagnostic procedure for vitreous study.

Tumors, retinal detachments, and foreign

bodies (including those that are nonmagnetic and radiolucent) in the vitreous all give distinct, high amplitude echoes. Vitreous (hyaloid) detachments, retinoschisis (usually bilateral), and asteroid hyalitis (usually unilateral) give the next most specific echoes. More variable, however, both in amplitude and chronology of change, are the echoes from vitreous degeneration, hemorrhage, and inflammation. Fresh or unorganized hemorrhage in the vitreous, early vitreitis, or inflammatory responses give irregular echoes at high decibel levels but, unlike tumors and retinal detachments, disappear at lower levels. Old hemorrhages or dense strandlike formations continue to give some echoes even at low decibel levels. Thus, the intensity and something of the duration of pathology can be determined by echo amplitudes

at different decibel levels. For example, the degree of inflammatory response about a chemically active foreign body in the vitreous gives evidence as to whether it may be drawn forward—with limited likelihood of detaching the retina—or should be removed by a posterior transscleral route; the former would be suggested by weak vitreous echoes and the latter suggested by strong echoes about the F. B.

Current advances in understanding of vitreous structure and interpretation of vitreous symptoms have brought entirely new and greatly increased significance to alterations in this body. The examiner now possesses instruments and understanding that did not exist a decade ago; with this armamentarium he may preside over distinctly lessened morbidity from vitreous and retinal disturbances.

The lacrimal system and its disturbances

Complaints relating to the lacrimal system primarily concern insufficiency of tear secretion or epiphora (excessive tearing caused by inadequacy or blockage of the tear drainage passages). Less commonly there are complaints of enlargement or tumor involving either the tear gland or the drainage passages, and least frequently there is hyperlacrimation or hypersecretion. The last is often psychic, voluntary, or hysterical in origin, though it may be neurogenic from trigeminal or facial nerve irritation.

Examination of the lacrimal system should first assess the anatomy of the lids and lacrimal details without any traction or digital manipulation. This affords notation of tear flow over the lid borders, positioning of the lids, cilia, and puncta, and any disturbance or enlargement of the tear gland (tumors, inflammations, or, rarely, foreign bodies) or tear passages (inflammation, foreign bodies, or tumors).

The most common foreign body of the lacrimal system is a broken cilium lodged painfully in the punctum and scratching the bulbar conjunctiva. Its diagnosis is aided by a history of abrupt onset, pain, and hyperlacrimation, with redness confined to the inner canthal area. Direct inspection confirms the diagnosis and immediate relief follows by lifting out the cilium.

The two major areas of functional examination, then, relate to inadequacy of tear secretion and inadequacy of drainage. Observation, acute and astute, as in every area of diagnosis, spearheads, the examination of the lacrimal system.

EXAMINATION OF TEAR SECRETION

A series of progressively quantitative techniques is available for the study of tear flow:

1. Preliminary inspection
2. Slit lamp examination of tear film
3. Vital staining (fluorescein and rose bengal)
4. Corneal wetting time or break-up time
5. Schirmer tests (I and II)
6. Provocative tests (irritative and drying)
7. Tear analysis
8. Gelatin rod test
9. Biopsy of the lacrimal gland

Preliminary inspection. As in all areas of examination, preliminary inspection should precede more detailed study. In focused oblique light, the cornea, conjunctive, and lid borders should be inspected for brightness and the quality of a moist glistening surface. A dull or dry-looking cornea is immediate but gross evidence of tear deficiency. Ropy or stringy secretions on the cornea, in the cul-de-sac, or on the lid borders also suggest deficiency of tears.

Slit lamp examination. More subtle and early changes in the precorneal film are revealed by slit lamp examination. Small round to oval areas of interruption in the normal layering of the precorneal film often precede actual staining and major reduction in lacrimal fluid formation. Similarly, one may note loss of the "prism" or meniscus of lacrimal fluid* that normally forms on the lid borders

---

*"Lacrimal river" of Norn.

posterior to the meibomian orifices and curves to the bulbar conjunctiva.

Vital staining. Vital staining is best done either with the familiar sodium fluorescein on sterile dry paper strips or with 1% aqueous rose bengal solution. Impregnated sterile papers eliminate the previously tragic problem of *Pseudomonas aeruginosa* contamination and growth in fluorescein solutions (this is curbed by incorporating 1% chlorobutanol as is done commercially in "Fluress" solution,* which contains the topical anesthetic 0.4% benoxinate). With brief application of a dry or moistened strip to the upper outer bulbar conjunctiva, it is not necessary to remove excess fluorescein by irrigation. Devitalized or desquamated epithelial areas on the cornea show greenish staining with this dye, whereas similar areas on the conjunctiva show a yellowish hue.

Rose bengal is not available in sterile strips, and the aqueous solution presents a threat of bacterial contamination similar to that of fluorescein solutions. It is available, however, in 5-ml. bottles. A small drop should be placed on the upper bulbar conjunctiva and permitted to course downward over the cornea and lower conjunctiva with the aid of a few blinks. Excess dye must be promptly irrigated away. Positive reaction is shown by small, round, point-to-dot–like, rose colored areas, particularly in the lower corneal epithelium and inferior bulbar conjunctiva. The rose hue is essentially the same over both cornea and conjunctiva. This will often be positive before there is definite fluorescein staining. In more advanced stages of drying, strands or filamentary coils of devitalized epithelium hang downward from these staining areas of epithelial damage.

Corneal wetting time or break-up time. This is another roughly quantitative index of the adequacy of the tear film. It is best seen with oscillatory illumination and the aid of cobalt filtered light. It should be measured in seconds with a stopwatch from a terminal blink to the first appearance of a "hole" or

break in the fluorescein stained precorneal film. Values range widely from a few seconds to 130 sec., but normal averages are 10 to 35 sec. It is decreased after the age of 70, by the instillation of topical anesthetics or by digital retraction of the lids from the globes. It is pathologically shortened in Sjögren's syndrome and marginal keratitis (Norn, 1969; Lemp and Hamil, 1973).

Schirmer test. The Schirmer test (1903) is the most quantitative clinical procedure available. No. 41 Whatman filter paper is cut into strips 5 × 35 mm. in size,* with the distal 5 mm. at one end folded into an angulation that may be engaged over the lower lid border. Care must be taken not to irritate the conjunctiva or touch the cornea as the folded end of the strip is put over the ciliary border of the lower lid. The eye should be kept open but without restraint of normal blinking movements. After 5 minutes, the strip is removed and the linear distance of wetting from the fold measured. The results are crudely quantitative, with normal young adults dampening 15 to the entire 30 mm. of strip. This is a few millimeters less in males and less with advancing decades of life. Dampening of only 10 to 15 mm. is suspect deficiency, and dampening of less than 10 mm. is distinctly indicative of deficiency. Dampening of 5 mm. or less is almost invariably accompanied by significant symptoms (Fig. 11-1).

The preceding standard procedure is sometimes referred to as "Schirmer I," to differentiate it from a modified technique called "Schirmer II." In this modification a topical anesthetic is instilled, the lower conjunctival cul-de-sac is wiped dry with a cotton-tipped applicator, and then the standard strip of Whatman filter paper is engaged over the lower lid border. A 5-minute reading under these conditions may demonstrate surprisingly distinct deficiency of tear formation in an eye that appears clinically *wet* due to irritation of the mucous glands or goblet cells of the conjunctiva. These unicellular mucous

---

*Barnes-Hind Ophthalmic Products, Sunnyvale, California 94086.

*Available in sterile commercial packets of five strips. SMP Division, Cooper Laboratories, Inc., San Germán, Puerto Rico 00753.

Fig. 11-1. Schirmer test showing filter paper properly engaged over lower lid border at junction of medial and temporal third in order to avoid corneal irritation.

glands are destroyed in xerosis of the conjunctiva, but in the presence of chronic inflammation their mucin production, which forms the deep or mucoid component of the tear film, is much increased.

Provocative testing. When the results of Schirmer testing are uncertain or indicate apparent inadequacy of flow, the findings may be verified and amplified by stimulation of the nasal mucosa. Any irritating chemical such as ammonia or the lowly onion may be used to evoke tear flow. In the absence of such agents, touching the nasal mucosa with a cotton-tipped applicator has similar evocative power. These procedures are nonquantitative, but, when failing to produce any added tear flow, may be taken as a reliable index of lacrimal gland impairment.

Tear analysis. Tear analysis for deficient

lysozyme,* which is an early finding in the Gougerot-Sjögren syndrome (deficiency of aqueous tears, saliva, and synovial fluid), may be done conveniently by two methods. First, the dampened filter paper obtained by Schirmer testing can be transmitted to the laboratory in a moist chamber (Fig. 11-2) and used directly for electrophoretic analysis of the protein content of the tears. About a dozen different protein fractions can be identified by separate bands between the cathode and the anode. They provide data on serum leakage, allergic responses, and antibodies to viruses. Second, a 5-mm. section of the tear-moistened filter paper may be placed on a standard blood agar culture plate previously streaked with a known culture of a common

*Normal 1,000 to 3,000 μg/ml.

Fig. 11-2. Moistened paper from Schirmer test sealed in glass test tube for direct transmission to laboratory for electrophoretic analysis of protein content.

pathogen such as *Staphylococcus aureus*. In the presence of significant concentration of lysozyme in the tears, there should be a surrounding zone of bacterial growth inhibition after incubation for 24 hr. at 37° C. Complete absence of inhibition is strong evidence of lysozyme deficiency as in Sjögren's syndrome. Contamination may be introduced with the moist filter paper and its localized growth distinguished from the more uniform plating with the known bacteria.

Gelatin rod test. The gelatin rod test procedure is infrequently indicated in established deficiency of tears when patient comfort has not been achieved after successive trials of various artificial tear solutions. The test is done in contemplation of elective sur-

gical occlusion of the lacrimal puncta. Small gelatin rods about 0.5 to 1 mm. in diameter and 1 cm. long are inserted with forceps through each punctum of the eye under examination and positioned within the canaliculi. These provide a test period of about 10 days to evaluate lacrimal fluid conservation and patient comfort before they are spontaneously absorbed. Even when the results are gratifying to patient and examiner, subsequent surgical obliteration of the puncta still must be evaluated thoughtfully because of the tendency for Sjögren's syndrome to undergo remission after a period of years.

Biopsy of the lacrimal gland. Biopsy is frequently necessary to establish the nature of tear deficiency in the presence of enlargement. This can be done easily under local infiltration anesthesia. If the gland is easily prolapsed on eversion of the lid with the aid of the patient looking down and to the opposite side, it is best to biopsy the smaller or palpebral lobe through a conjunctival incision above the outer fourth of the tarsal plate. If the gland cannot be easily seen in this fashion, and if the orbital or superior lobe can be palpated, it is then permissible to biopsy through a horizontal skin incision. Because of occasional bleeding, these procedures are done most wisely in an ophthalmic operating room.

Should a malignancy such as mixed tumor or adenocarcinoma be suspected, it is wise to have a frozen section read by a pathologist familiar with the lacrimal gland (or the almost identical pathologic variations that occur in the salivary glands). If the findings on frozen section are questionable, then the incision should be closed until a satisfactory reading is obtained from paraffin or other permanent sections.

EXAMINATION OF LACRIMAL DRAINAGE
Preliminary inspection

Preliminary inspection of the drainage apparatus should be both ocular and intranasal. Ocular inspection is done first and in strong oblique light, with the aid of magnification and without touching the patient or

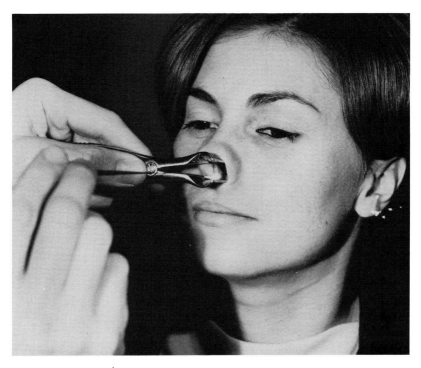

Fig. 11-3. Nasal speculum in position to visualize inferior nasal meatus and site of drainage from nasolacrimal duct. Excellent illumination may be obtained with standard indirect binocular ophthalmoscope.

lids. Observation should be made for (1) actual spillage of tears over the lid border, (2) maceration fissuring of the skin at the canthi or below the lower lid, (3) secretions on the lid border (ropy debris suggests keratoconjunctivitis sicca; frothy material suggests noninfectious oily meibomianitis; drying yellow debris suggests infectious conjunctivitis; oily scales suggest squamous blepharitis; collarettes about the lash bases suggest chronic staphylococcic blepharitis; and so on), (4) position of the lid border, (5) position and configuration of the lacrimal puncta, and (6) action of the lids for frequency of blinking and adequacy of both normal and forced closure.

Position of the lid borders and the lower puncta are often valuably verified, particularly in the elderly, with the head erect and then leaning slightly forward by about 20° or so. Diagnosis of early atonic or relaxation ectropion of the lower lids often is not apparent with the head slightly extended or reclining on a headrest. Only by flexing the head slightly forward are the lower lid borders seen to drop away from the lacrimal lake and reveal the cause of intermittent or reading epiphora.

In all cases of epiphora, there must also be evaluation for nasal disease, particularly allergy, polyps, injuries, or surgery. Every ophthalmologist should have a nasal speculum (Fig. 11-3) and should be comfortable in evaluating normal and altered intransal anatomy. Any binocular, indirect ophthalmoscope is an excellent illumination source for this purpose. Lateral angulation of the inferior turbinate may occlude drainage, or a major nasal septal deflection to the side of epiphora may similarly be at fault. The best dacryocystorhinostomy is doomed to failure in the presence of nasal polyposis, and it may be a lethal error in the presence of carcinoma of the antrum or ethmoids. Remember that tearing may be the presenting symptom in malignancy of a paranasal sinus.

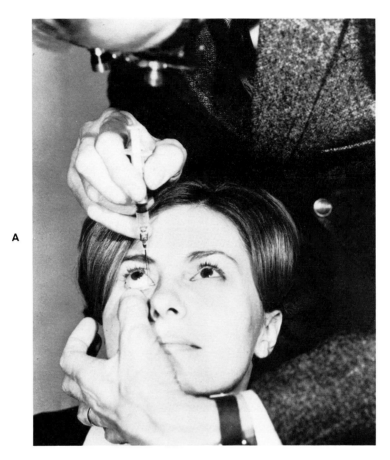

Fig. 11-4. A, Initial position of lacrimal cannula being introduced through inferior punctum into vertical segment of the canaliculus. Note slight eversion of the lower lid by thumb of examiner's opposite hand. B, Second position of lacrimal cannula, following passage through punctum and vertical segment of canaliculus. Cannula is now being advanced through horizontal canaliculus into the sac. Note gentle downward and lateral tension on lower lid from thumb of examiner's opposite hand.

Functional testing

Functional testing of the nasolacrimal pump and passages should proceed through the following steps:

1. Dye passage without assistance or force
2. Irrigation of the passages
3. Compression of the lacrimal sac
4. Probing of the passages
5. Roentgenographic examination
   a. Orbital and paranasal sinuses
   b. Dacryocystogram

Dye passage. A strip of tear fluid roughly triangular or prismatic in cross section is normally present along the posterior edge of both upper and lower lid borders. The nor-

mal punctum angulates posteriorly at about 45 degrees to dip into this meniscus of fluid rather than opening vertically, into air, or directly posteriorly, into physiologic occlusion by the bulbar conjunctiva. Normally both capillarity and siphoning action (Horner's muscle and the orbicularis oculi [pars lacrimalis]), aspirate tears into the lacrimal passages. Thus fluorescein, when instilled into the lacrimal lake, should appear within a minute or two beneath the inferior turbinate. This is best determined by direct visualization with the nasal speculum and indirect ophthalmoscope (the cobalt blue filter, if available over the light source, helps to re-

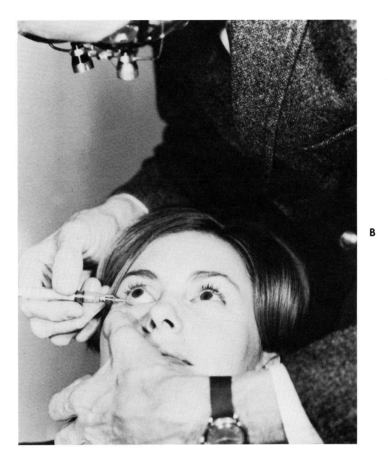

B

Fig. 11-4, cont'd. For legend see opposite page.

veal minute amounts of fluorescein). If nasal deformity makes direct inspection difficult, a malleable wire applicator carrying a small roll of cotton moistened in any topical anesthetic may be inserted for a depth of an inch or an inch and a half along the lateral nasal wall beneath the inferior turbinate. This can be used to wipe up or recover the fluorescein if it has traversed the passages. This is sometimes called the *primary* dye passage test of L. T. Jones, differentiating this passive test from active irrigation.

If fluorescein cannot be found in the nose, the passages may be blocked, or the siphoning action may be inefficient. A small percent of asymptomatic and clinically "normal" individuals, however, will have a negative spontaneous dye test.

Irrigation. Irrigation of the lacrimal passages should be done after instillation of a topical anesthetic. This is best accomplished with a plain, straight lacrimal cannula (these are traditionally gold-plated, for no apparent reason) attached to a 2-ml. syringe filled with sterile normal saline. If the puncta appear very small or tight, a sharp, pointed dilator (Simpson size 1 or 2; Ziegler size 1; Ruedemann; or a small safety pin) may be inserted before the cannula is used. Care must be exercised to avoid tearing the lacrimal papillae with large instruments or stretching maneuvers. Because such lacerations are functionally more incapacitating at the lower than the upper punctum, some physicians prefer to use the upper for routine access to the nasolacrimal duct. Before entering the punctum, eject a small amount of fluid through the cannula to be certain of its patency.

In examination of canalicular impairments or conjunctivitis secondary to lacrimal disease, it is necessary to enter *both* the upper and lower passages. The irrigating tip is advanced vertically into the canaliculus 1 or 2 mm. into the lower lid (Fig. 11-4, *A*) and slightly less in the upper lid. The syringe and cannula are then rotated laterally about 90 degrees to a horizontal position for traversing the principal length of this passage into the lacrimal sac (Fig. 11-4, *B*). Gentle lateral traction on the lid reduces any tendency for the canaliculus to invaginate or corrugate in front of the tip. Slight injection of saline should accompany the advance of the cannula just as during injection of local anesthetic. The examiner also palpates for roughness, strictures, or concretions as the cannula is advanced.

Diagnostic irrigation may be made with the tip at any point along the horizontal canaliculus, but if the cannula is a shouldered model, the added proximal diameter may be used to occlude the punctum and reduce any tendency for reflux. When more hydrostatic pressure appears needed and when there is normal, open communication between the upper and lower canaliculi, it may be necessary to occlude the opposite punctum with firm digital pressure against the orbital bone. If irrigating fluid cannot be delivered into the nose even with pressure sufficient to cause firm distension of the sac, it will be necessary to probe the passage.

Compression of the lacrimal sac. If the sac fills or distends, or if fluid regurgitates through the opposite punctum, there is obstruction between the sac and the nasolacrimal duct. This is a very common site for both congenital and acquired obstruction. The irrigating cannula should be removed and compression testing done by increasing pressure with the pulp tip of the examiner's index finger beginning deep in the inner canthal recess. Initial pressure is directed backward and medially compressing over the upper and lower or the common canaliculus. With increasing pressure directed more medially and down into the lacrimal fossa, fluid or secretions may rupture through a congenital web or inspissated debris may be discharged through the nasolacrimal duct. A

faintly audible "pop" in an infant may confirm the pathologic diagnosis and simultaneously cure the problem. This is less apt to scar the delicate epithelial lining or create a false passage than even the most gentle probing.

Probing. Probing of the passages should be done with a fine malleable probe of small diameter such as the Bowman 0 or 00 or the Williams 0 or 00. Entrance through the punctum and canaliculus should be with the same two-stage maneuver as with the irrigating cannula, but the tip is advanced farther horizontally until obstruction is palpated or the bony wall of the lacrimal fossa is felt through the medial wall of the lacrimal sac. Manipulations should be made to slip through or angle by moderate density obstructions, but heavy-handed pressure can easily cause additional damage to the epithelial lining of the passages. Pain is an indication that potentially damaging pressure is being applied. If the tip of the probe has reached the bone of the lacrimal fossa, a slight withdrawal should be made, and then the end of the probe in the examiner's hand should be rotated upward 90 degrees to a vertical position. In this alignment, it is advanced downward for passage through the duct into the inferior nasal meatus. A sudden fading of tissue resistance or a small amount of blood into the nose indicates completeness of passage, or unhappily a false passage if too much pressure was applied. In the infant, one or two passages such as this may entirely clear incomplete lumenization of the passages. In the adult with acquired stenosis, however, this may serve only to identify the level of cicatrization or to give temporary patency.

Probing or repeated attempts should not be done with the injection of regional block anesthesia. If the pain evoked on attempted probing is this severe, it is likely that probing will cause more disturbance than it will relieve.

Roentgenographic examination. Examination in a posteroanterior view such as the Waters view will identify areas of osteitis, traumatic bone compaction, or neoplastic involvement that can occlude the nasolacrimal passages.

Dacryocystograms of the membranous passages with the aid of contrast media can be more helpful. Emptying of secretions from the sac by digital compression should be attempted before instillation of contrast media. Injection of 1 to 2 ml. of slightly warmed 40% iodized oil (Lipiodol) should be done with the patient positioned at the unit for x-ray films of the skull. Iophendylate (Pantopaque), with

slightly lower viscosity, may be instilled more easily but tends to drain more rapidly. Ethiodol is even less viscous. Films should be taken immediately after injection (Fig. 11-5).

Normally, the sac is 10 to 12 mm. in length and the nasolacrimal duct extends 12 to 16 mm. below this. The most common area of obstruction, either congenital (caused by im-

Fig. 11-5. Roentgenographic dacryocystograms in **A,** posteroanterior, and **B,** lateral views showing Lipiodol filling immediately after injection.

perforation or incomplete lumenization) or acquired (resulting from infection or trauma) is below the sac or in the nasolacrimal duct. Proximal distension is then usually limited to the sac area because of relatively little constraining tissue resistance to expansion outward or upward between the anterior and posterior bony lacrimal crests. The tightness of lid tissues about the canaliculi and the firm constraints of bone about the membranous nasolacrimal duct preclude these levels from simple hydrostatic or nonmalignant enlargements. Infrequently, in the adult, there can be neoplastic growth producing obstruction in the canaliculi, the sac, or the duct.

Water soluble, more liquid, or lower viscosity contrast substances (such as iodopyracet [diodone, Diodrast, Umbradil, Oparenol]) approach the conditions of normal drainage physiology with lower injection pressures than are needed for the oily contrast media. They give slightly less contrast but are adequate to outline the passages.

Roentgenograms taken in the postero-anterior and lateral positions reveal any pathologic distensions and also visualize levels of obstruction.

This spread of examining procedures should always be confined to the fewest and simplest that will produce desired information concerning tear secretion or the nature and site of lacrimal obstruction.

REFERENCES

Jones, L. T., and Cinn, M. L.: Diagnosis of the causes of epiphora, Am. J. Ophthalmol. **67:**751-754, May, 1969.

Lemp, M. A., and Hamil, J. R.: Factors affecting tear film break-up in normal eyes, Arch. Ophthalmol. **89:**103-105, 1973.

Norn, M. S.: Desiccation of precorneal film: Corneal wetting time, Acta. Ophthalmol. **47:**865-880, 1969.

Diagnostic procedures relating to multiple disturbances

Ophthalmoscopy: visual examination of the retina, the optic nerve head, and adjacent structures

Ophthalmoscopy, the inspection of the interior of the living eye, fundamentally requires that a source of illumination and the observer's visual axis be brought into a straight line through the patient's pupil. This problem was first solved by the English mathematician Charles Babbage, who demonstrated his fenestrated reflecting glass to the distinguished London ophthalmologist Wharton Jones in 1847. The Jones-Babbage description, however, was not published until October, 1854, *(British and Foreign Medico-Chirurgie Review)* and in the meantime the modest but monumental German physiologist and physicist Herman von Helmholtz published his 1851 landmark description of *Augenspiegels.* Helmholtz's ophthalmoscope was essentially a series of superimposed glass plates angulated at 45 degrees both to his source of light and to the visual axis between his and his patient's pupils.

Within a year C. G. T. Ruete, Director of the Eye Infirmary of Leipzig, Germany, evolved the indirect ophthalmoscope. By 1853 essentially all of the major components of the direct ophthalmoscope as used today were developed.

The first binocular instrument was developed by the Parisian ophthalmologist M. A. L. F. Giraud-Teulon. Hundreds of variations in design were devised, eponymically christened, and committed to musty print during the next century. The incorporation of small electric bulbs into instrument design by William S. Dennett of New York led to development of other electric instruments during the twentieth century.

Miniature halogen bulbs, developed in the early 1970s, afford more than twice as much light per unit of electrical power and 2 or 3 times as much useful bulb life as conventional incandescent bulbs. Also, carbonization of filaments toward the end of useful life is less and, therefore, instrumentally produced changes in fundus color values are less.

BASIC TYPES OF MODERN OPHTHALMOSCOPES

Two basic instrumental variations, which supplement one another, are currently available in many modifications. These are the direct and the indirect ophthalmoscopes.

Direct ophthalmoscopes

Direct ophthalmoscopes (Fig. 12-1) use the refractive components of the patient's eyes as a magnifying system. A small, erect, and uninverted image is obtained under magnification of about 15× when the examiner and the patient are emmetropic. The hyperopic eye affords a larger area of visualization but under less magnification, whereas the myopic eye yields a more magnified image and a correspondingly smaller area of visualization. The fundal area in view at any particular moment, however, is increased as the examiner comes closer to the patient's pupil; this is similar to the principle of looking through a keyhole, in which the area of view is increased by coming as close as possible to the

Fig. 12-1. **A,** Portable direct ophthalmoscope. Long-life, zinc-cadmium battery in handle may be recharged hundreds of times. (Courtesy Propper Manufacturing Co., Long Island City, New York, and Heine designs by Optotechnik G.M.B.H., Herrsching, Federal Republic of Germany.) **B,** Euthyscope of Cuppers (improved model) may be used as a direct ophthalmoscope with large (30-degree) or small (7-degree) field. An auxiliary high intensity light source is included for use in amblyopia and afterimage testing (6 volts; 15 watts). (Courtesy Oculus Products, Dutenhofen, Federal Republic of Germany.)

opening. Moderate degrees of hyperopia or myopia in either patient or examiner can be neutralized by interposing lenses in the ophthalmoscope that, in effect, represent the net difference in spherical error between the patient's and examiner's eyes. Astigmatic errors yield axial distortion of the fundus image and cannot be compensated for by lenses in the ophthalmoscope; if these are of high order,

as is also the case in extremely high spherical errors, the appropriate spectacle or contact lens correction should be worn. Most ametropic examiners and all astigmatic examiners are wise to wear their own correction during ophthalmoscopy to obtain (1) a clear focus with fewer changes in the lens disc of the ophthalmoscope and (2) a qualitative estimate of the patient's spherical and cylindrical errors.

Many good hand ophthalmoscopes (Fig. 12-1) with battery or rechargeable handles are available.* The nickel–cadmium rechargeable battery, compared with the old carbon–zinc battery, offers brighter and better sustained illumination. These tend to fail rather suddenly and without a warning period of declining light. Remember, however, even the nickel–cadmium battery must be replaced. Most producers such as Welch Allyn guarantee rechargeable batteries for 2 years from manufacture. When recharging seems less well sustained, it's time for a change.

These instruments should generally be free of graticules, slits, and color filters, which only complicate their design and have little place in the small portable ophthalmoscopes. The major or giant direct ophthalmoscopes† with high intensity bulbs and transformer current supply are less portable but more versatile for precise office use and can be fitted with filters, grids, or polarizing discs of occasional value.

Direct ophthalmoscopy yields less clarity of details than indirect as examination moves from the posterior pole to the far periphery. This is caused by increasing distortion of oblique pencils of light passing successively through equatorial portions of the lens and peripheral portions of the cornea. It is practically impossible to visualize the ora serrata and totally impossible to visualize the pars plana with direct ophthalmoscopes.

Indirect ophthalmoscopes

Indirect ophthalmoscopy utilizes a supplementary, convex lens (+13 to +30 diopters aspheric) held a few inches in front of the patient's eye to focus the light reflected from the retina into a real, inverted, and laterally reversed aerial image between the lens and the examiner's eye. Though under less magnification, this affords a much larger field of view, distinctly less distortion in examination of the retinal periphery, and access (with the aid of scleral depression) to the pars plana and ora serrata. With progressively stronger condensing lenses the area of visualization is increased and magnification of details is reduced.

Much greater light intensity is required for indirect than for direct ophthalmoscopy. Probably the most contributing refinement in this technique has been development of the high light intensity head-mounted instrument by Charles Schepens of Boston (1947). Mechanical and optical modifications over nearly 3 decades, primarily by Mr. Oleg Pomerantzeff in cooperation with the surgical staff of The Retina Foundation in Boston, have made this MIRA instrument an engineering prototype. Two uniquely prime controls are the *viewing mirror adjustment* on the bottom of the scope, and the *illuminating mirror adjustment* in the middle of the right side. For orientation, each knob has a flat portion. These bring the two viewing axes and the illuminating axis closer together for small pupils or in other disposition as needed for special circumstances. The resultant instruments are somewhat bulky and weighty. Some simplification is available at twice the price with fiber optics illumination. Fiber bundles, however, are difficult to protect from staff personnel who roll them too tightly or attempt to fold them into small containers, thus breaking the glass fibers and destroying their light conductivity.

Schepens' refinements have also made true stereoscopic examination practical and valuable both at the posterior pole and the far periphery. This requires optic positioning of the observer's two pupils within the pupil of the patient by prisms or paired mirrors in front of each eye of the examiner. This is to be distinguished from older, table-model, binocular ophthalmoscopes with single objective lenses that present identical images to both of the examiner's eyes but do not afford the slightly disparate imagery necessary for true stereopsis.

Pupillary dilatation greatly aids stereoscopic indirect ophthalmoscopy by (1) affording a

---

*Keeler Practitioner; Welch Allyn halogen 3.5 v. systems; A-O Ful-Vue; Heine-Propper AutoFoc and bifocal; and others.

†Keeler 12 v. Pantoscope; A-O Vistadial and the successor Vistamaster Giantscope; Bausch and Lomb Professional Ophthalmoscope; Oculus Visuscope.

Fig. 12-2. Schepens Pomerantzeff small pupil indirect ophthalmoscope. Rheostatic control of illumination is mounted on right side of headband. Infrared filter removes light rays of 800 to 1,400 mμ. Weight: 20 oz. Three knurled knobs on top are to align lamp filament.

more easily accessible field, (2) displacing the dazzling effects of corneal light reflections, and (3) increasing the amount of stereopsis in proportion to the available width of the patient's pupil (that is, maximum separation of the examiner's pupils). The Schepens improvements necessitate good pupillary dilatation. Introduction of the Small Pupil Ophthalmoscope (Fig. 12-2) in 1967* made possible some, though reduced, stereopsis with pupillary diameters as small as 1.5 mm. The new Schepens instruments incorporate infrared filters over the high-intensity light source to reduce photic heating effects within the eye.

An excellently modified, light, and efficiently cool binocular indirect ophthalmoscope was introduced by the Keeler Optical Company† in 1969. This sturdy instrument has a pleasantly simplified headband. Mirror optics eliminate the weight of prisms and a Bi-Mirror viewing attachment is easily fitted

so that a student and second observer may see the fundus simultaneously with the examiner wearing the instrument. This is the result of refinement in design by L. G. Fison of London. Lambert and Cohen have also introduced (1970) a lighter (14 oz.) and somewhat simplified instrument of shock-resistant materials that appears to be very durable. This is manufactured by Frigiscopes Inc.*

The Australian-made Sola spectacle-mounted binocular indirect ophthalmoscope offers further lightness and portability with the maintenance of high intensity illumination. The unit utilizes front surface mirrors instead of prisms, and angulation of the light beam is directly adjusted by vertical movement of the light housing (Fig. 12-3). Either the Sola rechargeable power supply or the Weaver belt-supported transformer (5, 6.3, and 7.5 volts) may be used with this unit.† Subsequently Keeler introduced (1970) a lightweight spectacle binocular indirect oph-

*Medical Instrument Research Associates, Boston, Massachusetts 02114.
†London, England, W1M 6DS.

*Shelton, Connecticut 06484 (formerly, Frigi-Xonix, Inc.).
†Edward Weck & Co. Inc., Long Island City, New York 11101.

Fig. 12-3. A, Detail of Schultz-Crock spectacle-mounted indirect binocular ophthalmoscope, Mark III. Two models are made with mean interpupillary distances of 64 and 68 mm., which will accept examiner's variances of ±3 mm. Weight: 4⅛ oz. **B,** Compact or pocket-size, rechargeable battery power (6 volts) supply for Schultz-Crock spectacle-mounted binocular indirect ophthalmoscope. Rheostat controls intensity of light. (Both manufactured by Sola International Pty., Morphett Vale, South Australia 5162.)

thalmoscope that is convertible to a magnifying loupe by interchangeable plug-in components. Sola-Crock, in 1973, eliminated the cumbersomeness of two separate though interchangeable units by combining the loupe and the indirect ophthalmoscope in a single spectacle-mounted unit with interchange of the eye pieces by a simple horizontal control.

CONTRAST DYES AND VITAL STAINS TO AID FUNDUS EXAMINATION

Relatively nontoxic intravenous dyes* to aid in differentiation of fundus lesions have

*Kiton fast green; Geigy blue; merbromin (Mercurochrome); and others.

been explored for several decades, but not until the 1961 introduction (Novotny and Alvis) of modern intravenous fluorescein retinal angiography have any of these attempts yielded practical and useful information (pp. 259-263).

TECHNIQUE OF DIRECT OPHTHALMOSCOPIC EXAMINATION
The pupils

Direct ophthalmoscopy, like indirect ophthalmoscopy or looking through a keyhole, is best done with the largest possible aperture or maximum pupillary dilation. Principal reasons for not attaining good dilatation are (1) shallow anterior chamber or narrow iridocorneal angle predisposed to acute angle-closure glaucoma by mydriasis, (2) constriction or displacement of the pupils by adhesions, scars or congenital iris anomalies, and (3) iris fibrosis of advanced years or chronic miotic instillations. Inexcusable rationalization for not dilating the pupil are (1) visual acuity better than 20/20 and peephole glimpses of a normal posterior pole, leading to the hazardous assumption that "the rest of the fundus is probably OK," (2) insufficient time, (3) "I looked at the fundus on her last examination 2 years ago," or (4) the self-assuaging note appended to the end of an office examination record: "Check fundus on next visit."

The drops

Mydriatics for ophthalmoscopy should be rapid in onset, short in duration, and as free as possible from impairment of accommodation (cycloplegia). A drop or two of topical anesthetic facilitates corneal penetration and accelerates dilatation. One percent tropicamide (Mydriacyl) or 2.5% phenylephrine (Neo-Synephrine) are generally quite satisfactory with normal and light-colored irides. Darker irides may require a second or third instillation and sometimes a stronger drug such as 10% Neo-Synephrine. After examination, a drop of 1% pilocarpine should be instilled. If there is any question concerning marginal chamber depth, the physician should have the patient remain in the office until miosis is achieved, thus reducing the threat of induced angle-closure glaucoma.

In the presence of extensive trabecular pigmentation, dense Krukenberg spindles, or iris depigmentation, mydriasis may precipitate a transient high rise in intraocular pressure caused by liberated pigment temporarily plugging the trabecular openings.

The position

Patient and examiner are preferably seated with their eyes at similar heights. Room light should be very subdued, particularly in the presence of any opacities in the media; these cause irregular reflections of ambient light and distressing diffraction of the ophthalmoscope light in proportion to their number and density. Holders for ophthalmoscopes

should turn on the electricity when the instrument is lifted up and may be wired to turn off room lights at the same time. Generally, in binocular patients and examiners, the *right first* rule is extended to *all* right first. Thus the scope is held in the examiner's *right* hand before the examiner's *right* eye to examine the patient's *right* eye. The *right* index finger is positioned on the lens disc for rapid changes in lens power, and the examiner is a bit to the *right* of the patient who is fixing straight ahead. Initially, the aperture (zero) opening of the lens disc is rotated into position, the light intensity set at or near maximum, and the area of illumination adjusted to small or medium. Occasionally a dislocated lens (p. 167) shifting in the pupillary axis interferes with ophthalmoscopic view. This may be minimized by positioning the patient to one side so that gravity holds the lens out of the inspection axis.

The steps
Initial examination

Initial inspection is accomplished with the examiner 1 to 2 ft. away from the patient and the ophthalmoscope light directed into the pupil. The examiner should see a homogeneous or uniformly red reflection of light from the fundus. Any opacities from the cornea to the retina will appear as dark spots impairing this red reflection. A nuclear cataract appears as a central dark spot and cortical lens spokes appear as dark radial streaks toward the edge of the pupil. Corneal or vitreous opacities are distributed in the red reflection just as they are distributed in the pupillary axis. A bright and even reflection is general assurance of no significant opacities of the media that might impair acuity.

The location or depth of opacities can usually be quickly determined at this inspection by asking the patient to rotate his eyes up and down. The geometric center of rotation of the eye is usually just behind the posterior surface of the lens. Thus opacities in front of this center of rotation (lens, anterior chamber, and cornea) move upward with upward rotation of the eyes, and opacities behind the center of rotation (vitreous and sometimes posterior lens pole) move downward as the line of sight is rotated upward. An estimate of the freedom of such opacities or the fluidity of the medium in which they are contained is gained from their activity with eye movement. Opacities in a liquified vitreous thus are seen to drift or swirl when movement of the eye is stopped. Asteroid bodies in a normally gel-like vitreous recover their position in a somewhat spring-like manner, or as ornaments stop bobbing on a Christmas tree.

Fundus examination

Following inspection of the fundus reflex and identification of opacities in the media, the examiner then brings his ophthalmoscope and his eye quite close to the patient by approaching along the path of the bright red fundus reflection (Fig. 12-4). Details of the fundus are brought into optimal focus by rotating the lens disc to bring between the patient and examiner the suitable dioptric

lens to compensate for the net difference in their ametropia. With an emmetropic examiner and patient, no lens power may be needed. Commonly, however, the mere nearness of the examiner to the patient evokes accommodation and therefore the prepresbyopic examiner may need to interpose a −2 or −3 diopter lens.

The presbyopic examiner is spared the need for this extra maneuver and, if emmetropic or wearing his proper distance correction, can actually measure the patient's refractive error on the basis of the needed interpositional lens more precisely than can the prepresbyopic examiner. If either the examiner or patient is significantly nearsighted, then the appropriate minus sphere must be rotated into position. Similarly, if the patient is significantly farsighted or aphakic, the compensating plus sphere must be rotated into position.

If the patient is steady in maintaining straight-ahead fixation, the examiner usually will come somewhat directly onto the optic nerve head. If it is not immediately

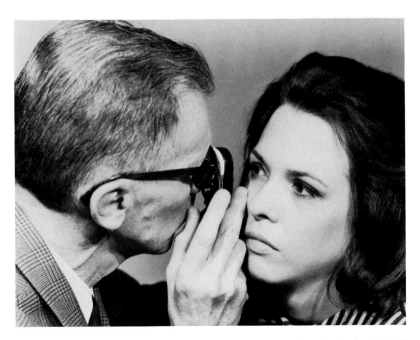

Fig. 12-4. Direct ophthalmoscope properly held in examiner's right hand with the index finger on lens disc and approaching patient's right pupil for detailed examination of the posterior pole. The second finger is used to maintain position with respect to the patient's face.

in focus, the examiner must follow progressive enlargement of the retinal vessels to the nerve head or rotate the lens disc of the ophthalmoscope to achieve clear focus.

Major ophthalmoscopic landmarks

With direct ophthalmoscopy the major points to be observed systematically are in the posterior pole and extend to the midperiphery. Indirect techniques are preferable for examination of the far periphery, and scleral indentation is usually needed in the nonaphakic eye to visualize the ora serrata and the pars plana.

Optic disc (optic nerve head)

The optic disc is the first and most conspicuous landmark. Its basic configuration and apparent distortions are closely dependent upon structural characteristics of the eye. Thus in a small and hyperopic globe, the posterior scleral foramen through which the optic nerve passes is generally small. This crowds the several hundred thousand axons of the retinal ganglion cells and tends to obscure the definition of the disc borders, reduce or eliminate the physiologic cup or depression commonly occuriring in the center of the disc, and give a somewhat hyperemic appearance to the disc.

Conversely, in a large, myopic globe the posterior scleral foramen may be large and the axon fibers may thereby be distributed over a greater disc circumference. This yields sharper definition of the disc borders, a large and sometimes saucer-shaped physiologic cup, and relatively less intense capillarity of the disc with the hazardous potential of diagnosing "myopic pallor."

Moderate to large amounts of astigmatism make the disc appear ovalized or elongated in proportion to the degree of astigmatism. Like every other structure in the body, the optic disc is subject to numerous congenital irregularities or anomalies that may (coloboma; congenital pits; large or multiple drusen; extensive medullation of the axons; inversion of the disc) or may not (oblique insertion of the optic nerve; small drusen; mild medullation of the axons; persistent Bergmeister's papilla or proximal segment of the hyaloid artery; congenital epipapillary veils) cause disturbances in vision.

Components of the optic disc that should be evaluated are the rim, the cup, the color, and the border. The *rim* is the healthy neural tissue between the physiologic cup or its excavation and the disc border. Normally this rim is somewhat narrower temporally than nasally and shows slightly less capillarity in the temporal portion. This is related to the crowding of large numbers of axons over the nasal half of the rim, whereas the temporal half serves almost exclusively the axons coming from the macular area. Even in the presence of myopia with normal intraocular pressure or of a documented and stationary large physiologic cup, there should be a healthy rim of normally colored disc.

The *cup* varies widely within physiologic limits, tending to be small in the hyperopic eye and large in the myopic eye. Its base is the sieve-like lamina cribrosa through which the axons pass into the optic nerve. This is mechanically a weak area of the sclera and yields to increased intraocular pressure by bowing posteriorly. This commonly is more marked in the temporal and inferior portions of the cup as it yields to pressure, and therefore nasal and superior field defects are among the earliest perimetric findings of nerve head damage. Except in moderate to highly myopic eyes, the lamina is normally not conspicuous. It does become more distinctly checkered in appearance, though, with the inroad of pressure.

The reddish *color* of the disc is normally somewhat more intense nasally than temporally. The *border* also tends to vary from usually clear definition temporally to slightly less definition nasally. Thus early changes of papillary congestion may appear as slight hyperemia or blurring nasally, whereas early changes of atrophy appear as pallor temporally.

Blood vessels

The vessels seen in the fundus are preponderantly of the *small* classification. Components of this arterial system are properly considered to be arterioles, except for the central retinal artery, its first bifurcation into superior and inferior papillary arteries, and occasionally proximal portions of the second degree (second bifurcation), which may be minimal examples of medium-sized arteries. Thus pathologic processes of medium or large arteries such as medial hypertrophy and atherosclerosis are generally confined to vessels on or near the disc or hidden proximal to the lamina cribrosa. Changes manifest in the vast majority of the arterial tree throughout the fundus are perforce the diseases striking arterioles (vessels without an internal elastic lamella and without a continuous muscular coat), such as arteriolosclerosis with its visibly conspicuous hyalinization and its close association with hypertension. Similarly, components of the vascular drainage system are properly considered venules and, in respect to the direction of blood flow, the lesser ones are tributaries rather than branches.

Vessel distribution and quantitation on the nerve head. Divisions and arrangements of blood vessels at the disc are highly varied, though striking similarity is seen in the majority of identical twins. Normally the largest vessels are positioned slightly nasalward on the disc. Kestenbaum (1946) introduced a reliable quantitation of these vessels by grossly dividing them into large or small and counting their numbers as they cross the disc border. The larger vessels normally number eight to ten and are rarely reduced, even in optic atrophy. The smaller vessels normally number a few more and are lost to visualization in atrophic processes (Kestenbaum count).

Vessel changes associated with papilledema. The reverse of atrophic changes and insufficiency in these vessels is seen in papilledema (congestion of the optic nerve head) or acute inflammatory disturbances (optic neuritis). The full-blown pictures of these conditions with the long preservation of central acuity in papilledema and the early loss of it in optic neuritis present little diagnostic challenge compared to the far more important identification of papilledema

in its earliest stages. The ophthalmoscopic signs of papilledema in order of their appearance are:

1. Venous fullness and tortuosity
2. Hyperemia of the disc
3. Slight blurring of the disc borders, vertically or nasally
4. Accentuated striations from the disc along the major vessels
5. Loss of venous pulsations, particularly in the presence of mild digital compression applied to the globe
6. Filling in of the physiologic cup
7. Blurring of the temporal disc border
8. Spontaneous arterial pulsations
9. Peripapillary edema and hemorrhages

In papilledema, tangent screen studies of the visual field show enlargement of the blind spot roughly proportional to the duration and intensity of the congestion.

Vessel changes associated with hypertension and sclerosis. Retinal vessels should be evaluated not only for their relation to optic nerve head pathology but also in terms of their general characteristics throughout the fundus. Particularly the changes of hypertension (spasm, narrowing, straightening, wider angulations at bifurcations) should be distinguished from those of arteriolosclerosis (increased light reflex, sheathing, arteriovenous compression, tortuosity, copper wire appearance, silver wire appearance) and each graded 1 to 4 in accordance with severity of the vascular changes and associated disturbances such as hemorrhages, exudates, and secondary papilledema.

Examination for grading of vascular changes must differentiate the hypertensive signs from those of arteriolosclerosis and must be based upon the most marked manifestations of each. Some vessels in the fundus may show distinctly less involvement than others, but it would be false assurance to base the quantitation on the least involved area. The following are usual grading criteria in arteriolosclerosis:

Grade 1 Early compression of vein at arteriovenous crossing; some limited disappearance of venule at either side of arteriole; slight increase in arteriolar light reflex

Grade 2 Similar crossing phenomenon as grade 1 and with early copperish light streak on arteriole

Grade 3 Distinct tapering, humping, or depression of vein at arteriovenous crossing; marked copper wire light reflex; early sheathing of arterioles; increased tortuosity

Grade 4 Pipestem sheathing and silver wire arterioles; blood column not apparent in most severely involved vessels; deflection of venules (Salus sign) at crossing sites; stasis in vein peripheral to crossing changes; marked tortuosity

The following are usual grading criteria in hypertensive changes:

Grade 1 Diffuse mild arteriolar constriction with infrequent area of focal constriction

Grade 2 Distinct generalized arteriolar constriction with scattered areas of severe focal narrowing; arteriovenous ratio of vessel diameters about 1:3

Grade 3 All of the above plus some straightening of the arterioles; scattered flame-shaped hemorrhages; small to medium-sized cotton-wool patches (small infarcts); some edema and edema residues

Grade 4 Vascular changes as above plus some areas of apparent obliteration of the arteriolar blood column; small and large flame-shaped hemorrhages; scattered areas of retinal edema and edema residues; many cotton-wool spots; papilledema from mild to massive

Vessel changes associated with diabetes mellitus and diabetic retinopathy. Ophthalmoscopy also offers a unique capability to diagnose and to quantitate the vascular concomitants of diabetes mellitus as revealed in early retinal changes and established diabetic retinopathy. Hopefully improving approaches to therapy of this retinopathy (such as photocoagulation and laser coagulation) demand careful notation of these changes with widely acceptable grading. To this end, the Airlie Classification of Diabetic Retinopathy (Davis, Norton, and Myers, 1969) represents a widely based, comprehensive approach. Details of this classification require not only direct ophthalmoscopy of the posterior pole but also the assistance of (1) binocular indirect ophthalmoscopy to evaluate peripheral and proliferative changes, (2) slit lamp biomicroscopy with a Worst or similar corneal contact lens to detect early retinopathy and disturbances in the vitreoretinal relationship, and (3) fluorescein fundus angiography to evaluate intraretinal microvascular abnormalities as well as early nonproliferative and early proliferative changes.

This classification emphasizes photographic grading in relation to five specific fields of approximately 30 degrees each: *1*, centered on optic disc; *2*, centered on macula; *3*, temporal to macula or nasal limit tangent to macula; *4*, above disc with nasal limit tangent to perpendicular line through center of disc; and *5*, below disc with nasal limit tangent to perpendicular through center of disc.

Each fundus photograph roughly equates in area with the view obtained with indirect ophthalmoscopy using a +14-diopter lens. By either technique this is considered a standard measuring area. Severity is specified in only three grades: *0*, no changes; *1*, mild to moderate; and *2*, moderate to severe.

Characteristics are graded under the following four headings as applicable:

A. Nonproliferative phase
   1. Hemorrhages and/or microaneurysms by number in a standard area
   2. Hard exudates by extent of fundus area involved
   3. Soft exudates by number in the total fundus
   4. Venous dilatation, beading, sausaging, or other abnormalities
   5. Intraretinal microvascular abnormalities as shunt vessels and dilated capillaries
   6. Macular edema by severity and area of extent
B. Fluorescein angiographic findings
   1. Changes seen in arteriovenous phase 15 to 25 seconds after injection (microaneurysmal changes)
   2. Changes seen in late phase 3 to 5 minutes after injection (leakage)
C. Proliferative phase
   1. Neovascularization within one disc diameter of the disc
   2. Neovascularization in areas other than centered on the disc
   3. Fibrous proliferation within one disc diameter of the disc
   4. Fibrous proliferation in areas other than centered on the disc
   5. Plane or forward extension of proliferation from normal level of retina
   6. Retinal detachment and elevation by extent of area
D. Vitreous hemorrhage
   1. Preretinal hemorrhage by severity

2. Vitreous hemorrhage by severity
3. History of previous vitreous hemorrhage by number of episodes in past year

Even though present therapy may carry disappointments, this is no excuse for the clinician to avoid some functional classification or grading of the disease process. Certainly many individuals and many institutions render good and adequate care, both clinical and research, with simpler methods than this evaluation. The clinician, however, must have some landmarks for overall evaluation of progress or failure and may add other and even more specific notations in areas where he has investigated interest.

The macular area

After studying details of the disc and vessels, the macula should routinely by examined. This vessel-free concavity normally appears slightly darker than the surrounding retina and in younger life presents a distinct yellowish center. This darkens and becomes less conspicuous with age. The radiating axons from the fovea constitute the nerve fiber layer of Henle. Because of their precise regularity of geographic arrangement, these axons have a polarizing effect on light and also tend to confine exudates (macular star) and hemorrhages into a radiate pattern when they present in this area. The prefoveal reflex normally is a pinpoint of light reflected from the ophthalmoscope by the concavity of the fovea interna. When this is bright and distinct, it indicates essentially no disturbance in the internal limiting membrane that lines this shallow concavity; loss or distortion of the prefoveal reflex is an early ophthalmoscopic sign of macular edema or distortion and should be studied further by slit lamp examination with the aid of an examining contact lens. Pathologic elevations here, when nondestructive, give rise to an acquired hyperopia that may range from 0.5 to 2.5 diopters. When caused by edema or similar transient insult, the artificial hyperopia subsides with resolution of the disease process.

The macular area has a very high metabolic rate and is quite vulnerable to minor vascular insufficiencies, contusion insults, or the induced gliosis of even minute amounts of retinal hemorrhage. Lipid deposits are a common cause of central visual loss in adult life, and patients with such macular deposits should have careful study of their serum cholesterol and lipid fractions.

Funduscopic lenses

Fundus lenses, particularly for examining the posterior pole with a slit lamp, are the early, narrow field and noncontact Hruby −55D, the flat front flange-retained Ruiz, the Kreiger direct lens, the four-mirror fundus lens of Thorpe (two opposing mirrors set at 64° for viewing from the ora to the equator and two other opposing mirrors at 70° for viewing the equator to the posterior pole), the handle-mounted biconcave lens of Lydapor, the finger-held Hruby-Friedman with flat front, the direct and flange retained, minus face lenses (Sarwar; Schirmer-Marie; Mandelbaum-Rynco), the Enger flange retained fundus lens, the Allen-Braley Indirect Central Fundus lens with flange retention and handle stabilization, the Worst LoVac flat front, nonflanged Fundus Lens that permits visualization to the equator, and the direct (nonmirrored) Enger. Of these, the most easy manipulation and widest fields are afforded by the smaller diameter, nonflanged, direct lenses, such as the Worst LoVac, the Enger, or the moderately minus faced contact lenses that permit visualization to the equator. The precorneal (noncontact) lenses, such as the Hruby-55D, have been superseded by these more maneuverable lenses, particularly those with corneal contact surfaces smaller than the corneal diameter.

The periphery

Even with good pupillary dilatation, direct ophthalmoscopy of the far periphery is distorted and that of the ora serrata and pars plana is precluded. These areas, which are vitally important in the problems of retinal detachment, sickle cell disease retinopathy, retinoblastoma of infants, the chronic inflammations of pars planitis, and contusion injuries, must be inspected by indirect binocular ophthalmoscope.

Diagnostic contact lenses adapted to the corneal surface with a small amount of 2 to 6% methylcellulose solution (Goniosol 2.5%) neutralize the high anterior corneal curvature and greatly reduce optical distortion in examination of the periphery. They afford much greater magnification than obtained with the indirect ophthalmoscope. The pupil should be well dilated. Contact lenses particularly suited for *peripheral* fundus examination are the Worst LoVac Peripheral Fundus lens, the familiar and larger Goldmann three-mirror, which largely permits binocular viewing and is aided by the Eisner Scleral Indentation Funnel, and the handlemounted Cordona Fundus Focalizing Lens. Of these, the large Goldmann three-mirror is the most versatile, but the other two have higher maneuverability and the advantage of direct rather than indirect visualization.

BINOCULAR INDIRECT OPHTHALMOSCOPY

PATRICK R. O'CONNOR, M.D.

Increasing facility of examining techniques and effectiveness of therapy have heightened interest in studying the *entire* retina. Binocular indirect ophthalmoscopy and slit lamp biomicroscopy permit access to the total fundus with detailed three dimensional view. The binocular indirect ophthalmoscope offers advantages of (1) true stereopsis, (2) a larger field, up to 42 degrees in diameter with a +30-diopter lens, (3) clearer visualization through hazy media, (4) easier access to infants and children because of the more remote position of the examiner, (5) less distortion and larger field when examining the high myopic patient, (6) better access to the peripheral fundus, and (7) reduced distortion in examining the far periphery of any eye. Its greatest advantage is achieved in combination with scleral depression both to bring the far periphery into view and to differentiate, by pressure or manipulation, the true retinal hole from confusing lesions such as cysts, small hemorrhages, or pigment disturbances. Disadvantages include the vertically inverted and laterally reversed image and the high light intensity that most patients endure unhappily (Figs. 12-2, 12-3, and 12-5).

The major optic accomplishment of the ophthalmoscope design is effectively to po-

Fig. 12-5. Conventional head-mounted binocular indirect ophthalmoscope with transformer power supply and two strengths of condensing lenses. Observer's pupils are brought to interpupillary distance of about 3.5 mm. within patient's pupil. (Courtesy Neitz Instruments Co. Ltd., Tokyo, Japan.)

sition both pupils or visual axes of the observer within the pupil of the patient. This is done by paired mirrors or prisms before each of the observer's eyes. Since stereopsis is proportional to the interpupillary distance, it is essential to have maximum pupillary dilatation, not only to gain widest access to the fundus but also to attain the maximum degree of stereopsis. The ophthalmoscope must be properly and securely adjusted with most of its weight supported from the strap over the crown of the examiner's head rather than by poorly endured tightness of the encircling head band. The oculars should be as close as possible to the examiner's eyes and centered for comfortable binocularity with gaze directed slightly downward and at a focal plane 14 to 18 in. away. The illumination mirror must be angulated to center the light in the upper half of the field of view or away from the line uniting the entrance images of the observer's pupils in the patient's pupil. The patient's pupil is the pivotal and fixed center of rotation for the examining axis on which the fundus point of regard, the examiner's eyes, and the condensing lens must always be kept centered.

Before purchasing an indirect ophthalmoscope, one should become familiar with the half dozen or more designs that are easily available. Most modern indirect scopes are similar but vary particularly in regard to light source, weight, head support, durability, ease of adjustment, and cost. A few small spectacle-mounted units have become popular for hospital rounds and survey use. The small pupil ophthalmoscope, introduced by Schepens and Pomerantzeff, with flexibility to spread apart or close together the triangulated positions of the illuminating axis and the examiner's two visual axes within the patient's pupil, is reproduced similarly in some other scopes, and allows low level stereopsis through small pupils or around opacities in the media.

A note of question was raised concerning intensity of indirect ophthalmoscope lights in 1968. Experiments in the rhesus monkey showed retinal and pigment epithelial damage from prolonged exposure to focused light of a clinical indirect ophthalmoscope. The infrared component of light was incriminated as a probable source of damaging radiant energy. Though the long-term effects of light damage to the human retina are unknown, infrared light should probably be filtered out and observation of the macular areas should be of short duration.

The room should be dark and the patient supine. It is essentially impossible to attain adequate peripheral examination in the vertical meridian if the patient is in the seated position. There must be access of about 270 degrees around the patient's head to align the 360 degrees necessary for inspection.

The condensing lens

The light reflected from the fundus must be brought to a real focus in front of the patient's eye and at a convenient anterior focal plane for the examiner's eye. This is done with a condensing lens held about 2 to 5 in. anterior to the patient's eye, depending upon the converging power of the lens. Generally, there are three ranges of powers to choose among: (1) a low diopterage of about +13 to +16, which usually is made as a large diameter (45 to 52 mm.) lens, gives high magnification of about 4×, presents a relatively small area of fundus view, and must be held farthest from the pupil (about 5 in.); (2) a high diopterage of about +25 to +30, which must be made as a small diameter (23 to 40 mm.) lens, gives low magnification of 2× or slightly more, shows the largest useful area of fundus view, and is held closest to the pupil (about 2 in.); and (3) an intermediate diopterage of about +18 to +22, which falls between the characteristics of the preceding lenses. The real, aerial image of the fundus is formed toward the examiner, at the focal length of the condensing lens—for example, at 4 cm. from a +25 diopter lens. Moderate latitude is available between the image and the observer to adjust his arm length, accommodative status, and slight gains in magnification afforded by approaching the image more closely.

For optimal clarity of imaging, the lens

surfaces are preferably aspheric or constructed of unequal front and back curves to reduce optic aberrations such as pincushion effect, coma, and astigmatism of oblique pencils. So-called "crossed lenses," as designated by English terminology of the previous century, are combinations of inexpensive spheric rather than aspheric lenses in which the radius of curvature on one surface is about six times greater than the radius of curvature on the other. This is scant improvement over the even cheaper plano-convex lens to reduce spheric aberration, and this method cannot be recommended in preference to condensing lenses, which add aspheric or conoid surfaces to the unequal powers of the two sides. Volk Conoid lenses* of crown glass have slightly aspheric front surface and a correlated spherical back surface. These are available in both large and standard diameters and at 14, 20, 25, and 30 D. The constant user will find the durability and scratch resistance of such lenses in glass preferable to the lighter weight plastic.

The lenses may be ground from crown glass, which has the disadvantage of weight and the high cost of hand-lapping aspheric surfaces. Lenses made of optical plastic (usually allyl diglycol carbonate, CR-39) have the advantage of lightness and the reduced expense of being injection-molded. The plastic lenses scratch much more easily than glass and can have their usefulness grossly impaired by careless surface scratches. In all events, the lens must be handled only by its mounting rim and kept carefully free of finger smudges or dirt.

The wide diameter glass, 3× Nikon aspheric lens, gives the beginning student, as well as the accomplished retinal surgeon, a high quality condensing lens that provides clarity of retinal image even with small pupil size. Its singular virtue is a useful compromise for most viewing situations. In general, aspheric surfaces are preferable to spheric because of reduced distortion, and glass is preferable to plastic for durability and lessened scratching. As the examiner gains automatic reflexes of positioning and movement, however, the diameter and diopterage of the lens are of subordinate concern.

Fundus sketching or drawing

In addition to mere inspection of the fundus, the examiner planning treatment of retinal disease should sketch with color-coded pencils the vascular details (landmarks) and pathologic changes. This promotes a discipline of thoroughness and exactness. Standards for color coding are listed on p. 206. The beginning examiner unfamiliar with binocular indirect ophthalmoscopy, particularly if he has not used scleral depression, will gain skill and confidence by practice with a life-sized plastic model (Bartener and Paton, 1971), which affords a stereoscopic view of simulated fundus pathology, and by study of comprehensive atlases. The student can become more familiar with actual disease in the clinical patient by observing a skilled examiner through a teaching mirror attached to his ophthalmoscopes. Most modern instruments offer such mirrors as an auxiliary item. The side of the lens toward the examiner should be the stronger or more convex as this affords greater reduction in spherical distortion and size of the light filament reflection from both lens surfaces.

In changing the area of fundus under examination, the observer's head and the condensing lens always move in the same direction and to the side of the fundus image toward which one wishes to shift.

The patient lies on a narrow, padded stretcher,* table, or fully reclining chair without a pillow and with his chin slightly elevated. The examiner begins from a standing position or seated on a high stool at the head of the table. The patient is instructed first to look straight up at the ceiling. The examiner holds the selected condensing lens in his nonwriting hand between the first

---

*Tech Optics, Inc., Mentor, Ohio 44060.

*Da-Laur, Inc. Ophthalmic Examining Table, Watertown, Massachusetts 02172.

Fig. 12-6. A, Thimble-mounted scleral depressor in position for examination of superior nasal quadrant in right eye. End of tip is obscured in upper lid fold. B, Thimble-mounted scleral depressor in position for examination of inferior nasal quadrant in right eye. Tip of depressor is obscured in lower lid.

two fingers and the thumb. The ring finger is used for retracting the lid and the little finger may be rested on the patient's face to assist in maintaining proper lens distance. The writing hand is kept free for scleral depression and drawing. The drawing chart on a clipboard may be placed on the chest of the patient, on the stretcher by his head, or on a small caster-based podium. The 12 o'clock position of the chart is toward the patient's feet.

The light from the scope is directed into the fundus while the patient is reminded (sometimes frequently) to keep both eyes open. There is a natural tendency to close the other eye. The condensing lens is first brought into the light path close to the patient's eye and then moved toward the examiner until the fundus image fills the entire lens. The annoying light reflections from both surfaces of the condensing lens can be avoided by slight tilting of the lens.

A brief explanation of the examining procedure is important and reassuring both to children and adults. Cooperation is essential for meaningful evaluation. Adaptation to the bright light is hastened by beginning the examination in the superior quadrants where helpful elevation of the eyes is assisted by the natural Bell's phenomenon. Examination then proceeds systematically to the inferior quadrants. The most light-sensitive area, the posterior pole, is ordinarily examined last and with slightly reduced light intensity.

Excessive tilting of the spherical power condensing lens induces cylindric effects or astigmatic distortion similar to that interposed by the normal cornea and crystalline lens when attempting to see peripheral details with a direct ophthalmoscope. Fortunately, planned tilting of the condensing lens can create a compensatory spherocylinder of variable strength and any axis. The lens must always be tilted or rotated about an axis at right angles to the axis of rotation of the eye in order to achieve this effect.

The inherent prismatic power of the lens can also be utilized (at a sacrifice of part of the field of view) by sliding the lens in its plane so that only the peripheral lens overlaps the pupil. This affords more angulation or peripheral view.

The examiner focuses critically on the aerial image only and draws it on the chart as he sees it. The inverted image drawn on the reversed chart yields normal anatomic correspondence when the drawing is righted and attached to the patient's chart. Initially, 2 to 3 hours may be required to draw all the retinal blood vessels of one eye. However, with practice this can be accomplished in less than half an hour, and when no pathology is discovered such detailed drawing is unnecessary.

All fundus details and pathology are drawn in relation to careful plotting of the retinal blood vessels. Landmarks like pigment deposits, nevi, and retinal folds should be drawn in proper relationships to facilitate later relocation of pathologic areas easily and quickly.

Use of the scleral depressor

Variously designed smooth, metal contact tips mounted on gently curved but rigid shafts are great aids to thorough examination. The scleral depressor, if thimble-mounted, is usually placed on the index finger of the writing hand with the remaining fingers kept flexed. It may also be used by grasping the thimble between the thumb and first two fingers. The latter hold has a slight advantage, especially if the thimble does not fit the finger snugly. The middle finger is actually the fine control finger in indentation, guarding against excessive wrist or hand pressure. The shaft and tip are kept tangential to the sclera with pressure applied only to the area of the globe that coincides with the examining axis through the patient's pupil, the condensing lens, and the examiner's eye.

If the area of scleral pressure is not seen, then the depressor tip is not in the axis of observation. The tyro examiner must resist the temptation to press harder—which the patient will find distinctly painful—and instead make corrective movement of the tip without interposition of the condensing lens.

The scleral depressor of Hovland, Tanenbaum, and Schepens (1968) has a hinged depressor shaft mounted with a spring action on a small stainless steel cylinder. The serrated and slightly concave ends of the cylinder may be held between the thumb and index finger, using the middle finger to press on a small post perpendicular to the depressor shaft in its proximal third. Any tendency to exceed the slight scleral pressure required to bring the ora into view is called to the examiner's attention by mild discomfort in the pulp tip of his second finger as applied to this post. Length of the depressor shaft has been increased beyond that of the Keeler (large or small) or Schepens American Optical Corporation's thimble and is an advantage in deep-set eyes.

To visualize the superior ora, the examiner moves beside the patient's midbody position; the patient looks slightly down, and the depressor tip is applied through the lid just above the tarsal plate. Pressure cannot be applied through the thickness of the tarsal plate because this is painful and because the pressure effects become unacceptably diffused. The patient is then asked to look up and at the same time the depressor tip is carried posteriorly, still tangential to the globe. The examiner looks into the fundus without the condensing lens and usually can see slight graying of the retina at the site of depression. The high-power condensing lens is again introduced close to the cornea and then brought toward the examiner approximately 2 in. or as needed to produce a sharp focus. Once the observer has noticed the position of scleral depression in the fundus, the depressor tip is moved anteriorly to bring the ora serrata in view. Only minimal pressure is needed to visualize the periphery. The depressor tip should hug the edge of the tarsal plate and not be applied too far above the upper tarsal border or the lid will drop over the upper cornea when the patient looks up and thus frustrate visualization of the upper pole (Fig. 12-6, A).

To examine the inferior ora, the examiner moves to the head of the table. The technique is similar to that for examination of the superior ora but is facilitated if the patient's chin is well elevated (away from his chest). A common mistake is to have the patient look too far down (Fig. 12-6, B).

The temporal periphery is most easily studied from across the patient's head.

The nasal periphery should be done last because the depressor tip must be applied to the bulbar conjunctiva and because topical anesthetics with their adverse effects of epithelial drying and hazing are usually needed.

Scleral depression to visualize any quadrant of the equatorial region can be done with the patient looking straight up (not away from the examiner), or at times slightly toward the examiner.

Examination of immediate postoperative retina patients

The new and sometimes heavy-handed examiner should avoid scleral depression in patients who have had retinal detachment or cataract surgery within 4 or 6 months because of possible mechanical opening of the wound. Remember that only the most gentle pressure is needed, never more than that required for tactile estimation of ocular tension.

The side of the patient to which the examiner stands is usually in accordance with the eye operated upon or the quadrant under particular study. The examiner rests one hand on the forehead of the patient and uses that thumb gently to retract the lid against the bony orbital rim. The condensing lens is held in the other hand. A common mistake is attempting to retract the lid with the middle finger of the hand holding the lens. Without good support of the hand, the extended finger can slide over the globe and cause discomfort to the patient.

Monocular indirect ophthalmoscopy

Monocular indirect ophthalmoscopy has recently been given instrumental attention by some manufacturers on the heels of increased interest in binocular techniques and use of the monocular indirect system in fundus cameras. The Lozano monocular indirect ophthalmoscope (1966) by Rossbach, Mexico City, Mexico, requires a fully dilated pupil. The American Optical Corporation's Monocular Indirect Ophthalmoscope (1968), affords fundus screening information through an undilated pupil. A possible justification for such an instrument is the one-eyed examiner, though a field of about 20 degrees and an erect (aerial) image are lauded by some of the producers.

The Cardona Indirect Ophthalmoscope* (1970) is a hand-held, single-unit optic system that presents a real and erect fundus image through either monocular or spectacle-mounted binocular eyepieces. It contains a heavy hexagonal prism in its lighting system that transmits from a fiber optic source, two bundles of light directed as semicircles on the fundus. The image returns through a 4-mm. diaphragm in the center of this illuminating prism. The objectives can be changed to provide 5.5× magnification in a 35-degree field or 2.2× magnification in a 55-degree field. The erect and uninverted image is familiar to the new user of indirect ophthalmoscopy, but the mechanical re-

---

*Edward Weck & Co., Long Island, New York 11101.

straint of a stand or hand-held unit a foot or two from the examiner have not made this unit popular.

Landmarks: physiologic and anatomic features seen by indirect ophthalmoscopy (Fig. 12-7)

The long ciliary vessels and nerves conspicuously divide the fundus horizontally. These can be recognized in the 3 and 9 o'clock meridians as yellow strips bounded by pigment on either side extending from midway in the fundus to the mid–pars plana.

The short ciliary vessels are considerably more difficult to see, particularly in brunettes, and are located near 6 and 12 o'clock positions, well anterior to the equator.

The scleral exits of the vortex veins form the best clinical landmarks for the equator. They are particularly conspicuous in blondes.

The equatorial region extends approximately two disc diameters on either side of the anatomic equator. The posterior limit of the equatorial region is formed by an imaginary circle passing through the posterior edge of the scleral exits of each vortex

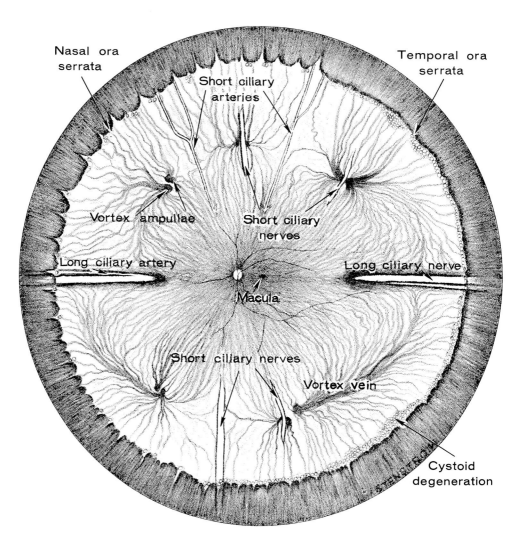

Fig. 12-7. Schematic representation of normal fundus landmarks (left eye) as seen with the indirect ophthalmoscope and the aid of scleral depression. (By Stenstrom and Tilden of the Retina Foundation; courtesy MIRA, Inc., Boston, Massachusetts 02114.)

vein. The anatomic equator is difficult to identify clinically but is approximately two disc diameters anterior to this circle. The vortex veins usually number four, but at times as many as seven may be seen. The peripheral fundus clinically is the area anterior to the exits of the vortex veins.

The ora is marked by distinct, peripherally pointing retinal extensions or teeth separated by variously wide oral bays nasally, but these are generally smoothed out in a more even ora temporally. There are about forty-eight teeth per fundus and they correspond approximately to intervals between the ciliary processes. The teeth are often the sites of peripheral termination of congenital meridional folds, and in about 10% of autopsy eyes zonuloid traction tufts 0.25 to 1 mm. long are found here. The clinical importance of these meridional folds and zonu-

loid traction tufts lies in the fact that holes can form at their posterior tips. Meridional folds are more common nasally than temporally. The bays are finely irregular and wavy convexities found directly posteriorly between two teeth. In many patients neither bays nor teeth appear in the temporal periphery. Cystoid degeneration is almost always located in the retina adjacent to the ora serrata and is seen more frequently in the temporal periphery. Small round retinal breaks near the ora are seen in 5 to 7% of the population. These seal spontaneously with formation of narrow pigment rings about their edges and do not lead to detachment.

Appearance of "white-with-pressure" seen on scleral depression represents cystoid degeneration of the retina which in most eyes is a normal finding, especially in mature years. When cystoid areas of degeneration become confluent they form a senile type of retinoschisis that also appears white-with-pressure on scleral depression, but which in advanced cases is white-without-pressure. White-with-pressure is also seen in flat retinal detachment. However, it is almost always seen in Negro eyes where it may not represent any pathologic change.

The occasional user will find indirect ophthalmoscopy frustrating. Only perseverance and constant use will make one a proficient indirect ophthalmoscopist.

Only frequency of use and intimate familiarity with technique will bring the indirect binocular ophthalmoscope into the widespread use it merits in protection of eyesight entrusted to each ophthalmic examiner. With its use, peripheral retinal breaks will be detected early and many patients will be spared later, more hazardous scleroplastic retinal repairs. Also, peripheral fundus malignancies will be detected while they are small and before metastatic hazards increase.

The instrument should be connected at all times and immediately convenient to the examiner. A dust-free plastic front cover and holder such as Fig. 12-8 is therefore very valuable in facilitating frequent use. Cradle actuated transformers are convenient

Fig. 12-8. Plastic front dustcover and support bracket for indirect ophthalmoscope. Hinged walnut finished cover is held in the up and open position by magnetic catch. Available for any specific indirect ophthalmoscope. (Jenkel-Davidson House of Vision, San Francisco, California 94103.)

Table 4. Standards for color coding of fundus drawings

Color	Condition
Blue	Detached retina
	Retinal veins
Red	Attached retina
	Retinal arteries
	Hemorrhage in retina
Red lined with blue	Retinal breaks
Black	Retinal pigmentation
	Choroidal pigmentation when seen through attached retina
Brown	Choroidal pigmentation seen through detached retina
Green	Opacities in media, including vitreous hemorrhage
Yellow	Chorioretinal exudation
	Macular edema

for holding single instruments, such as indirect or direct ophthalmoscopes without complex wiring. They turn the instrument on when it is lifted from the cradle, and immediately turn it off when the weight is returned to the cradle. Devices, such as the AO Cradle Instrument Transformer, can be mounted on any vertical surface.

REFERENCES

Bartener, H., and Paton, D.: An improved model for instruction in binocular indirect ophthalmoscopy, Arch. Ophthalmol. 85:530-533, May, 1971.

Hilton, G. F.: Accessories for binocular indirect ophthalmoscopy, Arch. Ophthalmol. 85:709-711, 1971.

Hovland, K. R., Elzeneiny, I. H., and Schepens, C. L.: Clinical evaluation of the Small-pupil Binocular Indirect Ophthalmoscope, Arch. Ophthalmol. 82:466-474, Oct., 1969.

Hovland, K. R., Tanenbaum, H. L., and Schepens, C. L.: New scleral depressor, Am. J. Ophthalmol. 66:177-178, 1968.

Lincoff, H.: Finding the retinal hole, Arch. Ophthalmol. 85:565-569, May, 1971.

Pericic, L., Crock, G. W., Parel, J. H., and Henderson, B. N.: The Commido: combined operation magnifiers and miniature indirect ophthalmoscope, Br. J. Ophthalmol. 58:766, 1974.

Ruete, C. G.: Th. Der Augenspiegel und das Optometer, Goettinger, 1852.

Schirmer, K. E., and Shea, M.: Wide-angle fundus contact lens, Arch. Ophthalmol. 84:66, 1970.

Ts-o, M. O., Fine, B. S., and Zimmerman, L. E.: Photic maculopathy produced by the indirect ophthalmoscope: Clinical and histopathologic study, Am. J. Ophthalmol. 73:686, 1972.

CHAPTER 13

Visual field examination

"Examining a visual field is as personal a matter as any other form of clinical examination; if full benefit is to be obtained the tests must be carried out by oneself and not delegated to an assistant."

BRODIE HUGHES, 1954

Perimetry, the investigation of indirect vision or visual fields, has been subject to countless refinements of instrumentation, but from its Hippocratic beginning in the fifth century B.C., it has been shackled by its subjective nature and dependence on the alertness, mentality, and cooperation of the patient. Simplicity of procedure plus direct observation of examinee by examiner are therefore vital to validity. The nearly 100 years of "morphologic ophthalmology" that characterized the nineteenth century were replete with ingenious devices to examine the outlines or periphery of the photosensitive area. Only at the end of that century did Bjerrum of Copenhagen discover that he could evoke more detailed and informative data from a black cloth stretched over a pair of large doors in his office. Thus evolved the valuable Bjerrum (tangent) screen, campimetry, and scotometry. Esoteric techniques of autoperimetry and afterimage perimetry have led to many publications by scotomatous ophthalmologists but are of almost no practical clinical value.

Examining techniques may be divided according to whether the target stimulus moves (kinetic method) or whether it increases in luminosity (static method). Office examination of the visual fields is conventionally a kinetic or topographic method in which fixed-brightness targets are moved from nonseeing to seeing areas. Light-sense or static (profile) methods, contrariwise, measure thresholds directly at various locations within the visual field; these are more particu-larly laboratory or research techniques requiring preadaptation, precisely controlled background brightness and target illumination, and much more time.

In the 1960s and 1970s the objective technique of visual field examination by visually evoked (occipital) responses or electroperimetry is offering a new approach to refreshing freedom from subjective methods. Such potentials are in the range of only a few microvolts and ordinarily are overshadowed by other electric activity in the brain and about the skull. Equipment requires all the components of electroencephalography, plus countless varieties of photostimuli and computerized averaging equipment to sift gestalt from the grass of higher voltage background noise. Compact and practical, though inescapably expensive, models of such equipment are currently available for hospitals and medical centers where many ophthalmic and neurologic patients are to be examined. Completely shielded rooms are necessary.

In the primary effort to prevent blindness from ocular disease or ocular manifestations of systemic disease, visual field examination is a vital step. This follows closely on the heels of preliminary inspection, the establishment of optimal visual acuity with refractive correction as needed, and ophthalmoscopy. Qualitative or preliminary perimetry is an important diagnostic step after the above procedures when acuity cannot be corrected to full 20/20 in each eye or when there is disparity between the two eyes, as 20/20 in one eye and 20/12 in the other, without firmly demonstrated reason. Perimetry is also needed for its diagnostic *and* localizing value when specific headaches, menstrual deficiencies, hemiparetic disturbances, papilledema, or other allied findings suggest central nervous system pathology encroaching somewhere on the long visual pathways from the orbits to the occiput. Perimetry may further be the only reliable measure of progression or control in chronic open-angle glaucoma or the elusive complex sometimes called "low-tension glaucoma."

No individual assuming responsibility for the sight of a fellow human being can meet this obligation without a thorough working knowledge of at least one accurate and standard perimetry method. The 1-meter tangent screen is the recommended minimum.

Visual field studies are particularly suitable on the basis of instrumentation for division into qualitative and quantitative tests, or preliminary and screening test versus detailed examinations.

A. Qualitative or preliminary procedures
  1. Autoperimetry (patient sketches)
    a. Amsler grids (1947)
    b. Afterimage projections
    c. Auto-ophthalmoscopic perimetry
  2. Tests administered by an office aide
    a. Harrington-Flocks (1954) ten-pattern tachistoscopic test
    b. Friedmann visual field analyzer
    c. Horizontal field of vision screener
    d. Automated or self-administered spherical perimetry and blind spot campimetry
  3. Tests conducted by the practitioner
    a. Confrontation or comparison test—simultaneous double confrontation (extinction, inattention, or suppression fields)
    b. Tangent (Bjerrum) screen tests; Auto Plot; Pantographic aids
B. Quantitative or detailed tests
  1. Arc perimetry
  2. Spherical projection perimetry: Goldmann; Harms
  3. Color perimetry
  4. Flicker fusion frequency fields
  5. Dark adaptation perimetry
  6. Stereocampimetry
  7. Angioscotometry
C. Scoring of visual fields

QUALITATIVE OR PRELIMINARY PROCEDURES
Autoperimetry

Autoperimetry is principally the patient's notation or informal sketching of his own field loss. This is usually evoked by sudden and major field losses and is often unnoticed in minor or slowly progressives losses. The patient's delineation of defect may afford lucid understanding of occupational handicaps, as for example the judge of thoroughbred horses or other animals who is completely incapacitated by a fixed homonymous hemianopia even though retaining 20/20 in each eye. The engineer patient may present himself with a detailed drawing of field impairment (or distortion in the specific axis of his astigmatism).

Amsler grids (1947-1949) have formalized such notations for the central 20 degrees of field by plates containing patterns of white lines each 1 degree apart when viewed at a distance of 30 cm. Distortions of these lines reveal and quantitate macular disturbances causing micropsia and metamorphopsia, but they have largely been superseded by slit lamp examination of the fundus and fundus photographs for both diagnosis and follow-ups. The advent of fluorescein fundus angiography since the early 1960s has added identification of vascular leaks and pathologic mechanisms amenable to photocoagulation therapy, further exceeding the almost negligible patient aid obtainable from Amsler chart demonstrations.

Afterimage fields may be evoked following timed exposure to bold, intensely transilluminated patterns. In a darkened room, positive afterimages of the same color or bright configuration can be seen. Against a bright background, negative or dark afterimages will be seen. Both positive and negative afterimages undergo a succession of changes influenced by secondary stimuli and colors but apparently related to retinal or photochemical alterations. An intelligent patient can describe and sketch these afterimages and defects in them indicating retinal disturbances, particularly from tumors, exudates, vascular occlusions, and similar locally destructive pathology.

Auto-ophthalmoscopic perimetry is an entopic phenomenon evoked with closed eyes in a dark room by continuously moving an electric light source to and fro across the lower lid with gentle pressure against the globe. Soon a magnified and inverted image of the retina appears in space before the patient. The network of branching vessels is usually identified first and then a perceptive patient may describe the optic nerve head area and the avascular macular area. Retinal lesions appear as dark or negative defects in this pattern. Contracted fields or quadrantic or sector defects can be identified, particularly if the patient has a good fellow eye with which to compare. This method is useful in the presence of opaque media, in order to assess the function of the posterior segment.

Tests administered by an office aide

Although an office aide is distinctly valuable in the conduct of preliminary screening or survey visual field examination, the ophthalmologist himself generally can evoke the most informative and diagnostic data with desirably minimum fatigue. This is because the ophthalmologist knows the areas in which there is possible trouble. He therefore concentrates immediately on the areas of significance and brings to bear the most appropriate stimulus and test distance. Thus in the presence of an enlarged pituitary fossa or menstrual impairments suggesting pituitary tumor, he examines particularly the bitemporal outer isopters and gives only brief survey attention to the blind spot. Conversely, in suspect or early glaucoma, he carefully seeks arcuate defects, minimal enlargements of the blind spot, or early nasal steps (Roenne) and gives only brief survey attention to the temporal isopters. In the presence of hazy or clouded media such as corneal dystrophies, early cataracts, or old vitreous hemorrhage, he avoids the small 2- or 3-mm. test objects and immediately turns to the larger 5- or 10-mm. objects.

Harrington-Flocks screening. The aide or technologist can easily accomplish specified techniques on first visit (preliminary) examination with the Harrington-Flocks (1954) campimeter screener.* This tabletop unit is self-contained (Fig. 13-1), with an ultraviolet light source shielded beneath the chinrest. Ten different cards, hinged at one edge, may be flipped open consecutively as a campimeter field and present abstract patterns of three to four dots and crosses.

The patterns are printed in white fluorescent sulfide ink on white cards so that in ordinary room light only a central 5-mm.

*Jenkel-Davidson House of Vision, San Francisco, California 94119.

Fig. 13-1. Harrington-Flocks ten-pattern tachistoscopic campimeter screener in use. Instrument is placed on table top, and ultraviolet light source is concealed beneath the patient's chinrest to left. Cards are hinged above.

black fixation point is visible. At the fixed testing distance of ⅓ meter, these cards, which are 12 × 17 in. in size, cover a field of approximately 25 degrees. Controlled test exposure of ¼ second is achieved by a fixed duration flash of ultraviolet light, which is adequate for visualization and registration of the stimuli on each card but too short to allow a shift of fixation. Errors are checked off on record charts that indicate the composite thirty-three stimuli of the ten charts. By removing the white cards, the dull gray supporting surface may be used as a ⅓-meter tangent screen; a fluorescent fixation spot is incorporated centrally so that wand-mounted fluorescent targets can easily be used with the ultraviolet light source. The complete ten-pattern screening test can be accomplished in 4 or 5 minutes and is desirable as part of general eye examinations, routine physical examination, driver license exam-

inations, moving equipment operator examinations, armed forces personnel examinations, and mass surveys.

Children under the age of 8 or 9 commonly present major difficulties in classical tangent screen, arc, or spherical perimetry. Often, however, the child of 6 or over will respond reliably to the Harrington-Flocks screener either verbally or by pointing.

In a similar effort to reduce the fatigue with perimetry, Mr. Allain I. Friedmann of the Royal Eye Hospital, London, introduced a prototype (Fig. 13-2) Visual Field Analyzer in 1962. His unit has been refined but continues as a small tabletop campimeter using a 33 cm. working distance and embracing a test radius of 25 degrees. Mr. Friedmann uses a flat disc with a series of 46 apertures measuring 1 to 3 mm. in diameter and carefully localized to test the most discriminating portions of the central field.

Fig. 13-2. Friedmann Visual Field Analyzer as it is seen by the patient. Flat disc screens contain 46 or 100 test apertures in manually-controlled sequence of 15 exposures.

Target groups of 2, 3, or 4 apertures are illuminated by a flash tube behind the disc. Intensity of the light source can be reduced by neutral filters. Fifteen stimulus groups are displayed in randomized sequence by manual control. A dark room is needed and mesopic adaptation is advised. It is possible to complete central field testing in 30 or 40 sec. and complete screening in 3 min. or less. A new 100-stimulus plate was added in 1976.

Horizontal field screening. Driver testing is creating increased need for quick and simple screening devices for horizontal form fields as well as other visual functions necessary in transportation. The American Automobile Association* has for more than 25 years been developing about eight sturdy and inexpensive devices for visual screening to be operated by vision technologists or police personnel. Their table model Field of Vision Tester† is 20 in. in diameter and encompasses approximately 220 degrees horizontally within a steel band finished on its interior surface in flat black. Under shielded illumination sources, black and white segmented disc targets rotate as they are moved from peripheral to central under lever control hidden from the subject. The subject, while looking straight ahead, advises the examiner as soon as he becomes aware of a target approaching from either the right or the left. Calibration of the arc in degrees is easily read immediately in front of the examiner. Only the horizontal meridian can be examined, but this type of information meets model criteria suggested by the American Committee on Optics and Visual Physiology as well as by the U.S. Public Health Service (1969).

The Titmus Push Button Perimeter is a 180° arc screener that fits on top of the Titmus Vision Tester to check horizontal form fields only. It may be supported separately by a spring-balanced arm (Luxo tabletop base or clamp) and rotated for testing in any meridian. Identical equipment is marketed by B & L for the "Master Ortho-Rater."

Similar horizontal arc screening attachments are available for the Tracor Vision Screener and the Keystone Telebinocular.

*Automated or self-administered spherical perimetry and blind spot campimetry.** Beginning with prototype perimeters and preliminary publications in 1962, J. A. Gans has evolved a practical and patient-operated visual field test system that frees both professional examiners and aides from physical presence during this part of ocular study. Maintaining and monitoring fixation have been chronic problems in all attempts at automated perimetry. The Ocutron Automatic Electronic Perimeter in its 1970 and 1976 models (Fig. 13-3) is a conveniently compact 30-cm. radius hemisphere. The number of sequentially illuminated targets has been reduced to ninety-one and these are placed every 10 degrees along twelve major axes. Targets are 1.5 mm. in diameter and white. Neutral density or colored filter sets are supplied to place before the patient's eye when such reductions in stimulus are desired. Constant fixation illumination is provided centrally and is monitored by a blind spot illumination, which is recorded as unseen so long as the patient maintains proper fixation.

Target illumination is sequentially pulsed at adjustable intervals of 1 to 4 seconds. The patient registers his awareness of the individual targets by pressing a hand-held button. This automatically makes a mark on the recording chart to correspond with the stimulus position in the visual field. Programmed stimuli directed into the blind spot, of course, will not be acknowledged by pressing the button and thus serve to verify fixation. When the machine has completed the cycle for one eye, it turns itself off and sounds a gentle alarm for the operator to return, transfer the patch to the opposite eye, or remove the patient.

The Ocutron uses no pantographs or mechanical linkage that may require adjustment. Special electroconductive chart paper

*Washington, D.C. 20006.
†No. 3535.

*Ocutron Co., Shaker Heights, Ohio 44122.

Fig. 13-3. Ocutron Automatic Electronic Perimeter showing special electroconductive chart being inserted at left side for marking by recorder. Pushbutton indicator at lower right side of instrument face is held in patient's hand during self-administered field examination. Control unit is built into self-contained cabinetry of this table model equipment.

4 × 5 in. in size is necessary for recording (Fig. 13-4). Electronic components are solid-state transistors and integrated circuits capable of years of trouble-free operation. The control panel is built into the table model design.

Though the instrument is sufficiently simple to be used as a time-saving screener, it does produce conventional type field charts. Patients needing serial fields over several years, such as those with chronic glaucoma, learn in a couple of visits not only to use the push-button recorder but also to seat themselves in proper position and place the patch over each eye successively.

Because the spherical perimeter does not analyze the blind spots in detail, Gans has more recently devised an Automatic tangent screen based on similar operating principles. This is based on Armaly's 72 points plus additional modifications.

In the early 1970s Auto-Field I was introduced by Biotronics, Inc.* This is a large bowl instrument that presents 99 targets in random sequence. Design and operation are somewhat similar to the earlier Ocutron. Fixation, however, presents a problem and monitoring by photoelectric control is not

*Santa Barbara, California 93103.

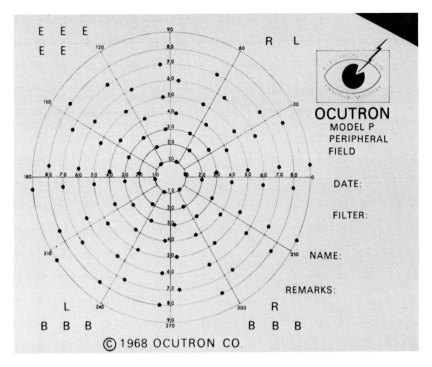

Fig. 13-4. Ocutron Perimeter Chart, 4 × 5 in., made of electroconductive paper shows distribution of the 91 sequentially presented test stimuli and gives a conventional portrayal of visual field.

completely successful. A high density of central test spots orient the instrument particularly toward studies of early glaucoma. A permanent record on heat sensitive paper is printed out as the patient indicates awareness of each stimulus by depressing a button on either side of the table-height base. The instrument is constructed of fiberglass, is 38 in. high, and weighs 38 lbs.

Along similar lines, Coherent Radiation has introduced a computerized bowl perimeter that automatically maps static or kinetic fields.

Tests used by the practitioner
Confrontation or comparison

The confrontation screening technique should be familiar to the ophthalmic as well as the neurologic examiner and the general physician. It is useful in handling young children of 4, 5, or 6 years of age as well as in emergency room situations and bedside examinations. Confrontation compares the (previously established) normal field of the examiner with the suspect field of the examinee, who should be seated or facing the examiner at a distance of about 1 meter.

Preferably the examiner is in front of a homogeneous and dull surface. Diffuse light comes from behind the patient. One eye at a time is tested; it is best to tie or tape an eyepatch over the eye not being tested rather than to rely on the patient to occlude manually this eye. The examiner similarly must close one of his eyes; initially this should be the right so that he is using his left eye, which is positioned directly in front of the patient's right eye. The patient and examiner maintain fixation on one another's eye.

The test object is brought, as usual, from the nonseeing area or periphery toward the center, testing each quadrant successively and checking such additional radii as the suspect defect indicates. The examiner's

Fig. 13-5. Electroluminescent Lumiwand III with battery handle and activating control button under examiner's thumb. Ten-millimeter diameter stimulus is shown; covers reduce stimulus diameters to 6, 4, 2, and 1 mm. Wand is 22 in. long.

fingertip or a cotton-tipped applicator are the most ubiquitous test objects; asking the patient to note whether one or two fingers are displayed adds a rough estimate of peripheral acuity. A semiquantitative aspect to the test is added by a suitably sized white target ball (5, 10, or 15 mm. in diameter, commonly) mounted on a handle. When vision is extremely poor, the exposed bulb of a small flashlight or hand ophthalmoscope may be used with crude validity. With an alert patient, it is even possible to identify the physiologic blind spot a few inches temporal to the imaginary line connecting the fovea of the examiner and examinee; it is essentially impossible, however, by this technique to estimate enlargement of the blind spot.

Failure to demonstrate a defect on confrontation must never be interpreted as a "normal field" but rather as "no defect to finger confrontation" (or to 5- or 10-mm. white confrontation, and so on). Defects of considerable size and density can be missed by this technique.

In the child of 4 to 6 or 7 years of age, the most useful field examination is generally the confrontation procedure. An activational accommodative target hooked over the bridge of the examiner's spectacles as in near-range motility examinations will often secure the child's fixation. Confrontation testing in various quadrants may then be accomplished engagingly with small toys or figures mounted on wands. The self-contained fluorescent Lumiwand (Fig. 13-5) also is often attractive to the child patient. Most department stores carry a variety of small figures or toys incorporating activity components; these should be part of the ophthalmic office equipment.

Extinction, inattention, or suppression techniques. Confrontation lends itself particularly to the eliciting of extinction (or inattention or suppression) fields by simultaneous double confrontation. With this variation, rel-

Fig. 13-6. Extinction (inattention or suppression) testing technique with identical Lumiwands in each hand of examiner.

ative or early defects may be uncovered or exaggerated. The technique may be used in monocular or binocular testing, and again patient and examiner face each other directly. Two identical stimulus targets (Fig. 13-6) are exposed briefly in diametrically opposite portions of the field, or they may be advanced from the periphery centrally. Depending on the patient's level of acuity and alertness, the targets may be as gross as the examiner's two index fingers or as subtle as 2-mm. white discs.

Better localization in degrees from fixation may be gained by displaying two targets against the background of an arc perimeter. If a tangent screen is used for display of the two stimuli, rather than as background for the physician, then two examiners are required to present the targets from opposite directions.

The physiologic effect is such that distinct perception evoked through one part of the visual field causes a similar stimulus in another part of the visual field to become imperceptible. In certain cases, when the stimulus is removed from the perceptual field, then the previously undetected stimulus is perceived. In some pathologic conditions, particularly neurologic disturbances of the cortex, extinction fields may reveal homonymous defects that cannot be elicited on single target examination.

Tangent (Bjerrum) screen tests. The tangent screen is the most essential, most flexible, most practical, most diagnostic, and least expensive of all available instrumentalities in visual field examination. The same screen may serve as a highly efficient preliminary inspection device or as a detailed and subtle verification tool. In the decades of retinal surgery before introduction of the binocular, self-illuminated indirect ophthalmoscope, the perimeter was hauled into service to outline areas of gross detachment and to plot holes. However, perimetry is no longer desirable in the study of detachments and even as an academic exercise is at best an incomplete one. A 1-meter distance screen (Fig. 13-7) (64 to 65 in. square) is the most practical, though the larger screen, useful at 2 meters, gives greater magnification of central details. The greatest usefulness—and with minimal edge distortion—is within 30 degrees from fixation. Practically any pe-

Fig. 13-7. One-meter wall-mounted tangent screen with author's folding steel bracket and chinrest preset for test distance.

ripheral field defect extends to within 30 degrees of fixation, and therefore probably less than 0.25% of neurologic patients will present with such a minute and early defect as to elude tangent screen detection, particularly if the small 1- or 2-mm. white test objects are used. The same screen can be used for (1) any size test object, (2) fluorescent techniques, (3) flicker fusion methods, (4) dark adaptation studies, or (5) examination with colored stimuli.

For individual adaptation, space, economy, and understanding of tangent screen mathematics it is well to construct your own tangent screen. Black felt is commercially available in rolls 50 in. wide. This slightly exceeds the needed width for a screen subtending 30 degrees at 1 meter and therefore allows a small amount of felt on either edge for hemming or tacking to a wooden frame. A commercial windowshade roller in this width will serve well if the screen is to be retractable above another wall testing back-

ground, such as the Lancaster red-green test. One- and 2-meter tangent screens for ceiling (8 ft.) mounting directly in front of the examining chair are commercially available.*

The technique of tangent screen examination is essentially the same as for confrontation, arc, sphere, and other instrumental methods. Basic principles are:

1. Equipment should be as close and accessible as possible to the patient to minimize patient movement or the setting up of equipment.

2. The patient should be seated as comfortably as possible, adjusting the equipment to him.

3. Explanations (like equipment) should be simple and should be tendered as the patient is moved into position.

4. The eye not under examination (re-

*Jenkel-Davidson House of Vision, San Francisco, California 94119; Richmond Products Inc., Somerset, New Jersey 08873.

member, the right eye is traditionally examined first) is occluded.

5. Test objects should be the smallest practical size based on preliminary evaluation of retinal function and mental agility. With near normal acuity, most intelligent patients from childhood to late life can recognize a 2-mm. white object, which makes a broadly suitable examining target. In the presence of moderate corneal- or lens opacity–reducing retinal resolution throughout, a 5- or 10-mm. white target may be necessary. Marked loss of central vision from a circumscribed macular lesion, however, may not affect the extramacular retina and in such cases, even with best central acuity below 20/200, the small target size should be used.

6. Test distance should be practical and adaptable to usual office floor space, though larger screens (2 meters) and spheres (1 meter radius) give greater magnification of field defects. A 1-meter working distance is excellent for most tangent screen diagnostic and follow-up studies. (Similarly ⅓ meter or 33 cm. has become the standard radius for office types of arc and sphere perimeters.)

7. Surrounding illumination should be low; distracting movements, light colors, and reflecting surfaces should be excluded to avoid dazzling and disturbing light.

8. Spectacles generally should not be worn during field studies because (a) the frames create a positive ring scotoma; (b) high plus lenses create both "pincushion" distortion of the field and, from their edges, a negative ring scotoma that widens in proportion to increasing dioptric power; (c) high minus lenses cause peripheral doubling or target jump; and (d) high-power lenses incorporate optic distortions such as marginal astigmatism and chromatic aberration. Bifocals add inferior field confusion and "target jump" in their area. High dioptric prescriptions, however, may have to be worn at times to study the central 10 or 15 degrees when a small target is required to elicit details. Contact lenses have very little effect on the central field and should be worn if the patient is generally adapted to them. Small diameter contact lenses, particularly in young or my-

opic patients with large pupils, may create aberration rings at their edges or in relation to peripheral bevels and may have to be removed under these circumstances. Rarely is it desirable to map out the ring scotoma from spectacles or high power lenses in order to demonstrate its hazard to a patient.

9. Pupillary size does not have major effects on kinetic (topographic) field studies, but dilated pupils tend to increase apparent field size by affording better light admission. Conversely, very small pupils tend to reduce apparent field size by reduction of light access to the retina and by excluding a few of the most peripheral rays by virtue of the large (opaque) iris diaphragm.

10. Fixation must be maintained by the eye under examination on an easily identified central marker and monitored by the examiner. When central acuity is grossly reduced, several methods are available to secure fixation:

a. Vertical and horizontal strips of ½-in. white adhesive tape may be placed on the screen intersecting at the fixation center. Even though the central portion of these strips may not be seen by a patient with a central scotoma, he can project their intersectional point by completion or "gestalt." This is suitable even for a one-eyed patient.

b. Where the opposite eye can be used, the simplest technique is to roll up a short paper funnel or cone 5 or 6 in. long and big enough in diameter at the large end to cover the eye not being examined. The patient holds this with one hand over the eye not being examined and maintains alignment on the fixation marker while the other eye is being tested.

c. Finger fixation can be used when acuity is extremely poor in both eyes and when testing is being done with 10- or 20-mm. diameter targets or a small light source.

d. More complicated procedures are (1) fixation through a mirror angulated at 45 degrees before the eye not being tested; (2) use of polarized light and polarizing glasses with axes at 90 degrees from one another over each eye; or (3) employing red-green glasses with a red fixation light for one eye and green test light for the other. These three methods, however, use not widely available office equipment, except for the last, which can be easily made from Lancaster red-green test equipment used in motility examination. The flashlights can be modified by a cap or opaque paper diaphragm to convert their streak image to a spot of known size.

11. Movement of the test object should proceed from a less sighted or sightless area to the visible area. It is best to make one or two introductory advances of the target from the periphery toward the center to demonstrate the outer isopter and the target size. The patient is instructed to report his first "awareness" of the "white" rather than waiting until the target outline can be clearly described. Similarly, if colored targets are used, the patient reports his first awareness of the *hue* or *color*—he may actually discern a form or colorless target before the color is recognized. The physiologic blind spot and all pathologic scotomata must be outlined by moving the test target from within the defect to the seeing area.

12. Blind spot outlining should be done immediately after eliciting the first point on the outer isopter. It is wise, in the absence of known temporal field impairment, to initiate the examination of each eye from the temporal periphery so that the examiner is in physical position to proceed to the blind spot. Outlining the physiologic blind spot (Mariotte) will (a) provide a sharp or steep edge of transition for the patient to identify, (b) instruct the patient in the appearance-disappearance behavior of the target, (c) give an index of the patient's mental alertness or responsiveness, and (d) accomplish an important element of the tangent screen examination, which is generally unreliable on a 33-cm. radius perimeter. If the patient cannot identify the blind spot disappearance of the 2-mm. white target at 1 meter, then for demonstration purposes the examiner should switch to a gross 10- or 20-mm. target, which

will, of course, completely disappear within the blind spot. This dramatic illustration enables the examiner to compliment and encourage the hesitant performer. The optimally small target should then be resumed.

13. Radial exploration should proceed in an orderly fashion at intervals of about 45 degrees. This is reduced in keeping with suspect areas of pathology and for the verification or elucidation of defects (contracture, depression, quadrantic, altitudinal, homonymous). After identifying the outer isopter, advancement of the target should be continued steadily on to the fixation point, looking for scotomatous defects (peripheral, central, paracentral, centrocecal, winging, arcuate, annular, junctional, or sector).

Pantographic aids. Pantographs are devices generally using mechanical, electric, optic, or magnetic components to move targets by remote control, coupled with a recording device to automate a precise outline map of patient responses. A simple and serviceable pantographic apparatus is manufactured for each of the three basic types of field testing equipment: (1) for the tangent screen, the Bausch and Lomb Auto-Plot projection device, (2) for the spherical or bowl perimeter, the Goldmann projection pantograph, and (3) for the arc perimeter, the AIMARK or Bausch and Lomb table-model, cable-driven projection unit.

Other pantographs for the tangent screen include the Gunkel wall-mounted screen and pantograph; the Allied Ophthalmic Corporations tripod-mounted Photo Field Plotting Unit, using multiple exposures on Polaroid film; the Guist magnetically controlled test object; and others. For the spherical perimeters, a mechanical pantograph is incorporated in the 2-meter diameter behemoth of Donaldson and Norton. For the arc perimeter there have been many self-recording and semi–self-recording devices led by the Maggiore and the Ferree-Rand.

Auto-Plot. The Auto-Plot projection device introduced by Bausch and Lomb in 1965 reduced projection equipment and pantographic charting to a small unit (12 × 21 in. base; 13 in. high) that eliminates extraneous optic or acoustical cues to the target. The unit is solidly built of welded steel. Though distraction of the examiner's arms and carrying devices are eliminated in common with all projection systems, this table-top unit allows the examiner to sit quietly at the patient's right, removing him totally from movements that could be disturbing and yet allowing necessary observation of the patient directly and without instrumental aid.

The Auto-Plot is fixed to the practical 1-meter test distance and provides finger control of the projection aperture to give targets of 0.5, 1, 2, 3, 6, 12, and 15 mm. in white, red, green, or blue light. A short, mechanical pantographic arm links the projection head to a pencil holder over the record paper. A completely unmarked gray vinyl plastic screen is furnished for consistent brightness and procedural uniformity, though a similarly light wall surface may be substituted. Room light should be low. In use the patient's chin is placed on a movable rest behind the projection light and adjusted

vertically until the eye under examination centers behind the eye ring (which is folded down during testing). A magnet and ferrous fixation target may be held on either side of the vinyl screen. The eye not under examination is occluded. Testing is rapid because the target stimulus is moved by the examiner's hand as it holds the pencil in the pantoscopic arm on the record chart; thus control and record marking are with the same finger-tip movements (Fig. 13-8).

QUANTITATIVE OR DETAILED TESTS
Arc perimetry

Arc perimetry is mechanically simpler than spherical perimetry and offers some operational advantages:

1. Less complex and less expensive equipment
2. Easy, direct observation of the patient for fixation, alertness, and so on
3. Smaller equipment requiring less phys-

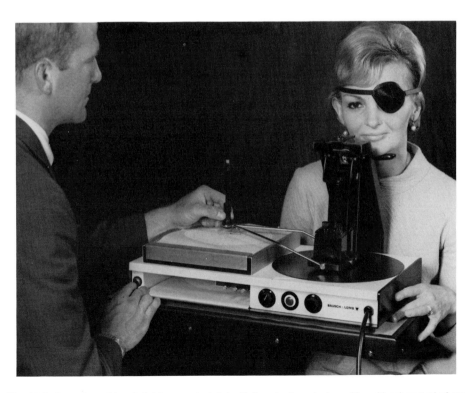

Fig. 13-8. Bausch and Lomb table-mounted Auto-Plot projection device with unitized control of projection light and recording stylus in examiner's hand. Examiner faces away from tangent screen to obtain constant observation of patient's fixation.

ical space and amenable to wall mounting, stand suspension (Fig. 13-9), or fold-up unit on caster-based floor stand*
4. Complete freedom and interchangeability of projection targets, mechanical target carriers, or hand-controlled targets

The disadvantages of arc perimetry in comparison to spherical or bowl perimetry are (1) less uniformity of background conditions and illumination, (2) difficulty of controlling preadaptation when desired, (3) more conflicting and distracting stimuli from both the

*Harrington 33-cm. cold cathode and ultraviolet illumination unit; formerly made by Jenkel-Davidson House of Vision.

examiner and the surrounding area, and (4) less certain relation of target to background intensity. However, for practical clinical screening of the peripheral fields between 30 and 100 degrees from fixation, the arc instrument affords an adequate working answer to most diagnostic problems.

Modern arc perimeters have been standardized with (1) radius of 33 cm., (2) arc exceeding 180 degrees, (3) rotation of 360 degrees, (4) uniform or coordinated rotating light source providing approximately 7 footcandles of illumination, (5) uniform matte black or dark gray finish for the arc surface, and (6) minimal arc width of 3 in. Much of the basic understanding of perimetric findings in the modern context of ocular disease was derived by H. Roenne of Copen-

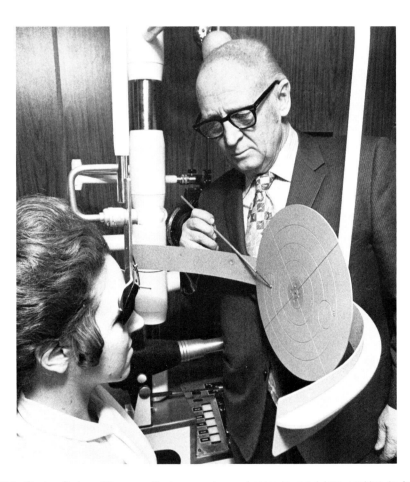

Fig. 13-9. Guyton-Carlson 33-cm. unified arc and campimeter lowered into position in front of patient.

hagen, as was much of the understanding of field changes in neurology by C. B. Walker of Boston. The practical and still simple perimeters of today's office have evolved from dozens of prototypes but largely from combined work on instrument and technique as accomplished by Walker, by C. E. Ferree with Gertrude Rand, and by the Italian ophthalmologist Maggiore.

The most useful and rugged arc perimeter commonly available today was designed by the Allied Instrument Manufacturing Company of England and called AIMARK (Fig. 13-10). It is also built in New York for the Bausch and Lomb Optical Company and sold under the designation Projection Perimeter. This ingeniously uses one light bulb to produce the target (variable in size, intensity, and color), the fixation point, and illumination for the recording form. Hand rotation of

a control knob simultaneously moves the projected light stimulus and a recording punch stylus, without any sound or movement of the examiner's arm—operational advantages not afforded by the Bausch and Lomb Ferree-Rand perimeter.

In use, instrument height must be adjusted comfortably to the seated position of the patient and then the chinrest elevated or lowered so that the eye under examination is directly centered on the fixation target or light. The eye not under examination is occluded. Distracting lights, sounds, and other stimuli must be excluded from the area and the examiner must be in position to observe the patient's maintenance of fixation.

Perimetric fields are traditionally outlined with the patient frontally aligned to the fixation point. This produces a variable nasal ob-

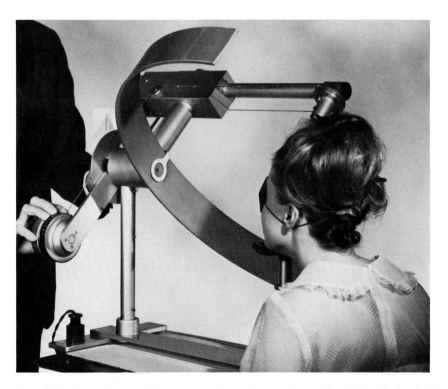

Fig. 13-10. Projection perimeter of the arc type with semiautomatic recording device. Patient is shown with right eye fixing. Fold-down auxiliary fixation ring surrounds the smaller illuminated fixation cross. Examiner's right hand is on rotating drum that controls the projection light and the marking stylus with same endless cord drive. Three knurled rings in bulb housing and control box at top permit adjustment of stimulus diameter, intensity, and color. (Distributed by Clement Clarke and by Bausch and Lomb.)

scuration artifact because of the relative prominence of the nose to the globe. Similarly a superior field artifact may be created by a protruding brow or deep-set globe. Studies made in this position should be designated *relative perimetric fields*. Fuller analysis of the outer isopters is obtained by turning the face approximately 30 degrees to the opposite side and slightly extending the chin, if needed, to see beneath a massive brow. (This may require the examiner, as with a ptosis patient, to elevate the patient's upper lid with his finger or a cotton-tipped applicator while exploring the upper field quadrants.) This may be called a *maximum perimetric field*. In the presence of marked latent nystagmus, strabismus fixus, bilateral nerve VI paralysis or in motor transport driver examination, practical evaluation of the functional field may require perimetry

with both eyes open. For this examination, the midline of the face should be centered on the fixation point and findings designated as *binocular perimetric field*.

The patient must not be involved in conversation during testing and should make only the simplest possible responses such as "yes," "no," or a tap on the table to advise the examiner. A few verification or confirmation runs are necessary to check consistency of response; all projection perimeters have a silent flicker or extinguishing device that may also be used to check the patient's accuracy of responses. Eight meridians usually constitute a maximum test unless specific defects require further exploration. The examination should be kept as brief as possible consistent with securing minimally adequate data. Fatigue of either patient or examiner greatly reduces accuracy of field findings.

Fig. 13-11. Schweigger or Spiller bedside arc perimeter showing patient aligned on mirror fixation device for her left eye. Patient holds perimeter in left hand with cheek support resting on lower orbital rim.

For bedside, emergency room, or home examinations the 15-cm. radius Schweigger or Spiller hand perimeter (Fig. 13-11) is quite serviceable, easy to carry, and provides testing meridians through 360 degrees. In use the patient (or the examiner) holds the instrument by its handle with its cheek-rest against the inferior orbital rim. Fixation is maintained on the reflected image of the patient's own eye in a small central mirror. A short, wand-mounted test object 3 to 5 mm. in diameter is desirable, but a cotton-tipped applicator may be used for less exacting or urgent diagnostic steps. This instrument affords better observation of the patient and manipulation of the test object than can be achieved with any of the collapsing umbrella-type bedside devices.

Spherical projection perimetry
Goldmann Perimeter* (Fig. 13-12)

The Goldmann Perimeter, a rather imposing though table-top instrument, was introduced in 1945 and has undergone only minor modifications, which are incorporated into the current Model 940. It is uniquely accurate for both kinetic and static perimetric techniques and affords unusual speed of operation for the familiar examiner. When the patient can maintain fixation with the eye under examination, the observer merely watches the patient's pupil through a telescopic observation tube immediately above the illuminated recording surface. The examiner, who is seated behind the bowl, has complete control of the silent recording pantograph, movement of the target, and adjustment of its size (1/16 to 64 mm. in diameter) and brightness (1.0 to 0.0001).

Auxiliary color filters are not incorporated but can be supplied on request. The radius is 30 cm., and theoretically a patient under examination should have ametropia corrected for this distance (a supplemental lens holder is provided). Diffuse background illumination of the bowl provides excellent control both of preadaptation and surrounding light conditions during actual examination.

A central scotoma device may be added to increase the area of display and accuracy of plotting minute central defects. The patient is freed from necessity of talking (and moving his head) by an electric buzzer system under his fingertip control with which he notifies the examiner of his target awareness. An automatic recording system with electronically controlled pantograph was introduced in 1972.

Harms (Tübinger) Perimeter*

The somewhat massive Harms Perimeter console unit (Fig. 13-13) was introduced by H. Harms and Aulhorn in the mid 1950s and is particularly useful in elaboration of static (light-sense or profile) perimetry. Moreover, it also has full capacity for conventional kinetic or topographic examinations. It has a unique facility in examination of the foveal area, because the observation system enabling the examiner to monitor the patient's fixation comes through the area of the normal blind spot rather than centrally as in the Goldmann instrument. The blind spot area is also used to introduce dazzle or glare for simulation of testing of night-driving conditions. This instrument affords capacity for special testing of (1) dark adaptation curves, (2) central and peripheral visual acuity, (3) flicker fusion frequency, (4) motor sensitivity of the pupil, and (5) color perimetry. With this equipment and a careful technologist, is may be possible to diagnose such disease processes as primary pigmentary degeneration of the retina (retinitis pigmentosa) before ERG reductions or ophthalmoscopic manifestations appear.

Color perimetry

A controversial aspect of perimetry, color perimetry reflects much difficulty in achieving standardized color test objects (both pigment and light), maintaining their color

---

*Manufactured by Haag-Streit Co., Berne, Switzerland. Adaptations of the basic design are Rodenstock Projection Perimeter, Topcon SPB-11, and Marco.

*Manufactured by Oculus Products, Dutenhofen, Federal Republic of Germany.

Fig. 13-12. Goldmann spherical projection perimeter made by Haag-Streit; pantographic arm is shown projecting stimulus to left of dark fixation spot. Examiner monitors patient fixation in primary position. Electric buzzer operated by patient's right thumb is used to indicate appearance of target. Available for kinetic testing only (Model 940-K7) or for both kinetic and static testing (Model 940-ST).

values, controlling preadaptation, obtaining proper background illumination, establishing absolute luminous flux values for targets, and ensuring proper recognition responses by the patient. The peripheral retina normally has a dyschromatic zone of variable width in which a patient may detect the presence of a colored test object before detecting its hue or color.

Color fields are generally a function of stimulus intensity, but they do present a method for reducing stimulus brightness or simulating a type of mesopic testing without other luminance variables. Harrington and Hoyt (1955) reported careful identification of a normal, minute central scotoma for monochromatic blue light (450 to 475 nm) when testing with a stimulus under 2 mm. in diameter.

Most careful perimetrists feel that any

Fig. 13-13. The Tübinger (Harms-Aulhorn) spherical projection perimeter is shown from the examiner's side. Table-model unit may be placed on any convenient height stand.

type of defect elicited with colored test objects can be demonstrated with small and carefully controlled white test objects. As a matter of convenience, however, when ambient and stimulus light cannot be as well controlled as in a Goldmann spherical perimeter, the use of a large red test object 15 or 20 mm. in diameter (preferably Heidelberg red paper) may at times elicit a conduction defect before it is demonstrated by the conventional 2-mm. white object at 1 meter.

Similarly, the use of a blue test object may elicit macular pathology before it is revealed with small white test objects. The patient is always asked to report his awareness of color (hue), not the target per se, which is often detected as a neutral stimulus considerably beyond the isopter of color recognition. Minimal and small test objects in color are of essentially no practical use.

Generally in clinical testing, precision and repeatable findings with color perimetry are more difficult to obtain than with white perimetry. Therefore color testing is usually an adjunctive procedure.

Flicker fusion frequency (FFF) perimetry

FFF perimetry is a static technique of plotting sensitivity at various areas in the visual field on the basis of the latent period between the light stimulus and response, plus the time required for groups of percipient cells to recover from the inhibitory phase following a stimulus and thus to become sensitive to a subsequent stimulus. Individual sites in the field are quantitated numerically on the number of flashes per second required to make flickering light appear continuous. For practical purposes of testing, this method has only been in use since the early 1930s.

Equipment for the background commonly is the 1-meter tangent screen, though larger screens and large bowl perimeters may be used. A small, portable stroboscope* is an easily adaptable stimulus source. The strobe flashbulb is modified and covered with opaque black paper, conventionally leaving open a target area of 3 to 5 cm. in diameter. Latitude of several degrees in target size will not alter clinical findings, but FFF does increase with the log of the stimulus area (Granit-Harper law).

The exposed target area should be covered with white translucent paper as used for typing so that the light is diffused. The four-wire electrical cable connecting the flash tube is passed through a rigid steel or aluminum tube 2 or 3 ft. long, which constitutes the supporting wand. This should be covered with black felt matching the tangent screen, or at least painted dull black.

The Gans (Ocutron) Flicker Wand is a commercially available yellow light emitting diode with adjustable pulse frequencies from 15 to 85 cycles per second (Fig. 13-14).

A conventional outline chart for noting tangent screen findings is used for record purposes, and the numbers in flashes per second representing FFF are written in for

*Strobotac, manufactured by General Radio Co., West Concord, Massachusetts 01742; or Photo Stimulator, manufactured by Grass Medical Instruments, Quincy, Massachusetts 02169.

the macula and at appropriate locations corresponding to each site tested. The eyes are tested separately, and normally a few flashes per second difference may be found between the two eyes, particularly in the macular area. Testing may well be confined within the central 30 degrees from fixation because (1) most pathologic depressions appear within this area, (2) testing beyond 30 degrees is mechanically difficult except with a major spherical perimeter manufactured to include

Fig. 13-14. Gans (Ocutron) Flicker Wand provides light pulses at frequency variables from 15 to 85 per second.

flicker, and (3) findings in the far periphery tend to be variable and less reliable.

FFF testing, like auto-ophthalmoscopic perimetry (p. 208), is particularly indicated in the presence of opacities in the media, poor vision, high refractive abnormalities, and suppression amblyopia. It may also present an advantage in testing patients with limited intelligence or poorly sustained attention. The technique is suited to detection of early or subtle field depressions, which may be widespread. Small scotomata, however, may be easily missed.

Macular or central fusion frequencies normally tend to be quite consistent at about 42 flashes per second. The midperiphery, however, has greater sensitivity to flicker and therefore rates in this area normally climb to 50 or 55 flashes per second, with slightly lower frequencies temporally. Beyond 20 degrees from fixation, the FFF drops progressively through the midforties at 30 degrees and to frequencies as low as 20 in the extreme periphery. Minor variations from these normal frequencies are physiologic, but pathologically reduced frequencies are usually distinct. The FFF rate or the "end point" in testing may be determined either from ascending or descending changes in frequencies, with some questionable variation in significance. Therefore the selected alternative in technique should be noted on the record. Changes in rate of flicker (ascending or descending) during the examining run at each test site should be just slow enough for patient awareness and fast enough to avoid fatigue.

Angioscotometry

From the 1890s through the 1930s, many morphologic studies and plots were made of the vascular shadows radiating from the optic nerve head, particularly about the posterior pole and macula. In the United States, however, John Evans went beyond academic interest in these minute shadows to describe (1926-1938) pathologic widening phenomena of angioscotomata under such conditions as increased intraocular pressure, increased jugular pressure, fright, extraocular congestion, and cervical sympathetic irritation. The technique is laborious, requires excellent fixation, and needs minute silver bead targets 0.25 and 0.50 mm. in diameter. A 1-meter tangent screen can be used for demonstration of these vascular shadows, but rigidly solid "short range" (190-mm.) instruments with appropriate aspheric collimating lenses (+5.25 diopters) are much more efficient.*

Improvements in tonometry and tonography have superseded the particular role of angioscotometry in detecting widening of the vessel shadows as a sign of early open-angle glaucoma or inadequate control. Fluorescein angiography of the optic nerve head also provides better differentiation and analysis of the several vascular groups involved in blood supply to the disc.

SCORING OF VISUAL FIELDS (TANGENT SCREEN AND PERIMETRIC)

Attempts at scoring visual fields quantitatively by some numerical or percentage system are as old as this century and gen-

erally have relied upon comparing serial fields, hopefully obtained under similar conditions, in order to assess improvement or loss. Increasing needs for accuracy in establishing compensation for permanent loss, or establishing criteria for transport licensure, led Ben Esterman* to develop and validate (1967-1968) two scoring grids, one for tangent screen and one for perimetric studies, each of 100 units. Component units, however, are of unequal size and unequal distribution, recognizing the unequal functional value of different parts of the field. Though each unit is valued at 1% and therefore a simple count of included units yields the functional score in percent, this relative value scale weighs central units above peripheral units, inferior units above superior units, and horizontal units above those in other meridians (Fig. 13-15).

In use, the outer isopter is first recorded in the standard fashion (2-mm. white test object at 1 meter for the tangent screen; 3-mm. or 0.5-degree white test object at 33-cm. radius for the perimeter). The grid,

*Lloyd Stereocampimeter, formerly manufactured by American Optical Corp., Instrument Div., Buffalo, New York 14215.

*Esterman, B.: Grid for scoring visual fields, Arch. Ophthal. **77**:780-786, 1967; ibid. **79**:400-406, 1968. Approved by the American Committee on Optics and Visual Physiology, October 27, 1968.

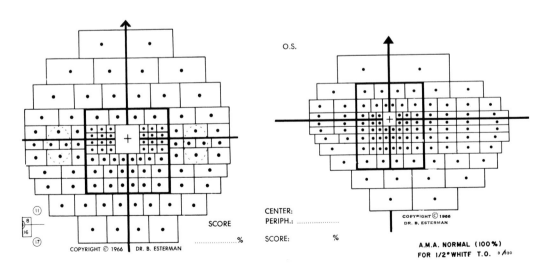

Fig. 13-15. Esterman 100-unit scoring grid for tangent screen (left) and for arc perimeter (right) in "relative perimetric position." (Courtesy Benjamin Esterman, M.D.)

printed on transparent Mylar, is superimposed on the field record; alternatively, the field outline may be transferred by carbon paper to the appropriate grid. A central dot is printed in each of the 100 grid squares. The dots within (not touching) the field outline are merely counted in order to obtain the score. The percentage score thus derived (1) eliminates guesswork of significance, (2) reduces total calculations to be made in determining field efficiency, and (3) yields a numerical expression that is computer-compatible.

FINAL RESPONSIBILITY

The conscientious examiner will maintain an easily accessible tangent screen or other favorite perimetric device for frequent and quick use both in clinical diagnosis and in follow-up evaluation. All perimetric findings must be interpreted in the light of ophthalmoscopic findings. The examiner must recognize normal variations and pathologic changes in the fundus that alter the visual fields. In the absence of fundus pathology he should be prepared to make appropriate central or neurologic interpretations, see that the patient has proper neurologic studies (examination, x-ray films of the skull, electroencephalogram, spinal tap, air, or EMI studies as indicated), and interpret the localizing specifics of visual field defects to the neurologist or neurosurgeon planning definitive care.

"There is an art to proper examination of the visual field which is being more and more neglected in recent years. With increasing sophistication of the instruments there is a tendency to view the examination as wholly scientific. These subjective examinations require a degree of psychic evaluation which will often determine their validity. Flexibility is the key to accurate diagnostic perimetry."

DAVID O. HARRINGTON, 1975

REFERENCES

Gans, J. A.: Considerations in the design of an automatic visual field tester, Med. Res. Eng. **10:**7-11, 1971.

Greve, E. L.: Single and multiple stimulus static perimetry in glaucoma, Dr. W. Junk N. V., Publishers, 1973, The Hague.

Ivanoff, N.: A new method (Friedmann's Visual Field Analyzer) of investigating macular function, Klin. Monatsbl. Augenheilk. **164:**213-271, 1974.

Sloan, L. I.: The Tübinger Perimeter of Harms and Aulhorn, Arch. Ophthalmol. **86:**612-622, Dec., 1971.

CHAPTER 14

Tests of color vision*

Color depends upon hue (wavelength of light), brightness (intensity of light), and saturation or chroma (homogeneity). When either the intensity of light is reduced or the specific spectral components are missing, coloration disappears. Thus when the amount of white light (a mixture of radiant energies of all the visible wavelengths or approximately 400 to 750 nm) is reduced or when, for example, wavelengths for red (650 to 750 nm) are excluded from the light, it will not be possible to perceive the color red. Testing for color vision must be done with fully adequate illumination and with full spectral representation in the light used.

High filament temperature of about 6,750° K. may be used to produce illumination that simulates the full spectral range derived from the sun. More economically and with longer filament life, a conventional 100-watt light bulb (which operates at a tungsten filament temperature of about 2,854° K.) may be used if provided with the bluish appearing "C" filter of C.I.E. (Commission Internationale de l'Eclairage) illuminant standards. This filter removes a disproportionate amount of the long or red wavelengths. A New London Easel Lamp of table base design and yielding a desirable 15 to 35 footcandles of illumination† has been made particularly to meet these specifications for color vision testing. If resort is made to fluorescent bulbs of the "daylight" type, care should be taken to ensure that full and proportioned spectral representation is present. The Duro-Test Corporation* produces a Vitalite tube that yields unusually full representation in the short (violet) wavelength end of the spectrum.

Color vision defects may be either congenital or rarely acquired. Most congenital defects are inherited as sex-linked recessive dyschromatopsia with the genetic loci on the X chromosome being different for the protanopes (red deficient) and the deuteranopes (green deficient). These dichromatic defects are the most common specific defects but minor irregularities, known as anomalous trichromatism, are frequent. The blue insensitive tritanopes are rare. The true monochromats are extremely rare and usually present poor central acuity with congenital nystagmus. Acquired impairments of either the optic nerve or the macula cause defects in color vision but pseudoisochromatic tests are of little value in differentiating these sites. Though some lead may be obtained from the Nagel anomaloscope or the Farnsworth-Munsell 100 Hue Test, it is more direct to differentiate retinal (blue-yellow) defects from optic nerve (red-green) defects on the basis of ophthalmoscopy and fluorescein angiography of the retina, or ultrasonic examination of the optic nerve.

Testing is generally of two types: (1) pigment tests based on matching, identifying, or arranging pigment samples or (2) spectral instruments based on light sources and adjustment of the components of different wave lengths. The former are relatively less expensive, require less time, and can be done either by the patient himself or by a technician.

A useful and preliminary inspection of

*Lewis, M. F., and Ashby, F. Y.: Diagnostic tests of color defective vision, annotated bibliography, 1955-1966, Washington, D.C., May, 1967, Federal Aviation Administration Office of Aviation Medicine.
†Manufactured by the Macbeth Corp., Newburg, New York 12550.

*North Bergen, New Jersey.

color vision is accomplished by a self-testing procedure such as the Rosner "Do-it-Yourself" wall-mounted color test. This 24 × 30 in. walnut-framed display of sixteen pseudoisochromatic plates can be hung—possibly—in some area of the office where it may attract the patient's attention. Two legend areas within the bottom portion of the frame give interpretation for the patient. (Though solid and substantial, it will tax a decorator's ingenuity to work this into attractive office appointments.)*

Of more immediate usefulness is the unlearnable Hardy-Rand-Rittler† (HRR) (Fig. 14-1) booklet of twenty-four plates of gray versus color-confusable dots. The introductory four plates demonstrate, even to the color defective, the three types of colored test figures (O, X, and Δ) immersed within the field pattern of gray dots. These are followed by six plates specifically for preliminary screening to separate the red-green defectives, the blue-yellow defectives, and the normal trichromates. Ten further test plates quantitate the red-green failures and four final plates evaluate the blue-yellow failures, thus yielding qualitative classification of the defect and quantitative degree of impairment as mild, medium, or severe. Scoring and interpretation sheets are supplied with the booklet of test plates. The older Stilling (1883), Ishihara (1925, thirty-eight plates; 1968, twenty-four plates), Dvorine (1953, twenty-one plates; revised 1955), and similar sets of plates are based on pseudoisochromatic dots but are less specific in their differential capability and, by using learnable series of Arabic numbers, are subject to the disadvantage of memorization.

The Ishihara pseudoisochromatic test is a very exacting screen that no one with a color vision defect can read without making some mistakes. A person who does not make a single mistake on the Ishihara plates can be confidently labeled as color normal. American Optical Corporation introduced in 1971 an abridged series of fifteen numerical color

test plates based on the Ishihara pseudoisochromatic principle but designed primarily for rapid screening of red-green deficiencies. T. Okuma et al. of Yokohama have issued one of the most recent (1974) sets of plates hopefully adding to the Ishihara principles, new test plates of qualitative and quantitative differential capabilities. Murakami and Umazume of Tokyo Medical College have also produced a book of thirteen hand-painted pseudoisochromatic plates for screening and classification (seven plates) or quantification (six plates) that is divided into three degrees of mild, medium, and severe. Clinical validation of any newly-introduced test plates, however, is complex and may be misleading unless done by a careful color physiologist familiar with statistical methods.

Because the precise physical basis for color perception remains obscure, and because nonspectral cues and psychologic factors affect testing procedures, visual literature contains dozens of other color tests based on spectroscopic matching (Helmholtz; Abney; Nagel), pigment or dye matching (Wilson; Holmgren; Jeffries; Farnsworth), or lantern identification (Donders; Edridge-Green, 1920; Williams, 1903; Farnsworth New London Navy Lantern).

For critical accuracy and quantitation, the spectral matching technique as utilized in the Nagel anomaloscope (1899-1907) continues as the most definitive instrument.* This consists essentially of a telescopic tube directed at a light source. The lower half of the field of view is filled with a sodium yellow color that can be adjusted by the examiner both in brightness and in components of red and green. The subject then attempts to match the yellow of the lower field as preset by the examiner with the upper field where he may adjust the proportions of red, green, and yellow. Settings of the subject's controls then indicate the relative amounts of red, green, or yellow that he needs to match the test setting.†

---

*House of Vision, Chicago, Illinois 60602.
†American Optical Co., revised 1957, but subsequently discontinued.

*Manufactured by Schmidt and Haensch, West Berlin, Federal Republic of Germany.
†Rayleigh Equation (1881): x red + y green = k yellow.

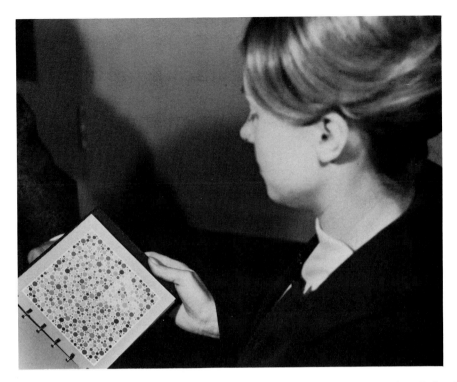

Fig. 14-1. Hardy-Rand-Rittler booklet of 24 plates of gray versus color-confusable dots. Patient is requested to identify only three test figures: O, X, and △.

The time-consuming Nagel precision test is of less ready practicality than a good lantern test such as that of F. W. Edridge-Green (or the simplified Giles-Archer Lantern with only 5 standard color filters). Twenty-one variously colored glass filters on three rotating discs can be combined in front of a standard luminance source. A fourth rotating disc contains seven variously sized apertures that can be used as diaphragms to reduce the stimulus intensity. The fifth rotating disc contains modifiers such as ground glass to simulate mist, ribbed glass to simulate rain, or neutral densities to simulate fog. For usual requirements in the transport industry, examining is restricted to the control colors of yellow, red (A or B), and signal green. The compact unit takes considerably less table space than does a Macbeth easel lamp.

Less subtle tests to identify patients with functionally limiting color deficiencies are lead by such pigment matching tests as the practical Farnsworth D-15 test (1943). This test does not identify minor degrees of anomalous trichromatism but does identify significant anomalous trichromatism and true dichromatism (protanopia or deuteranopia). The D-15 test is simple, inexpensive, and easily accomplished by children or those with reduced acuity. Illumination requirements are less exact than with the Ishihara dots. A fixed reference chip of color is presented along with fifteen movable and numbered chips of hue progression. The subject is asked to align the fifteen movable chips in an order of color progression, matching their colors to that of the fixed reference chips. Scoring sheets as provided identify handicapping degrees of anomalous trichromatism or dichromatism but neither separate the two nor identify the quite rare blue-yellow defective. Patients may fail the HRR or Ishihara plates but, if able to pass the Farnsworth D-15 test, may be considered functionally color adequate.

This test is to be differentiated from the

Fig. 14-2. Farnsworth-Munsell 100-hue test of color discrimination (1943, 1949, 1957). Four wooden cases contain 93 discs, each of a different hue, mounted in protective plastic rings. Subject arranges discs of different hues in progressive series. Errors, mismatches, or transpositions are coded on a radially arranged diagram.

more time-consuming, costly, and complex Farnsworth-Munsell 100-hue test* (1943), which is not dependable for classification on a quantitative basis. Cost is 5 to 6 times that of pseudoisochromatic plates (Fig. 14-2).

Color vision testing has not been a routine facet of eye examination in many clinics and offices because there is essentially no treatment for color defects after they are diagnosed. Industry, the military, and public carriers, however, maintain various standards of color perception that must be met by individuals in these fields. Distress at the time of a later request for such information may be avoided by incorporating some simple color screening into usual routine. Having such information in a diagnostic form will also avoid embarrassment at the end of an eye examination when a patient inquires about the significance of his previously unmentioned difficulty with colors.

*Munsell Color, Baltimore, Maryland 21218.

Identification of deficiency in color vision will occasionally aid greatly in the diagnosis of specific congenital defects such as the nystagmus accompanying congenital achromatopsia. Notation of color defects in family members will be of frequent value in genetic counseling and in career planning for young individuals.

The exacting or compulsive examiner in this field can invest much time in complex testing systems that are of both research and genetic importance. Only rarely are such tests of value in identification of toxic damage to the retina. For usual purposes, however, the Ishihara test plates presented in proper light give secure diagnoses or clinical data and should be an easy working part of most eye examinations.

REFERENCES

Color vision, a symposium, Washington, 1973, National Academy of Sciences.
Lakowski, R.: Theory and practice of color vision testing: a review, Br. J. Indust. Med. 26:173-189, 1969.

Light sensitivity and dark adaptometry, mesopic and scotopic vision

Evaluations of vision under reduced illumination fall into four sets of contrasting conditions:

1. Laboratory versus clinical
2. Absolute minimum thresholds versus practical levels for seeing in dim light
3. Minimum threshold of appearance versus course of dark adaptation
4. Objective versus subjective techniques

Complicated tests requiring preconditioning, such as for absolute minimum thresholds and minimum light differences, like quantum physics of the light-sense, are time-consuming labors primarily of the pure or laboratory-oriented examiner. They have suffered from insufficient control of the many variables that affect such examinations. Similarly, diagnostic attempts oriented to practical needs of assessing working vision under dim light (as a watch at sea) or under variable low intensities (as in night driving) are largely empirical, do not yield absolute values, and are subject to considerable latitude in reproducibility.

McFarland (1960) has disquietingly quantitated what most presbyopic examiners know, that man needs essentially doubled amounts of illumination every 13 years of life for objects to be seen under dim light. Thus presbyopia not only calls for a quantitative addition of plus spherical diopterage for near acuity but also presents a quantifiable need for progressively increasing illumination. The grandparent who puts larger bulbs in his reading light understandably remonstrates with the young teen-ager who

reads happily and healthily in "poor" light that would be impossible for the oldster.

Finally, there is a peculiar lack of correlation between performance of an individual under mesopic illumination (0.01 to 0.5 foot lambert) and tests of dark adaptation. This is a curious result of psychology, fatigue, motivation, alertness, and technique of visual use at night.

Empirically, there are three factors of night vision that are clinically important and amenable to some practical quantitation: (1) mesopic acuity or acuity under reduced illumination, (2) glare tolerance, and (3) glare recovery time, which is usually expressed in seconds. Preadaptation (photostressing) for standardized periods of 10 seconds to 3 minutes, followed by 10 to 40 minutes of dark adaptation, adds an element of laboratory quantitation to any of these procedures. Similarly, the use of repeated pilocarpine instillation to fix the pupillary diameter and to reduce this great variable makes test results more comparable, but these steps introduce abnormal conditions that will not be present in actual working or environmental situations.

Several practical devices are available to the practitioner for office testing of mesopic functions. The Feldman adaptometer (1937) has been produced by the American Optical Corporation in several compact, table-model versions, but essentially it permits only a measurement in minutes between standardized photostressing (3 minutes) and recognition of a dimly illuminated bar. The scotometer of Henkind and Siegel (1967)* is a smaller, hand-held, monocular instrument that affords an optically simulated distance Snellen reading followed by 10 seconds of dazzling glare. After extinguishing the glare, the patient continues fixation on the reduced Snellen chart (through the fading afterimage) until attaining his preglare level of Snellen recognition. Under these conditions, glare recovery time in normal individuals under age 40 should be less than 40 seconds, but this may be prolonged by age or disease to 180 seconds or more. This self-contained instrument also may serve as a bedside test for visual acuity (Fig. 15-1).

A screening instrument widely used by driver license examiners in North America is the table-model Night Sight Meter† (1953) (Fig. 15-2). This unit is built in a light-tight box 30 × 10 × 7 in. Below the viewing point is an illumination source that may be reduced by rotation of two sheets of Polaroid film over it. At the far end of the box, a motor-driven target wheel presents Landolt C's at the rate of 45 per minute (angular displace-

ment of 18 degrees per second), requiring the patient to identify the direction of the opening in the C and announce one of four possible positions (up, down, right, or left) every second and a half. The size of the C's simulates 20/300 acuity. In use, the patient is

Fig. 15-1. Medin hand-held scotometer with optically simulated distance Snellen type and built-in dazzle source. Batteries are in handle.

*Medin Corp., Wallington, New Jersey 07055.
†Manufactured by the American Automobile Association, Washington, D.C. 20006.

Fig. 15-2. American Automobile Association Night Sight Meter, 30 in. long, for testing central acuity under reduced illumination, glare tolerance, and glare recovery time (Stock No. 3538).

asked to report the direction of the openings as the illumination is reduced under dial control. At the lowest level where he recognizes the openings, an empirical unit reading from the dial is recorded as mesopic acuity. Two glare sources (approximately 1 footcandle) are then presented at an angle 9 degrees to the left of the targets, thus simulating a car approaching on the left side of a 20-ft. wide pavement at a distance of 150 ft. Target illumination is then increased to a level necessary for recognition again of the Landolt C's; the dial reading is now a measure of glare tolerance.

For the third phase of the test, the glare source is extinguished and target illumination simultaneously decreased to the last visible level as determined in the first part of the test. The patient maintains fixation on the target area, and the examiner watches the interval timer reading in seconds. When ability to see the moving targets under his previously established mesopic acuity illumination is just regained, the elapsed seconds are recorded as glare recovery time.

These three procedures can be done by an office aide in 5 minutes with no more preconditioning than exposure to usual indoor ambient illumination. Results are generally repeatable, though a small percentage of patients, even with apparently normal eyes and a few pretest runs, seem too slow in interpretive ability to report the necessary discriminations.

About a dozen sophisticated modern test instruments for testing minimal thresholds are available. The French Jayle-Blet adaptoperimeter (1955) is almost as large as a Link trainer and also capable of flicker, chromatic, and glare testing. At the other end of the size scale is the small, compact Comberg nyctometer with only a preadapting lamp and a 25-cm. diameter sphere in which test letters are exhibited after photostressing. Intermediate in size are projection devices to give controlled target stimuli developed by Beyne in 1952 or to present full cinemas of actual environmental conditions developed by Jayle in 1957.

Of the modern, absolute value type instruments the Goldmann-Weekers adaptometer (1950)* is the most accurate compromise between research laboratory equipment and office devices. This hemispheric instrument, though elaborate and only slightly smaller than the Goldmann table-model spherical perimeter, is uniquely flexible and simple to use. Determinations can be made of minimal thresholds, differential thresholds, visual acuity at any level of adaptation, sensitivity to dazzle, response to color, and time course of light adaptation, both through the rapid alpha phase (measured in tenths of a second) and the slower beta phase (measured in seconds and minutes). Brightness steps are controlled in logarithmic units. Both subjective and objective measurements, with automatic drum recording of data, and examination of all or any portion of the retina, either central or peripheral, are possible (Fig. 15-3).

Though most adaptometry relies on subjective responses of the patient,† objective methods (including electroretinography) are adaptable and commercially available. The Rieken principle (1941-1943) of utilizing optocokinetic nystagmus is incorporated in the Goldmann-Weekers and also the Jonkers (1947) adaptometer. Deviating from the precontrolling technique of fixing pupillary size with topical pilocarpine, Alpern (1959) incorporated pupillometry as an objective index, recording the intensity of light required to keep the pupil at a given diameter during an initial 12 minutes of dark adaptation. The relationship between sensory response and

---

*Haag-Streit, Berne, Switzerland.

†The Hartinger Recording Adaptometer, built on the basis of two Ulbricht spheres, and the simpler Recording Nyctometer, which automatically proceeds through a 4-phase, 10-minute cycle, are manufactured by Carl Zeiss of Jena, Democratic Republic of Germany. The Aulhorn projection mesoptometer, made by Oculus Products of Tubingen, Federal Republic of Germany, is designed for a 3-meter test distance in a totally dark room and is therefore cumbersome and space-consuming. It utilizes Landolt ring optotypes to quantitate (1) acuity at nine preset luminances, (2) night myopic shift, (3) glare recovery time after a 10-second simulation of oncoming headlights, and (4) acuity in the presence of glare.

pupillary diameter becomes less correlated after the first 12 minutes of adaptation as the visual process becomes mediated primarily by rods (below the level of 0.1 meter candle [lux]). This objective technique, however, requires an infrared viewing or photographing system and is not easily integrated into office routines.

In general, test equipment for dark adaptation and mesopic vision is usually very complex and expensive or empirical and less reproducible in results. Compared to equipment for visual field studies or color discrimination, it is relatively unavailable in the offices of most eye practitioners. Therefore,

as recently as 1969, both the American Committee on Optics and Visual Physiology as well as the A.M.A. Committee on Medical Aspects of Automotive Safety advised that practitioners evaluating night vision capabilities place primary reliance on detecting the disease entities and morphologic variations known to reduce visual capability in low illumination. Those especially reducing mesopic acuity and glare recovery are glaucoma (particularly when requiring miotic therapy), primary pigmentary degeneration of the retina (retinitis pigmentosa), retinal and choroidal arteriolosclerosis, retinal abiotrophies, retinitis punctata albescens, cho-

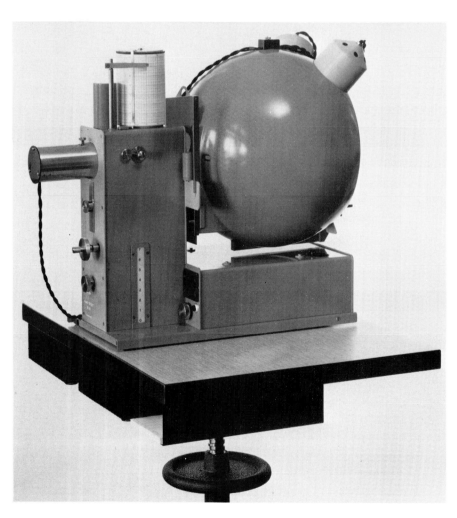

Fig. 15-3. Goldmann-Weekers adaptometer manufactured by Haag-Streit. Hemispheric bowl is shown from the rear (to the right), and automatic drum recorder is shown to the left.

roideremia, diabetic retinopathy, aphakia, degeneration of the macula, optic atrophy, Oguchi's disease and other forms of familial or congenital night blindness, chronic hepatic disease, and avitaminosis A. Reduced glare tolerance or increased dazzling may similarly be predicted in the presence of opacities or diffraction alterations in the media such as corneal irregularities, scars, opacities or dystrophies (particularly affecting the central portion), lens opacities or vacuoles, and vitreous floaters. Dirty, pitted, and scratched spectacle lenses or windshields create similar effects and present a further handicap compounding any pathology in the patient's eye.

REFERENCES

Henkind, P., and Siegel, I. M.: The Scotometer, a device for measuring macular recovery, Am. J. Ophthalmol. **64:**314-315, Aug., 1967.

McFarland, R., Domey, G., et al.: Dark adaptation as a function of age, J. Gerontol. **15:**149-154, April, and **15:**267-279, July, 1960.

Miller, D., Jernigan, M. E., Mainar, S., Wolf, I., and Newman, J.: Laboratory evaluation of a clinical glare tester, Arch. Ophthalmol. **87:**324-332, March, 1972.

Ryan S. J.: Diagnostic tests employed in macular lesions, Survey Ophthalmol. **17:**94-100, Sept.-Oct., 1972.

CHAPTER 16

Exophthalmometry

Instrumental exophthalmometry need not be performed as a routine on every patient; rather, it should be done in keeping with the patient's complaints, ocular history, and preliminary findings. Every examiner should also remember that the complaint of exophthalmos on one side may actually be enophthalmos on the other. Critical attention should therefore be given also to the possibly normal or relatively enophthalmic fellow globe. Sometimes the concealed history of a blow or the omitted diagnosis of a previous orbital floor fracture initiates orbital fat atrophy or herniation and possible incarceration of extrabulbar soft tissues. At times all the clinical wit of the examiner plus x-ray films, ultrasound, ear, nose, and throat examination, medical studies, EMI scan and biopsy are needed to attain a satisfactory diagnosis in exophthalmos.

Preliminary inspection should evaluate each eye in relation to the other eye (orthophoria to heterotrophia) and also in relation to other facial landmarks (exophthalmos, enophthalmos, displacement). This inspection should not only be in frontal view of the patient but also by examination from above (Fig. 16-1), where it is easier to note the relative position of the lateral orbital rims and the relative position of the zygomatic arches (Fig. 16-2). The examiner should palpate the orbital rims with equal pressure in the pulp tips of each index finger. Holding the fingers in straight extension augments, by aligning power, the ability to discriminate small differences in anteroposterior position. Similar positioning of the fingers over the zygomatic arch indicates their relative anteroposterior position. This physical inspection can be supplemented with a submentovertex x-ray view (Fig. 16-3),

which displays the angulations and relative depths of the orbits.

It is important to record any relative anteroposterior asymmetry of either lateral orbital rim in reference to the other, because these sites are reference points for essentially all exophthalmometers, except for the Mutch proptometer, which compares a plunger depth setting on the closed lid over the corneal apex, with vertical reference points on the orbital rim at 12 and 6 o'clock.

The simplest exophthalmometer is the Luedde rule (Fig. 16-4), made of transparent acrylic and vertically etched in millimeters from zero at a notch on one end. The observer places the notch firmly against the lateral orbital rim and, from his lateral position, aligns the etch marks on both sides of the rule with the anterior-most limit of the corneal curvature while the patient fixes straight ahead. Usually it is necessary to direct a bright penlight beam onto the cornea from below with the other hand or else this essential distal line is lost in the shadows of the inner canthal recess. Ordinarily the Luedde measurement ranges from 16 to 20 mm., but scale markings extend to 40 mm.

This instrument is available in double form by mounting two of the single Luedde rules onto a connecting crossbar of similar plastic.* Each rule can be moved laterally or medially on the ungraduated crossbar to position the notched ends of the exophthalmometer scales on the lateral orbital rims. When viewed from above, this arrangement helps to identify symmetry or asymmetry of the anteroposterior position of the lateral orbital rims.

More complex instruments with right and

*Clement Clarke, London, England, W1H ODH.

238

left prisms (Rodenstock), or right and left double mirrors (Hertel) (Fig. 16-5), enable the observer to make readings of each corneal limit while maintaining a frontal position to the patient. The design of these instruments is based on an assumed mean distance (usually 20 mm.) between the corneal apex and the lateral orbital rim. In small children or broad-faced individuals accuracy of reading may be compromised. Parallax errors of 0.5 to 1.5 mm. in alignment of the corneal apex, orbital rim, and examiner's visual axis plague the instrumental purist, but constitute a lower order of magnitude than anatomical variations in the facial bones.

A scale measuring the distance of separation between right and left units of these exophthalmometers is etched on the carrier bar; this figure has no bearing on the exophthalmos reading but should be noted in order to set the reading surfaces in the same relative position on subsequent examinations.

The Copper* orbital tonometer (1948) (Fig. 16-6) is an elaboration of exophthalmometry using a slotted aluminum bridge with fixed height-supporting legs against each lateral orbital rim and a third or cen-

*Lameris Instrumentum, Utrecht, The Netherlands.

Fig. 16-1. Inspection from above to evaluate symmetric position of lateral orbital rims. Direct extension of examiner's fingers gives added assistance of aligning power to differentiate small irregularities.

Fig. 16-2. Examination from above to evaluate symmetry of zygomatic arches. Examiner uses equal pressure of fingertips against midpoint of lower orbital rim. Extended fingers again afford advantage of aligning power in estimating small differences.

Fig. 16-3. Submentovertex x-rays showing marked difference in width of orbital angles and position of lateral orbital rim. **A** shows broad or flat facial configuration; **B** shows narrow or slender facial configuration.

ter leg adjusted in height to the glabella. The patient must be recumbent. The unit is secured by an elastic band adjusted to stay around the occiput with minimum tension. Topical anesthetic is instilled and a clear plastic contact shell bearing a female receptacle on its convex surface is inserted between the lids onto the cornea. A spring-loaded dynamometer is then introduced through the slot in the aluminum bridge while the patient steadily fixates through the slotted bridge with the other eye.

For the initial or base reading, the tip of the dynamometer is rested in the receptacle of the contact lens. The position of the cornea is read in millimeters from the point

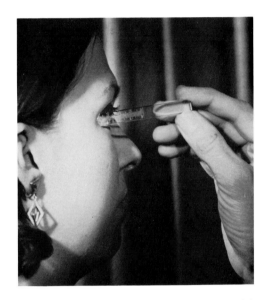

Fig. 16-4. Luedde exophthalmometer placed on right lateral orbital rim to measure linear distance from rim to corneal apex.

where an etched scale on the plunger of the dynamometer appears above the bridge. This figure should be recorded by an aide and then successive readings made with plunger loads of 100, 200, 300, and finally 400 gm. If the readings are done quickly, most patients do not find this uncomfortable, except for the maximum or 400-gm. pressure. A compression curve should then be plotted on the patient's record to indicate the reduction in exophthalmos in relation to increasing pressure. Expression of blood or soft edema fluid in the first 100 or 200 gm. of compressions usually accounts for a proportionately greater initial reduction in exophthalmos than is achieved with succeeding weights. In the presence of scirrhous orbital neoplasm, the compressibility curve may be quite flat from 0 to 400 gm.

The Copper instrument is a very accurate exophthalmometer and, as a piezometer, may theoretically aid in the differentiation of soft or vascular retrobulbar lesions (showing early, steep drop in the orbital compressibility curve) from hard neoplastic or infectious processes (showing flattening of the orbital compressibility curve). Thus a cavernous hemangioma or thyrotoxic exophthalmos might be expected to show distinct retrodisplacement of the globe with light pressure of 100 and 200 gm., whereas a meningioma, thyrotropic exophthalmos, or orbital cellulitis might show relatively less retrodisplacement (flattening of the curve) with the 100- and 200-gm. forces. However, just as in Mulvany's effort (1943) to categorize thyrotropic and thyrotoxic forms of Graves' disease, there are transitional or unclear

Fig. 16-5. Hertel reflecting exophthalmometer. Millimeter marks apparent on front surface of horizontal carrier bar should be noted after contact points of instrument are adjusted to lateral orbital rims; this facilitates same separation of reflecting mirrors on subsequent examinations. Millimeter scale indicating actual position of corneal surface anterior to orbital rim is read on sighting through the mirrors at each side. Rodenstock (Krahn) modification built with angled prisms instead of mirrors.

cases both to clinical and to orbitometric evaluation.*

Graves' disease itself suffers from a confusion of nomenclature including toxic diffuse goiter, Basedow's disease, and Parry's disease. The hyperophthalmic form of Graves' disease or endocrine exophthalmos has also lead to a century and a quarter of eponymic ecstasy since Dalrymple's name was attached to the appearance of upper lid retraction in 1852. Many other eponymic signs confound the literature. Among the more signal are von Graefe's upper lid lag on downward gaze

*J. M. Elsby has produced a modification of the Copper tonometer substituting a series of four 50-gm. weights for the spring dynamometer that may develop variations through the years. The Elsby scale—50, 100, 150, and 200 gm.—is thus just half of the Copper scale.

and von Stellwag's reduced frequency of blinking. Less compelling eponyms include Mobius' weakness of convergence, Gifford's difficulty in everting the upper lids, Rosenbach's lid tremor on gentle closing, Mean's globe lag on looking up, Baston's jerking downward motion, Suker's inability to hold fixation in extreme lateral gaze, Joffroy's absence of forehead creasing, Sainton's contraction of the frontalis with elevation, Snellen's bruit over the closed lids, Jellinek's (Rasin's, Tellais's) pigmentation of the upper lid, Enroth's puffiness of the lids, Kocher's increasing lid retraction of fixation, and others.

A more important functional classification of eye changes was developed by the staff of Columbia Presbyterian Medical Center, improved by the American Thyroid Associa-

Fig. 16-6. Copper orbital tonometer secured in position with elastic strap around occiput. Right contact lens is in place, and spring-loaded dynamometer is inserted through slot in bridge to engage in receptacle of contact lens.

Level	Mnemonic	Findings
0	N	No eye signs or symptoms
1	O	Only signs (lid retraction or stare, no symptoms)
2	S	Soft tissue involvement (tearing photophobia, lid or conjunctival edema)
3	P	Proptosis
4	E	Extraocular involvement (limitation of rotation, diplopia)
5	C	Corneal involvement
6	S	Sight loss caused by optic nerve involvement

tion, and published in 1969.* Further, a mnemonic NO SPECS has been adopted to indicate zero through six levels of eye changes. The first or zero level is "No signs" and each of the other six are subdivided into minimal, moderate, and marked.

In diagnosing very slight or questionably pathologic exophthalmos, it can be helpful to make measurements with the patient in the recumbent position in addition to the seated position. A slightly prominent globe in the absence of orbital pathology will normally show a bit less exophthalmos in the recumbent than in the sitting position. In the presence of endocrine ophthalmopathy

*Werner, S. C.: Classification of the eye changes in Graves' disease, J. Clin. Endocrinol. 29:982-984, July, 1969.

or orbital infiltration, such reduction does not occur.

The conscientious though sometimes puzzled diagnostician must be prepared from time to time to defer diagnosis and recommend reexamination in a few weeks. Repeating detailed measurements and studies may then yield far more information as to both basic nature and activity of a suspect process. Exploratory orbitotomy, differing from the more flexible confines of exploratory laparotomy, is a hazardous and significantly traumatic procedure. Generally it will not clear up deep enigmas unless they have been localized preoperatively to specific orbital depths, quadrants, and relationships to such structures as the extra-ocular muscle cone.

"Frequently a definitive decision must go by default until such time as the clinical evaluation of the case or its response to therapeutic assays makes tentative diagnosis possible or the opportunity arises for microscopic examination of the tissues. Even then the certainty is by no means always realized."

SIR STEWART DUKE-ELDER

REFERENCES

Copper, A. C.: Measurement of the retrojoulbar resistance (orbitonometry) in the clinic, Trans. Ophthalmol. Soc. U. K. 69:219-235, 1949.

Davanger, M.: Principles and sources of error in exophthalmometry, Acta Ophthalmol. 48:625-633, 1970.

Elby, J. M.: Orbitotonometer, Br. J. Ophthalmol. 52:355, 1968.

Ophthalmodynamometry and the diagnosis of carotid artery insufficiency

In the presence of amaurosis fugax, occlusion of the central retinal artery or its branches, or suspect carotid artery system impairments, it is diagnostically important to compare ophthalmic artery pressure on the two sides. Diastolic readings can be made first, but if significant difference (exceeding 20%) is not found, systolic readings should also be made. Other diagnostic evidence of arterial insufficiency disease may be gleaned by (1) auscultation for bruit in the ipsilateral neck or over either eye (Fig. 17-1), (2) palpation of the carotid arteries (Fig. 17-2) in the neck for thickening, reduction of pulsation, or thrill, (3) tonography for reduction of pulse waves, (4) x-ray examination of the skull for carotid system calcifications, (5) carotid system angiograms, (6) studies of the Doppler effect by continuous or nonpulsed, transcutaneous ultrasound, or (7) thermography.

Auscultation of the carotid artery is best done in the lateral aspect of the neck just anterior to the sternomastoid muscle. The patient should be asked to stop breathing briefly during auscultation so that breath sounds do not interfere with the detection of subtle murmurs. Localization is also enhanced by using the open-bell or Ford type fitting of small or pediatric diameter rather than a diaphragm type chest piece on the stethoscope (this instrument, of course, should preferably be called a stetho*phone*).

The absence of any carotid artery bruit means either no encroachment on the lumen or else complete occlusion. If the bruit is best heard high in the neck, this suggests stenosis in the area where the common carotid bifurcates into the internal and external carotid arteries. If the bruit is only heard low in the neck, it may represent transmitted cardiac sounds. Bruits heard primarily in the posterior triangles of the neck generally are not specific for carotid impairments but rather represent vertebral artery stenosis when heard on the right, or subclavian-vertebral artery stenosis when heard on the left. Murmurs heard best over the globes suggest stenosis in the intracranial portion of the carotid artery.

Palpation of the carotid arteries serves not only to compare the strength of pulsation and the vascular firmness or thickening on each side but may also yield tactile evidence of thrill when there is advanced stenosis. A thrill is a vibration or fremitus tactually detected by the fingertips and probably caused by eddies in the bloodstream beyond an area of narrowing. Thrills in carotid impairments are generally synchronous with cardiac systole and become increasingly apparent with increasing degrees of vascular narrowing. The thrill is most commonly related to the carotid system when felt high in the neck; its presence low in the neck may represent transmission from the heart (aortic valve stenosis) or aortic arch (coarctation or patent ductus). Generally it is not possible to palpate the *internal* carotid artery in the neck, but in a cooperative patient or with the assistance of topical anesthesia it is possible to feel this major vessel through the tonsillar fossa. Rarely a bruit or tactile thrill will come from an atheroma in the *external* carotid; usually this is without symptoms and surgery would be useless.

Tonographic tracings may be quite indicative of disturbances in the carotid lumen and wall. Narrowing of the lumen and reduced mural pulsations are manifest in the homolateral tonogram by reductions in pulse wave amplitude. Conversely, tonography in the presence of carotid cavernous fistula yields wide excursion in amplitude.

Conventional PA or lateral films of the skull show shadows of calcific accumulation in the carotid arteries in many mature and elderly individuals. Though frequent, these are always significant signs of serious pathologic alteration in the vessel walls. In older patients who are generally asymptomatic and without major impairments or physical findings, these bits of roentgen evidence may not call for further studies. In the younger patient, however, where there are symptoms and associated physical findings, such x-ray evidence may make further studies obligatory for potentially lifesaving interventions.

Carotid system angiograms are neuroradiologic studies that may now be done with high selectivity of vessels to be demonstrated by intra-arterial contrast injections. There are still, however, threats of mild morbidity and slight mortality (p. 251), so that a refer-

Fig. 17-1. Auscultation of the common carotid artery. Patient turns head 15° to opposite side and holds breath while an open bell or pediatric stethoscope is placed just anterior to the sternomastoid muscle.

ring ophthalmic examiner should have specific findings on which to support the request.

Doppler effect or frequency shift studies using ultrasound reflections from moving blood cells detect different velocities within the blood column. These are usually maximal in the center of the column and minimal near the vessel wall. They also detect alterations in blood flow rate as surge characteristics resulting from cardiac action. These compressions and rarefactions of ultrasonic waves are transferred to visual display on an oscilloscope, or the differences between emanated and reflected frequencies may be used as audible signals. The nonpulsed or continuous-wave ultrasound required for Doppler studies necessitates energy delivery at several logarithmic units greater than is used in time-amplitude (A-mode) diagnostic studies and therefore should be used for minimum periods of exposures. Since Doppler studies of vessels beneath soft tissue, such as the carotids, are qualitative rather than quantitative, it is necessary to compare right and left counterparts. Equipment, though simpler than that for time-amplitude ultrasound, is relatively expensive and more readily available in medical center settings than in clinical offices.

Thermographic apparatus* may run into investment of $15,000 to $45,000 and is primarily of investigational status in ocular diagnosis at present. It graphically creates thermal portraits in shades of gray or maps isothermic "contour lines" connecting selected heat levels. Temperature variations over the face commonly range through 10° C. from the

*Manufactured by Barnes Engineering Comp., Stamford, Connecticut, 06904; AGA Corp., Secaucus, New Jersey 07094.

Fig. 17-2. Palpation of carotid artery pulsation from behind, showing correct positioning of examiner's three fingers on the course of the artery. Right and left are compared simultaneously with gentle touch and never bilateral compression.

cool lashes and tip of the nose to the warm inner canthal area. It will record differences as slight as 0.1° C. and shows both focal and diffuse patterns of thermal increases (uveitis, arteritis, infections, neoplasms) and decreases (hemorrhage, retinal detachments, contusion edema, vascular occlusion) in tissue temperature. Ischemic areas as well as the specific paths of dilating collateral vessels can be quantitatively shown with complete objectivity (Fig. 17-3).

Ophthalmodynamometry produces more dynamic information and has less likelihood of dislodging emboli than either palpation or angiography. It is prerequisite for the patient to have two eyes, each with visible fundi, in order to accomplish this examination. Brachial artery sphygmomanometry should precede ophthalmodynamometry for comparative reference.

Under normal conditions of intraocular

Fig. 17-3. Normal thermogram of the orbits and midface. Relative heat scale shown across the lower edge indicates warmth (represented as darkness) and coolness (represented as lightness). The brows and nares can be seen as white or cool. The lips and inner canthal recesses appear as dark or warm. Corneal surfaces appear as intermediate grayness or coolness. Warm paths of the supraorbital vessels are indicated by dark lines extending upward through the nasal portion of the brow. (Thermogram produced on AGA Thermovision equipment, Secaucus, New Jersey 07094.)

pressure, intracranial pressure, and carotid system sufficiency, pulsations are not seen in the retinal arteriolar tree. Because the retinal vessels, however, are subject to an intraocular or tissue pressure of 15 to 20 mm. Hg rather than the much lower tissue pressure elsewhere in the body, a paradoxic venous pulsation is created during diastole in more than half of all normal persons. When intraocular pressure is increased by digital pressure, compression instruments, or glaucoma, rhythmic constrictions synchronous with cardiac diastole appear in the retinal arterioles. Conversely, when diastolic arterial pressure drops below intraocular pressure because of syncope, peripheral collapse, or aortic valvular insufficiency, pulsations also appear in the retinal arterioles. Further, a significant number of patients with increased intracranial pressure as from brain tumors, will show arterial pulsations as part of developing papilledema.

These physiologic principles underlie the measurement of ophthalmic artery pressure with the ophthalmodynamometer as developed by Paul Bailliart in 1917. In use, a topical anesthetic is instilled and ocular tension is measured by indentation or applanation. Dynamometry readings should first be made with the patient in the seated position. The patient is instructed to maintain steady fixation. The direct ophthalmoscope may be preferred to the indirect because of its greater magnification. With the ophthalmoscope in the hand corresponding to the patient's eye under examination, the dynamometer in the other hand is aligned with a diameter of the globe. The footplate is brought into contact with the lateral sclera, and pressure is evenly increased at the rate of about 20 gm. per second while the major retinal arterioles on the disc are kept under clear observation. Care must be taken not to angulate the dynamometer away from a position corresponding to a diamter or radius of the globe. This is often helped by steadying the instrument gently against the angulation of the outer canthus (Fig. 17-4).

Initial readings from the dial or scale may be made the moment an arterial pulsation is

Fig. 17-4. Linear type Bailliart ophthalmodynamometer aligned in use with an equatorial diameter of the globe and steadied against the outer canthus. Examiner watches central retinal artery pulsation as pressure is increased.

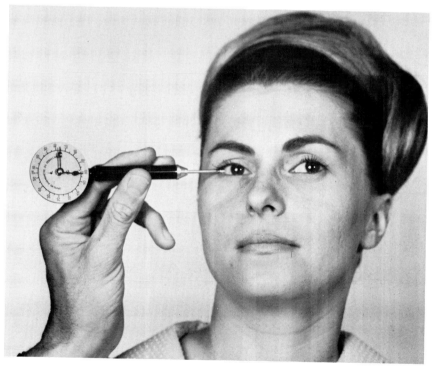

Fig. 17-5. Dial type Bailliart ophthalmodynamometer shown in correct radial position with footplate against right eye. Slave or passive indicator is resting above 80-unit mark and active indicator is shown lower near 40-unit level as pressure is being decreased from systolic to diastolic level.

evoked. A gross difference between right and left at this level may be quite diagnostic. This is an early or prediastolic value and some investigators prefer not to correlate readings with full diastole until the first completed arteriolar collapse is seen. Sustained arteriolar collapse indicates that systolic pressure has been reached.

The Bailliart spring dynamometers come in two designs: dial and linear. The dial type (Fig. 17-5) has two indicators—one active pointer connected to the spring load and equipped with a finger-controlled stop, and one passive or "slave" pointer, which remains at the highest reading. The cylinder or linear registering type reads directly from engravings on its piston and has a single stop button that can hold only one reading after removal from the eye. With either type, if the diastolic or low reading is made first (as the pressure is being increased) it is necessary for an assistant to note the diastolic reading while the examiner watches the retinal artery. The dial model offers an advantage if the systolic (higher) reading is made first; then the slave pointer will remain at this value and, on reduction of dynamometer pressure to the diastolic level (last pulsation), the finger-controlled stop can be engaged to hold the lower value. Thus both readings may be retained without the use of a second observer. Some examiners elect only to make diastolic readings, but this will miss a percentage of carotid insufficiencies.

The greatest difficulties in ophthalmodynamometry are maintaining perfectly radial position of the instrument to the eye and avoiding displacement of the eye from ophthalmoscopic observation. Because even slight inclinations of the instrument away from the radial position introduce gross errors, it is customary to make about three separate readings and to record the average.

Direct readings are in grams of pressure, but by plotting them against Schiøtz indentation tensions on the Magitot-Bailliart nomogram (1922), pressure in the ophthalmic artery may be derived in millimeters of mercury.

With Goldmann applanation tonometry values it is necessary to use the Bedavaija nomogram (1960). These figures, however, are subject to errors, and the comparative or relative values are of greater significance. Average normal systolic pressure in the ophthalmic artery as indicated by this technique varies between 60 and 85 mm. Hg. Average normal diastolic pressure varies between 30 and 40 mm. Hg or about one-half of brachial diastolic pressure.

If the diastolic pressure as found in each eye is more than 10 or 15 mm. Hg higher than the brachial diastolic pressure, it suggests increased intracranial pressure. Readings of the two eyes should agree within 10% to 15%. If either systolic or diastolic pressure is reduced by 20% or more on one side, this is excellent evidence of carotid system insufficiency proximal to the origin of the ophthalmic artery. If ophthalmic systolic and diastolic pressures are equal in the two eyes and in balance with brachial pressure, carotid system insufficiency can be excluded almost with certainty.

Slightly higher pressure readings and slightly less marked differential reductions may be found in the supine position, whereas slightly lower pressures and more marked differential reductions may be found in the standing position. When differences between right and left readings are borderline as determined in the sitting position, then examination in the standing position is often more definitive.

The Mueller recording electronic tonometer may also be converted to ophthalmodynamometry merely by inserting the appropriate transducer tip in place of the tonometer head. This automatically changes the recording scale units to read at an appropriately higher range for systolic and diastolic ophthalmic artery pressures. The Durham Applamatic Tonometer (Bausch & Lomb) is scaled only to 50 mm. Hg and therefore is not suitable for systolic readings in the present commercial form.

Applanation loading principles under slit lamp control offer new accuracy in observation of the larger retinal arterioles by a single examiner. The Sisler Dynoptor* (1974) offers undistorted slit lamp visualization of the disc along the same axis on which precise radial pressure is applied. This is an ingenious and simple modification of the

*American Optical Corp., Instrument Division, Buffalo, New York 14215.

Fig. 17-6. Sisler Dynoptor Ophthalmodynamometer evolved from Goldmann principles of applanation loading directly on corneal surface. Transparent −60D contact applanating head affords direct slit lamp view of optic nerve and major vessels during the process of loading. (American Optical Corp., Buffalo, New York 14215.)

Goldmann tonometer in which an 8-mm. diameter, −60 D contact lens for fundus examination replaces the contact biprism (Fig. 17-6). Spring resistance of the applanator is increased to deliver graded pressure to 150 grams. The Mackay-Marg Electronic Tonometer may also be adapted for ophthalmodynamometry and in any position but without the advantage of visual and pressured coincidence. For dynamometry the Mackay-Marg transducer tip must be applied to the cornea peripherally so that ophthalmoscopic visualization of the disc is not blocked. Use of a corneal rather than a bulbar conjunctival and scleral site for force application increases the precision of pressure transmission particularly in the Sisler unit. As in tonometric use, it is essential that the axis of pressure be maintained radially on a true diameter of the globe; otherwise a degradation of the force valve occurs.

In 1975 Berkeley Bio-Engineering modified their recording Mackay-Marg tonographer, adding a large Krieger type direct contact lens with a temporally placed receptacle for the transducer tip (Stepanik 770). The lens and tip, coupled in a rim-like collar, are held between the thumb and forefinger of the examiner's left hand for the patient's right eye (or right hand for the patient's left eye) at a slit lamp. Strip recorder and digital readout are presented. Both the Sisler Dynoptor and this instrument can be used only with the patient in the sitting position.

These applanators offer more accuracy and consistency than do spring loaded devices and are more conveniently verified. Such applanators require variable rather than fixed force, and thus rule out Halberg, Barraquer, or the Heine-Bruun-Jensen type instruments even with the use of heavier gravitational weights. Available applanation pressures must be able to exceed average systolic pressures in the ophthalmic artery and these normally are approximately 85 mm. Hg.

Other procedures, better described as "orbital plethysmography," have been evolved using water-filled goggles ("pulsensors") or latex balloons against the lids and orbits that sense resultants of many forces within the eye and orbit. Sometimes their use is referred to as "ophthalmodynamography," but the figures derived are difficult to relate to any single vascular component. Further validation is needed.

Suction ophthalmodynamometry is a variation in technique that increases intraocular pressure by the use of a perilimbal suction-cup apparatus of hemispheric configuration attached to the lateral aspect of the globe. By use of a built-in 50-ml. syringe, vacuum force is created and measured up to 600 mm. Hg. Suction of 500 mm. Hg will raise intraocular pressure to approximately 140 mm. Hg with some accompanying corneal distortion.

Generally, values obtained by the suction technique are higher than those obtained by the Bailliart method. This technique is less well established than is compression ophthalmodynamometry.

Careful history of arterial occlusive episodes plus physical examination by palpation, auscultation, and ophthalmodynamometry often yield a definitive working diagnosis of insufficiency disease of the arterial supply to the globe or localization to a major carotid arterial component. However, more specific and graphic localization is generally desired by a vascular surgeon before electing to do corrective surgery. The most finite step in diagnosis is carotid angiography by injection of radiopaque contrast medium, usually through the brachial artery. Because there is mild morbidity (conjunctival hemorrhage, transient contralateral weakness in the extremities), or infrequent mortality, the indication for such x-ray studies should be appreciated and organized by the eye examiner. The following general principles should be met before undertaking angiography:

1. The patient should be relatively well, without suffering a major stroke or other life threatening disease.
2. Transient ischemic attacks should correspond to the area of suspect arterial insufficiency.
3. Bruit or thrill should be present in the suspect artery to suggest a pathologic compromise but not complete occlusion of the vascular lumen.
4. Ophthalmodynamometry should be low on the involved side.
5. No other diseases that could explain the symptoms exist.

Increasing representation of older persons in the population is producing an increasing incidence of vascular insufficiency diseases, arterial occlusions, or ischemic disturbances. With a high coefficient of correlation, such disturbances in the ocular fundus indicate carotid system insufficiencies. As a working dictum, central retinal artery occlusion should be considered carotid system insufficiency disease until proved otherwise, as should the presumptive diagnosis of "ischemic optic neuritis" in a patient of advanced years. Thus ophthalmodynamometry is more frequently needed now than it was a few decades ago to achieve optimal interpretative value from fundus findings. With these techniques, the examiner again not only achieves diagnostic information concerning arterial supply of the eye but may also gain lifesaving information from a grossly uninvolved eye.

REFERENCES

Best, M., and Rogers, R.: Techniques of ocular pulse analysis in carotid stenosis, Arch. Ophthalmol. 92: 54, 1974.

Bronner, A., et al.: Thermography of the oculo orbital region, Klin. Monatsbl. Augenheilkd. 160:13, 1972.

Guibor, P., and Keeney, A. H.: Thermography and ophthalmology, Trans. Am. Acad. Ophthalmol. & Otolaryngol. 74:1032-1043, Sept.-Oct., 1970.

Hyman, B. N.: Dappler ultrasonography for assessment of carotid artery disease, Am. J. Ophthalmol. 77:227-231, 1971.

Knox, D. L.: Ocular pressure studies in the diagnosis of carotid artery disease, Trans. Am. Ophthalmol. Soc. 71:459, 1973.

Sayegh, F.: Comparison of ophthalmodynamographic and dynamometric measurements, Ophth. Research 1:201-210, 1970.

Sisler, H. A.: Optical corneal pressure ophthalmodynamometry, Am. J. Ophthalmol. 74:964-966, Nov., 1972.

Fundus photography and fluorescein angiography

Patrick R. O'Connor, M.D.

Fundus examination in its ophthalmoscopic aspects now benefits from the many advantages of photography such as (1) detailed permanent record, (2) magnification of 2.5× to 10×, (3) recording in monochromatic light for occasional accentuation of aspects that may otherwise be inapparent, (4) study of contrast dye injection angiography, (5) rapid sequence recording of dye passage or active vascular changes, and (6) later and leisurely study of the fundus after the patient's visit.

Ease, economy, and excellence have been introduced into this phase of examination, particularly since World War II, by vast technologic improvements in cameras and light sources, by refinements in speed and detail capacity of both black and white and color film, and by clinical need for fundus information on which to base treatment decisions concerning photocoagulation, laser intervention, vitrectomy, or enucleation in questions such as subretinal hematoma versus malignant melanoma of the choroid.

THE PHOTOGRAPHER

Fundus photography may be particularly beneficial in finding and focusing significant pathology or in bringing out precise details if the clinician makes the pictures himself. More commonly, however, in university centers, schools, or clinics serving several or more examiners, a skilled photographer is given full responsibility for this work including loving, dust-free maintenance of equipment and, at least, supervision in processing of the film. This photographer should be an expert with both the direct and indirect ophthalmoscopes. He must be familiar with the normal topography and landmarks of the fundus as well as the types and characteristics of alterations produced by pathology. Investment of a few moments from time to time by the clinician to demonstrate pathologic changes to the photographer will yield, over the months and years, steadily increased excellence of photographic records and conservation of time for the patient, the clinician, and the photographer.

Incidentally, the clinician must be certain that the photographer has and wears any appropriate refraction correction that he needs. Young and nonpresbyopic photographers, as well as those having even mild or modest refractive errors, will often have marked difficulty in attaining or maintaining maximum focus of the viewing lens. Their spectacles should be prescribed under cycloplegic examination and then the distance correction consistently worn for this work.

The photographer must be intimately familiar with the working controls and variations in the camera settings. He should have a knowledge of basic photographic principles and a working understanding of the optics of fundus cameras.

High quality and consistency in fundus photographs are determined more by how the camera is maintained and used than by which make of camera is employed. A systematic routine both considerate of the patient and technically complete must be followed.

THE CAMERA

After a few decades of unsuccessful attempts in many countries, the first satisfactory fundus photographs were presented by Friedrich Dimmer of Vienna in 1899 (IX International Congress of Ophthalmology). Unfortunately his apparatus was very cumbersome, being literally as large as a grand piano. Dimmer's technique was not published until 1911 and his process was not functionally repeated.

In 1922 J. W. Nordenson of Uppsala presented his compact table-top camera based on the Gullstrand principles (International Congress of Ophthalmology, Washington, D.C.). After more than 9 years of refinement, this self-contained, carbon arc camera was marketed in 1926 and was widely ac-

claimed. The first English language atlas of fundus photography was published in 1928 by Arthur Bedell using one of these cameras (Mann, 1970).

Another great dimension in fundus photography was added by the introduction of Kodachrome film in the early 1930s. The Bausch and Lomb camera (1950) served to maintain some capability in fundus photography until 1955 when G. Littmann developed the modern Carl Zeiss fundus camera (Fig. 18-1). This camera is now essentially the basic standard of all other instruments in the field, such as Topcon (1971) model TRC-F1 and the three-times faster TRC-F3, Nikon Retinapan, Maniya, Olympus, and the Clinitex 100° field. Two reliable hand-held fundus cameras—the Kowa RC-2 (Fig. 18-2) and the Nikon Retinal Hand Camera—are also available.

Details and instructions in this chapter re-

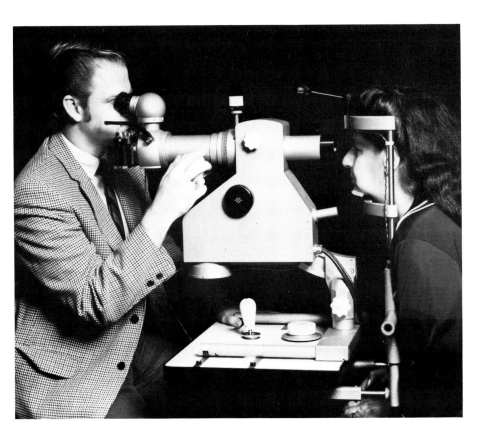

Fig. 18-1. Carl Zeiss fundus camera in use showing photographer's right hand on fine focusing adjustment and patient properly seated with fixation device before her right eye.

Fig. 18-2. Kowa RC2 Fundus Camera is useful as hand-held instrument or it may be mounted on slit lamp base. Power pack unit is shown at right.

Fig. 18-3. Light path through the standard Carl Zeiss fundus cameras. *1,* Electronic flash bulb; *2,* double filament incandescent illuminating system; *3,* glass plate; *4,* diaphragm disc to rotate different apertures into illuminating beam; *5,* mirror; *6,* aspheric objective lens; *7,* patient's eye; *8,* spherical corrective lenses; *9,* cross cylindrical lenses to compensate for astigmatism in patient's eye; *10,* collecting or focal lens system; *11,* tiltable mirror; *12,* camera back; *13,* eyepiece reticule; *14,* fixation target attachment.

late primarily to the Carl Zeiss fundus camera* (Fig. 18-3), because it has become a standard of excellence, and secondarily to the Kowa RC-2† hand-held camera, because of its excellence and originality in this type of equipment.

ROUTINE TECHNIQUE
Preliminary preparation of patient

As in all procedures requiring patient participation and ocular fixation, it is essential to explain briefly what is to be anticipated and to build confidence with soft, courteous words coupled with sure and direct actions. Topical anesthetics should be avoided before fundus photography since they tend to soften the epithelium or disturb the precorneal tear film and in turn interfere with the necessary corneal clarity for sharp imagery. This precludes manipulations such as retinography, tonography, gonioscopy, lacrimal probing, or corneal staining before photography. Similarly, protracted examinations by indirect ophthalmoscopy with scleral depression, or even repeated direct ophthalmoscopy by multiple examiners, may cause some drying or subsequent epithelial disturbance and should not be done immediately before photographic sessions.

The pupils must be dilated to at least 7 mm. in diameter (somewhat more if stereoscopic photographs are to be made). Dilatation is necessary to transmit the illuminating ring of light into the fundus, and complete cycloplegia is also necessary to stabilize the position of the image. The Zeiss fundus camera, like most instruments of this type, utilizes indirect ophthalmoscopy and a real aerial image that is focused by the ophthalmoscopic lens of the camera. Thus accommodative action by the patient will shift the aerial image of his fundus forward and backward to the frustration of the photographer trying to maintain a sharp focus.

Cyclopentolate (Cyclogyl) alone gives ex-

cellent mydriasis and cycloplegia without undesirable disturbance of the corneal epithelium, but it may take more than a half hour for maximum effect and cause some accommodative impairment for 3 or 4 hours. A more rapidly acting combination of drugs with shorter duration is 1 drop of 1% Mydriacyl repeated in 3 minutes and followed in another 3 minutes by 1 drop of 10% viscous Neo-Synephrine. The viscous solution of Neo-Synephrine should be used instead of the aqueous, which may disturb the epithelial clarity, or the emulsion, which may leave disturbing bubbles in the precorneal film. The usual precautions must be observed in the presence of a shallow anterior chamber or of a history of angle-closure glaucoma. When dilatation is elected in this situation, a weak miotic such as 1% pilocarpine should be instilled several times after photography and the patient retained in the office until miosis is achieved.

The use of mydriatics and cycloplegics is time consuming and uncomfortable to the patient, especially when serial photographs are used to record retinal changes. In this situation Choromokos and Kneeper (1973) have described a sometimes useful technique of retinal photography through a pupil that is dilated by darkness. After dimming room lights, the camera is focused with minimal illumination of the observation light. All light sources are then extinguished and the pupil is allowed to dilate in the dark room for several seconds before photographs are taken.

The patient should be seated comfortably on a sturdy chair of adequate size. A secretarial posture chair is quite satisfactory. When using the hand fundus camera, better control and patient comfort are secured with the patient lying down.

Preliminary preparation of equipment

Before the patient is brought into the darkened camera room the equipment should be checked. The proper camera back should be attached and contain adequate amounts of the desired film. Kodachrome II (ASA 25) is excellent for color transparencies. High-

*Carl Zeiss, Inc., Oberkochen, Federal Republic of Germany.
†Kowa Co., Ltd., Nagoya, Japan.

Speed Ektachrome (ASA 160) is desirable when using the Kowa RC-2 because of its lower flash intensity. Kodak Plus X (ASA 125) is adequate for black and white photography.

Color Polaroid film type 108 is useful for immediate documentation, side by side comparison of right and left fundi where there are borderline changes, or demonstration of ocular pathology to the patient or referring practitioner.

Dallow (1974) has demonstrated clinical application of color infrared sensitive film. Its unique properties of altered contrast, increased penetration through tissues, and color changes (elimination of the blue end of the spectrum) enhance the definition of pigmented tumors and choroidal vasculature.*

The photographer must be sure that the relay circuit or flash synchronization cord is properly inserted into the "X" receptacle on the camera back, and must check to see whether or not the 2× magnification lens is in place, depending on the planned use. This magnification accessory, which locks between the objective lens system and the camera, increases the image size from a standard 22.5-mm. diameter to utilization of the entire 24 × 36-mm. film area, but also increases the light intensity requirements. The lower magnification should be used on all initial and survey photographs.

The photographer should focus the eyepiece to bring the cross hairs into maximum sharpness for his own eye. He should set the control knobs on the top of the camera for cross cylinder astigmatic correction to 0 diopters and axis 90 degrees, except for the occasional patient with high astigmatism who requires interposition of compensatory lenses to attain sharp focus throughout the image field. On the right side of the camera, the control knob for the Rekoss disc (−16 to +17 diopters) should be set at the red printed number or alternate spherical diopterage range as needed to compensate for high myopia, hyperopia, or aphakia.

The diaphragm selector knob on the left side of the camera should be set to bring the

largest aperture, No. 7, (the 14-mm. diameter opening on the older models or the bull's eye opening of newer models) into the light path.

The power supply should be turned on at this time and the focusing light intensity placed at the medium or No. 2 setting. Flash number intensity should be correspondingly set at II when Kodachrome II is being used without the magnification attachment or at IV if the attachment is used. For color Polaroid film type 108 the intermediate flash setting III is used. The photographer must make knowledgeable adjustments in flash intensity for extremely light or dark fundi. In an albino patient or one with a large coloboma of the retina and choroid, flash brightness would be reduced to setting I while using Kodachrome II film. In a Negro or darkly pigmented eye, flash intensity must usually be increased to No. III.

Final positioning of patient

With the patient comfortably seated, elevation of the table and chinrest are adjusted to the height and position of the patient. A few moments of adjustment here will generally yield both a shorter and a more suc-

Fig. 18-4. Fundus photograph of posterior pole with Carl Zeiss fundus camera showing fixation target. This auxiliary device is particularly helpful in securing fixation of the one-eyed patient or the individual with poor vision in the other eye. It also serves to document the pattern of monocular fixation.

---

*Kodak Ektachrome Infrared ARO film type 8443.

cessful photographic session. Extraneous lights should be eliminated to reduce possible disturbances in the patient's fixation. In keeping with the usual dictum, the *right* eye is photographed first. Therefore the camera base is displaced to the photographer's left and the fixation device is placed 2 or 3 in. in front of the patient's left eye. Final adjustment in position of the eye being photographed is secured by moving the fixation light before the opposite eye.

The one-eyed patient or the patient with loss of central vision in the opposite eye must concentrate on maintaining his fixation in the center of the camera barrel. This difficulty can be reduced by installation of an auxiliary fixation target into any model of the Zeiss camera. This creates a small black shadow on the final picture (Fig. 18-4). Its use, however, is limited to posterior polar photography, where it is particularly valuable in documenting fixation patterns. It is not a helpful stimulus or target for photography of the peripheral retina.

The patient should not be instructed to hold both eyes widely open until the photographer is completely ready to trip the shutter. The overly cooperative patient can develop epithelial drying by volitionally refraining from blinking during the preliminaries to actual film exposure.

Final focusing of camera

The lens cap, which is kept in place as much of the time as possible to minimize dust and finger smudges, is now removed.

The joy stick, located in the center of the instrument table top, is the most important control in positioning of the illuminating light ring. The joy stick should never be completely free nor forced into tight lock. With slight release, the entire system can be moved in any horizontal direction. Final vertical positioning is secured by manually rotating the large horizontal control knob in front of the joy stick. Fine focusing in depth to and from the patient is controlled by the coupled, large knobs on either side of the camera barrel.

For these adjustments the photographer must look around or to one side of the camera using his direct visualization of the patient's eye to control centering of the light ring—or bull's eye—in the dilated pupil. The light ring is brought into sharp focus on the cornea over the pupil and then the joy stick partially snugged by rotation toward the locking position.

Final verification of uniform illumination and critical focusing is done through the camera eyepiece. If the desired field is not in focus, this is corrected by movement of the fixation device. Edge blurring in any one meridian suggests astigmatic distortion that may require correction by adjustment of the cross cylinder as controlled through the knobs on top of the camera. Crescents of light reflection (limbal catoptric image) at any edge of the field indicate that the illuminating ring is eccentrically displaced over the limbus at that area. Correction is made by tilting the joy stick to the opposite side if the bright crescent is lateral or by moving the camera vertically away from the crescent if it is apparent at the upper or lower edge of the field. If such bright reflection completely encircles the field, the camera is too close to the eye and must be withdrawn slightly. A diffuse gray haze over the entire field occurs when the camera is too far away from the eye. When illumination is proper and even, final snugging of the joy stick is completed. The photographer now makes final adjustment of the camera position to be certain that both the structures of interest and the cross hairs in the eyepiece are in crisp focus.

The patient is now asked to make a final blink to smooth his tear film and then to hold both eyes widely open. The shutter is tripped with the right hand, and then the film is wound or advanced for the next exposure.

Photographing the peripheral fundus

Focusing the extreme periphery often calls for ingenuity. Moderate displacement of the field can be achieved merely by rotating the eye, the camera, or both. A vertical arc adjustment affording 20 degrees of upward or downward camera angulation is available for the table-model Zeiss camera. Often it is

Fig. 18-5. Detail of vertical arc adjustment in left side mounting of the Carl Zeiss fundus camera. This affords 20 degrees of upward or downward angulation, in five-degree stops, from the horizontal position. (Allen Stereo Separator [1964] is shown attached to camera back for optic production of stereo-paired photographs.)

necessary to angulate the patient's face for access to the periphery. Aperture No. 7 should still be used for these oblique positions, but often there will be meridional distortion when focusing beyond the equator. Trial and error use of the cross cylinder astigmatic correction system will usually improve focusing in the far periphery (Fig. 18-5).

At times the hand-held camera offers an advantage in photographing the far periphery in the presence of spinal deformities or under anesthesia in the operating room.

EXTENT OF THE PHOTOGRAPHED FIELD

The Zeiss and most other cameras of this type encompass a field of about 30 degrees. This is displayed as a 22-mm. diameter disc on the film when no auxiliary magnification is used. The photographer should realize,

however, that all of the light that will form the real aerial image emerges through a 2-mm. diameter spot in the center of the pupil and within the larger ring of illuminating light. The image as formed on the film is magnified about 2.5× to 10×.

Clinitex, Inc.* introduced in 1974 a fundus camera for wide-angle retinal photography of 100° and which will automatically recycle at one frame per second. This is a progressive development above the Nikon Retinapan, which in the early 1970s offered an approximately 50% increase in coverage of the retina as compared to the standard Zeiss unit. Pomerantzeff and his Medical Instrument Research Associates of Boston have developed a prototype ocular contact camera capable of retinal photographic breadth of 180°.

*Clinitex, Inc., Danvers, Massachusetts 01923.

FLUORESCEIN FUNDUS PHOTOGRAPHY (FLUORESCEIN ANGIOGRAPHY)

In 1961 the medical student H. R. Novotny and the budding young intern D. L. Alvis of Indiana University published their original and now classical report on "Photographing Fluorescence in Circulating Blood in the Human Retina" by the use of a sterile sodium fluorescein solution injected into an antecubital vein. Fluorescein is one of many compounds that absorbs light principally of one wavelength and subsequently emits part of this light as fluorescence at a longer wavelength. Novotny and Alvis' spectrofluorometric data on blood-fluorescein mixtures indicated that the wavelength of maximum absorption or activation is in the blue range of the visible spectrum at 490 mμ. The emanation maximum is in the green-yellow range at about 520 to 525 mμ. Because of its molecular weight, 332, it does not diffuse out of the retinal vessels, but rather will reveal pathologic leaks. Fluorescein, however, normally diffuses throughout the choroid and therefore is not specific for delineating pathologic diffusion in this level.

Filters and films

For fluorescein fundus photography, two additional filters must be inserted in the camera. A blue gelatin filter (Wratten No. 47 or Baird Atomic* interference filter B4) is placed in the light path of the illuminating system to eliminate the longer wavelengths from both the electronic flash and the incandescent viewing lamp and yet to allow the maximum amount of appropriate, exciting light to reach the fundus. This is called the *exciter filter*. The second filter is a yellowish color† (Wratten No. 15) and is placed directly in the camera back to cut out the reflected blue light and yet transmit the maximum amount of greenish yellow fluorescence to the film. This is called the *barrier filter*.

Of the many types and brands of film, Kodak TRI-X (ASA 400) is readily available, relatively inexpensive, and highly sensitive in the fluorescent wavelength. When properly developed it will yield fine detail. When immediate documentation and analysis are desired Polaroid type 107 can be used.

Timing and recycling

Because timing of the various phases of fundus fluorescence is of differential diagnostic importance, there is increasing need for rapid exposure rates. Cardiovascular physicians also have interest in measures of circulation times from antecubital injection to appearance in the eye. Because of the higher flash intensities needed, standard power packs are relatively slow in recycling and may require as much as 15 to 30 seconds for some instruments. This is far too slow for photographic recording of circulatory events in the fundus as indicated by dye passage.

Many modifications and adaptations of power supply have been evolved to meet the needs for rapid recycling, including motion picture recording. The Robert Bussey unit, essentially custom-made in Kendall, Florida, will recycle the standard Carl Zeiss camera to one exposure per second. The 1973 Carl Zeiss Fundus Flash III provides a speed sequence selector to 2 c.p.s. Dyonics* now produce power systems for the Zeiss camera.†

Cooling of the power supply is a progressively more demanding task as the rate of recycling is advanced. These power units therefore have become table-height, caster-based consoles more suitable to special photographic laboratories than to private offices.

A Data Box Clock Module is available from

---

*Baird Atomic Inc., Bedford, Massachusetts 01730.
†Formerly a greenish Wratten No. 58 was used as a barrier filter, but it allows more of the blue exciting light to reach the film and gives less contrast than can be achieved with the No. 15.

*Woburn, Massachusetts 01801; successor to ULE, Inc., 1963-1968, and also Iota-Cam Corp.
†Auxiliary Charging Units (ACU) were also introduced in 1974 by Lepa Electronics Products (LEP), Scarsdale, New York.

Dyonics or Zeiss to print the time on each film frame optically.

Many thousands of dollars can be invested in these elaborate refinements of fluorescein fundus studies, and high precision records may thereby be produced. The attentive clinician, however, can gain much fundamental information, particularly about the presence and localization of vascular leaks, the identification of hemangiomata, differentiation of "pseudo-optic neuritis" from true papilledema or malignant tumors from hematomata, and other similarly important distinctions merely by ophthalmoscopic observation of the fundus events as the dye passes through its various phases of circulation. It is, of course, necessary for the ophthalmoscope to be fitted with the appropriate exciter and barrier filters.

The dye

Though other contrast dyes have been used experimentally, sodium fluorescein has now been administered to thousands of patients in many areas of the world and is well understood as to both its optic properties and its very low incidence of toxic reactions.

A few variations in amounts and concentrations of dye have been employed. Thousands of studies have been done using a 5-ml. injection of 10% sodium fluorescein solution in an aqueous buffer.* This is a low volume injection affording distinct arterial identification. Others use a 5- or 10-ml. injection of 5% sodium fluorescein or a lesser volume of 25% fluorescein. Dosage is reduced for small children. A following injection of sterile saline may or may not be given.

Transient nausea occurring 15 to 20 seconds after injection is reported in about 5% of patients. This seems particularly associated with rapid injection. Vomiting or sweating occurs in less than 0.5% of patients; hives and syncope each may occur in something less than 0.2% of patients. Localized throm-

bophlebitis has been noted, and a repeat coronary occlusion during such study has occurred.

The syringe containing fluorescein may be connected to a short sterile plastic extension tube with attached needle. A 0.1 cc. test dose of fluorescein may be injected intravenously at least 2 min. prior to angiography to rule out anaphylactic sensitivity. The entire system is taped in place on the patient's arm for 10 min. after dye injection to facilitate any possible emergency drug administration.

Patients should be advised of yellowish discoloration that will be noted in the urine for about 48 hours following injection. Inquiry should be made concerning dye, drug, or chemical sensitivity and also any history of marked allergy or anaphylaxis that might predispose to fluorescein reaction.

An emergency tray containing sterile syringes, epinephrine (Adrenalin), an antihistamine such as diphenhydramine hydrochloride (Benadryl), morphine sulfate, or similar preparations should always be available in the camera room.

Extravasation of the dye about the injection site will cause some pain and local reaction, but this subsides within a few days.

Phases of dye manifestation in the fundus

Appearance of the fluorescein dye either under direct visualization or by serial photographic record can reveal details of ocular pathology completely undetectable by other clinical means. Fluorescence may be *intravascular* (choroidal, arterial, venous), *transmitted* (through defects in normally opaque overlying structures, as is the case in early arterial fluorescence through angioid streaks), *staining or leakage* (as through localized vascular defects in central serous retinopathy or widespread vascular defects in diabetic retinopathy), or *pseudofluorescence* (artifactually apparent over nonpigmented areas of the fundus late or several hours after injection).

The time phases are, first, the very early or *choroidal* phase (Fig. 18-6, *A*), which appears 8 to 10 seconds after injection and

*Funduscein (10%) SMP Div. of Cooper Labs, Inc., San German, Puerto Rico 00753.

progresses to a diffuse mottling throughout the posterior pole (Fig. 18-6, *B*), except for the macular area. Cilioretinal arteries, if present, are usually seen in this phase or in the early arterial phase, which follows. In the *early arterial phase* (Fig. 18-6, *C*) the retinal arteries are beginning to be outlined. Drusen, if present, light up in this phase and persist as bright dots of fluorescence as long as there is much circulating dye. Retinal pigment epithelial defects, if present, light up in this phase and persist as

bright dots of fluorescence as long as there is moderate circulating dye.

The *late arterial phase* (Fig. 18-6, *D*) shows all of the retinal arteries in bold contrast. This filling is usually completed in 1 or 2 seconds but may be delayed 5 to 20 seconds in central retinal artery occlusion. The *arteriovenous phase* (Fig. 18-6, *E*) 15 to 25 seconds after injection shows filling of all the retinal veins, but the arteries are still visible though with reducing brightness. In the early part of this phase the veins may

Fig. 18-6. Normal fluorescein fundus angiograms in left eye with cilioretinal artery. **A**, Early choroidal phase (8 to 10 sec. after injection). **B**, Choroidal background filling in full choroidal phase. **C**, Early arterial phase with filling of a cilioretinal artery. **D**, Late arterial phase with early lamellar flow in venules.

Continued.

Fig. 18-6, cont'd. **E,** Arteriovenous phase with lamellar flow in venules. **F,** Full arteriovenous phase. **G,** Late arteriovenous phase. **H,** Late venous phase with residual lamellar flow in veins and choroidal flush; this may persist for 10 to 15 min. after injection.

manifest lamellar variations in brightness, whereas later in the phase such findings occur in the arteries (Fig. 18-6, *E*).

The next or *venous phase* (Fig. 18-6, *G*) is marked by fading of the arterial fluorescence. Diabetic neovascularization and disciform macular lesions of low-grade chorioretinal inflammatory origin begin to be apparent at this time. The *late venous phase* (Fig. 18-6, *H*) beginning 3 or 4 minutes after injection shows less arterial pattern and intense staining about disciform or ap-

parently inflammatory macular lesions, which may persist for 15 to 30 minutes after injection.

The *recirculation phase* persists 10 to 12 minutes after the venous phase and presents even distribution of dye in all vascular components. The background or choroidal fluorescence also continues up to a total of about 25 or 30 minutes after injection.

Pseudofluorescence is a variously interpreted expression that should be reserved for luminescence after filling, which may persist for many hours against a nonpigmented or reflective background, such as an atrophic nerve head or a coloboma of the choroid and retina. This is caused by blue light excitation of fluorescein particles normally remaining in the vitreous and aqueous for a day or so after injection. Very little incident light returns through these particles except over white or high reflection areas.

Color fluorescein angiography, differential fluorescent angiography, and angiography of the iris and limbus extend the usefulness of this technique. Gass has made significant contributions toward understanding a wide range of choroidal and retinal diseases through fluorescein angiography; his stereoscopic atlases are standard references.

Fundus photography is an excellent method of keeping accurate documentation of disease and objective evidence of response or progression. The addition of vital contrast studies with intravenous fluorescein gives new dimensions to identification of pathologic processes and places us a step closer to fundamental understanding of disease mechanisms. Without question, the use of intravenous fluorescein techniques has saved eyes that might have been enucleated for choroidal hemorrhages or hemangiomata of the choroid. Similarly it has identified localized extramacular vascular leaks now suitable for photocoagulation therapy and has postponed major visual loss in some such eyes.

REFERENCES

Choromokos, E. A., and Knepper, P. A.: Retinal photography without mydriatics and cycloplegics, Am. J. Ophthalmol. **76**:1008-1009, 1973.

Flower, R. W. and Patz, A.: A viewer for correlation of fluorescein and color fundus photographs, Invest. Ophthalmol. **13**:398-401, 1974.

Hayreh, S. S.: Recent advances in fluorescent fundus angiography, Br. J. Ophthalmol. **58**:391, 1974.

Mann, W. A.: History of photography of the eye, Survey Ophthalmol. **15**:179-189, 1970.

Novotny, H. R., and Alvis, D. L.: A method of photographing fluorescence in circulating blood in the human retina, Circulation **24**:82, 1961.

Diagnostic steps in dyslexia and reading retardation

"Reading retardation" and the unmodified term "dyslexia" are generic designations covering a host of etiologic mechanisms, both endogenous and exogenous, that play adverse roles in accomplishment of the reading task. Inability to read may further be a developmental defect associated with subtle disturbances in neurologic growth, or it may be an acquired defect from a clearly recognizable lesion of the parietotemporal lobe. In the latter case, the loss of a previously existing function should be termed "alexia."

Because the eye is the major sensory input route for the cortical process of symbol interpretation and association, it is understandable that parents and patients alike request ocular examination when faced with these problems, even though the eye itself rarely is the primarily offending organ. In order to organize proper diagnostic steps, the following classification will remind the examiner of the many mechanisms that can be involved.

All classifications in biology and medicine are provisional in character, by nature of the evolving science. Until every etiologic mechanism is identified and isolated, it will be helpful to continue some functional nosology.

Comprehensive classification of the dyslexias

A. Specific (primary) developmental dyslexia (strephosymbolia or dyssymbolia): inability or difficulty in the cortical process of symbol interpretation appearing in individuals of average or high performance I.Q. and with functionally adequate sensory input mechanisms; appears predominantly in males and has a dominant genetic inheritance

B. Symptomatic (secondary) dyslexia (secondary reading retardation)
   1. Secondary to organic brain pathology (brain damage, cerebral dysfunction, other encepha-
lopathy, cerebral palsy, mental retardation, low I.Q., visual agnosia, anomia, soft neurologic stigmata)
      a. Genetically determined
      b. Posttraumatic (prenatal, natal, postnatal)
      c. Postinflammatory (intrauterine or extrauterine encephalitis, meningitis)
      d. Asphyxic (intrauterine, extrauterine)
      e. Prematurity
      f. Other specific brain lesion (aneurysm, meningioma, porencephalic cyst, others)
   2. Secondary to slow maturation (late bloomer, developmental delay)
   3. Secondary to emotional disturbances (hyperactivity, depression, anxiety)
   4. Secondary to uncontrolled seizure states
   5. Secondary to environmental disturbances (cultural deprivation, poor motivation, poor instruction)

C. Slow reading (handicap without symbolic confusion)
   1. Ocular impediment to sustained visual use (hyperopia, heterophoria, astigmatism, partial cataracts, retinal and macular abiotrophies)
   2. Auditory impairment
   3. Hypothyroid state

D. Alexia or acquired dyslexia: lesions usually in the region of the angular gyrus of the dominant hemisphere

E. Mixed types

DIAGNOSTIC STEPS
History

At least one additional question must always be asked in examination of the seemingly healthy child: "How is he doing in school?" Parents are occasionally reluctant to indicate that they are seeking consultation because of an inability to read, and they nearly always minimize or deny any reading difficulty in the father or older generations, though they will acknowledge it in the patient's siblings. Scholastic achievement in arithmetic as well as in reading and spelling should be delineated, because the dyslexic child will usually have more difficulty with reading than with arithmetic and most trouble of all with dictated spelling. It is a rare dyslexic patient, however, who has no trouble at all with arithmetic, and his difficulty is enhanced in higher grades of school when mathematic problems are posed in words.

Though predictor factors are being sought at the age of 5 (de Hirsch, 1966), dyslexia, of course, cannot be diagnosed until the patient is at an adequate age and culture for reading.

Ocular examination

The usual steps of preliminary inspection, preliminary examination, determination of acuity, refraction, and ocular motility, as well as fundus examination, must be done as in any case. In measuring acuity, the perceptive examiner can usually tell if the child is unable to identify letters or is unable to see them. This should be recorded. Usually reading is not possible without an underlying ability to handle the individual building blocks of words.

Optic defects (hyperopia, astigmatism, impairments of the media, and so on) have been shown to have no relation to symbol interpretation, but they must be identified. If of significant magnitude, they may lead to ocular fatigue or asthenopia, which reduces the effective learning and attention span. Under these conditions they merit conventional therapy. Similarly, moderate degrees of heterophoria that may occasionally break into heterotropia can have a limiting effect on educational application and should be corrected where they are significant in their own right, particularly where difficulties in the reading-learning process coexist.

Although it is true that man reads with his brain and not with his eyes, patients presenting for evaluation of the visual system in relation to dyslexia or reading problems will be found to have a high incidence of modest or usually insignificant ocular irregularities. These include myopia, heterophoria,

astigmatism, amblyopia, strabismus, nystagmus, poor lateralization, and others; but they appear to represent "soft neurologic signs" of associated disturbances rather than causative factors.

Graded reading

Graded reading paragraphs of some type* should be included in the examination to (1) note directly the level and facility with which the patient attacks and accomplishes reading, (2) obtain a numerical reference point familiar to educators and psychologists, and (3) afford an index for comparison on subsequent examinations.

Paper and pencil tests

Constructional apraxia. Constructional apraxia, the inability to arrange geometric components, is a specific manifestation of parietotemporal lobe impairment, usually in

*Durrell: Analysis of reading difficulty; Gray: Oral reading paragraphs; Slosson: Oral reading test; Gilmore: Oral reading test.

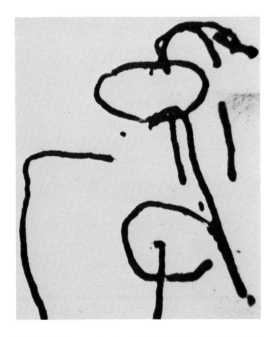

Fig. 19-1. Example of patient with acquired dyslexia, normal acuity, and right homonymous hemianopia attempting to draw a man. Disorganization of geometric units indicates constructional apraxia.

the dominant hemisphere. Its presence is a rather objective measure of neurologic deficit with which symbol confusion can be expected. The patient is asked to draw a few simple figures on a fresh office form or unlined piece of paper. These may be limited to a bicycle, a person, or the face of a clock. Hesitancy in starting to draw these familiar objects, inability to relate two wheels into a bicycle, and poor distribution of numbers, especially crowding to one side or quadrant on the face of the clock, are positive findings. These may be augmented by asking the patient to write his own name at the top of the paper. The examiner must have some knowledge of the expected drawing skill of children, which may vary widely within normal limits at each age level.

Specific dyslexia, like poliomyelitis, appears in all degrees of severity. Significant amounts of this impairment are almost always associated with some constructional apraxia, and only the very mildest case may escape wtihout it (Fig. 19-1). Quantitative testing or grading of constructional apraxia has been established by Eric Denhoff in his Meeting Street School Screening Test.

Lateralization. Poor lateralization or right-left confusion is generally concomitant with constructional apraxia. Information about impairment of lateralization as well as constructional apraxia is obtained by asking the patient to draw a few simple arrows. The dyslexic patient will often be unable to arrange the barbs at the end of the shaft and to orient the arrow to right or left on request.

Dominance

Dominance is of interest in dyslexia primarily because there has been confusion about its interpretation and its importance. In neurologic immaturity, ambidexterity, mixed dominance, or delayed right-left orientation are often apparent. Statistically, there is a slightly higher percentage of right-left orientation difficulty in the dyslexic population than in the comparable school-age population. This is now accepted to be accompanying rather than causative.

Hand and foot preference should be tested and noted, as should eye preference. Ocular lateralization, ocular preference, or so-called ocular dominance, however, should not be compared specifically with dominance or preference in the extremities. Because each eye is bilaterally represented in the cortex, rather than unilaterally as is true for the extremities, ocular "dominance" is primarily a peripheral quality (the better eye, the master eye, the sighting eye) easily subject to transient or prolonged alteration. Extremity dominance, conversely, has a central or hemispheric basis. Although studies have failed to identify or implicate ocular dominance or preference with impairments of the reading-learning act, some test should be made for completeness in studying the patient.

There are more than two dozen tests relating to ocular dominance described in the literature. A simple sighting test—such as handing the youngster a paper with a tiny hole in it and asking him to look through it at a designated distant object, first with the paper at arm's distance and then instructing him to bring the paper close to his face as he continues to sight through the hole—is often sufficient. The child will ordinarily align the hole over the preferred eye. Other suggestions of eye dominance already ascertained are: (1) the eye with better vision is generally preferred, (2) the eye that first breaks from near point of convergence testing is usually the nonpreferred eye, or (3) the eye that is difficult or impossible to blink separately.

Indications for related examinations

Most children presenting for ocular examination in relation to dyslexia have already had thorough and competent pediatric or general medical examination. If such has been omitted, it should be done both as an appropriate periodic examination and to search for any subtle disturbances of consciousness (petit mal seizures, temper tantrums, grand mal), metabolic function (diabetes, hypothyroidism), neurologic impairment (porencephalic cysts, slight hemiparesis originating in the dominant hemisphere), or hearing aberrations (nerve deafness, chronic middle ear infections). Where uncertain or borderline diagnoses occur, there should be detailed consultation with the neurologist, otologist, or other indicated specialist.

The visual examiner and those in related medical fields are obligated to obtain for the educator the healthiest possible student with best visual function to facilitate his learning experience. Many a child with extremely limited vision, however, has progressed through school on schedule and with high academic attainments. It is important to show true interest, encouragement, and reward to the dyslexic child who faces a world of unintelligible symbols and written directions.

Though emotional or psychiatric factors rarely cause specific dyslexia, many children with this problem certainly become candidates for emotional disturbance, distractive behavior, and even delinquency. Psychiatric approaches are generally neither to diagnose nor to cure the dyslexia, but in the long-neglected, irrationally treated, or late case, psychiatric treatment may be truly needed.

SPEED READING

The problems of sensory or cortical interpretation and their therapy by visual association or sensory augmentation drills must be differentiated from the field of speed reading. The later relates to nondyslexic individuals entirely. Speed reading is usually built up by teaching rapid scanning techniques and using tachistoscopic exposure drills with progressive reduction in display times. These techniques are aimed at increasing visual span, shortening fixation times, reducing the number of fixation pauses per line or page of reading, eliminating subvocalization, and developing phrase reading and selective skimming. Electrical or mechanical pacers are frequently used as home or classroom devices for speed reading. These may be utterly devastating to the true dyslexic child particularly if he is primarily an aural learner.

REFERENCES

Adams, R. M., Kocsis, J. J., Estes, R. E.: Soft neurological signs in learning disabled children and controls, Am. J. Dis. Child. **128:**614-618, 1974.

Benton, A. L.: Developmental dyslexia: neurological aspects, Abstracts in Neurol. **7:**1-47, New York, 1975, Raven Press.

Durrell, D. D.: Analysis of reading difficulty, New York, 1937 and 1955, Harcourt Brace Jovanovich, Inc.

Hainsworth, P. K., and Siqueland, M. L.: Early identification of children with learning disabilities: the Meeting Street School Screening Test, Providence, R. I., 1969, Meeting Street School.

Michaels, D. D.: Ocular dominance, Survey Ophthalmol. **17:**151-163, 1972.

Ultrasonography: A-scan and B-scan

Ultrasonography is an exploration with narrow beams of acoustic energy at frequencies far above the limits of hearing for the purpose of identifying alterations in acoustic echoes that localize and quantitate tissues of varying density within the orbit. Ultrasonic waves, both as emanating from an original source and as returning echoes, travel at measurably different speeds through the various ocular tissues. Thus differences in ultrasonic velocity and energy ("time-amplitude" function) can be recorded and displayed on suitable oscilloscopic tubes as the waves strike interfaces of different acoustic density (refraction of ultrasonic waves at sites of acoustic mismatch) or as they pass through structures of varied tissue characteristics that affect acoustic impedance and thereby the velocity of such energy passing through them. The speed of sound through the lens* is distinctly greater than through the vitreous,† though all such figures are altered by temperature. Ultrasound passing through dense and irregular tissues such as neoplasms or organized blood clots yields sustained irregular echoes of generally high amplitude, whereas ultrasound passing through homogeneously filled, cyst-like lesions (such as mucoceles or serous retinal detachments) yields distinct high-amplitude echoes at the faces or surfaces of such lesions and relatively little disturbance within the fluid mass.

INDICATIONS

Ultrasound may be considered a diagnostic modality for soft tissue study, somewhat comparable to x-ray study for bony tissue. Principal indications for diagnostic use are (1) evaluation of intraocular tissues obscured from visualization by opaque media such as corneal, lens, and vitreous opacities, (2) identification of solid or nonhomogeneous tissues from cystic or homogeneous masses, (3) determination of size, length, or thickness in ocular components, (4) investigation of retrobulbar soft tissue masses as in the presence of unilateral exophthalmos, and (5) identification, localization, and measurement of nonradiopaque foreign bodies.

EQUIPMENT
Components

Equipment for ultrasonic examination consists of three components: (1) a piezoelectric generating system supplying electric current to a transducer crystal such as barium titanate, which responds with high-frequency mechanical oscillations producing the ultrasound beam, (2) a piezoelectric receiving crystal onto which the returning ultrasonic echoes impinge and in turn generate electric potentials, and (3) an amplifier to convert these minute electric impulses into adequate magnitude for visible display on an oscilloscope. Significant echo displays may then be recorded by a Polaroid camera. Usually the same transducer crystal serves as generator and receiver because the ultrasonic energy is pulsed in brief bursts lasting about .000001 second, occurring about one thousand times a second. Thus the transducer crystal serves as a passive receiver for nearly a thousand times longer period each second than the time during which it is actively generating ultrasound.

*1,645 m/sec.
†1,532 m/sec.

Linear or A-scan (time-amplitude) ultrasound and two-dimensional or B-scan (intensity-modulated) ultrasound

The unidirectional A-scan is practical, accurate, flexible, and very suitable for quantitative studies. Like a flashlight in a large barn at night it is essentially a single beam and must be understandingly directed in a systematic exploration of the globe or retrobulbar orbit. It is certainly possible to miss significant masses, such as a small malignant melanoma under a large retinal detachment, unless the probe or scanning is done knowledgeably and methodically. On the other hand, false positive echoes, such as ringing, are few with good equipment that has been checked and standardized, particularly when the operator is clearly aware of intensity levels and the gain or amplification characteristics of the equipment.

Until 1973 two-dimensional or B-scan equipment was large, costly, and relatively inflexible; required water-filled goggles or other unpleasant liquid coupling; and was available in only a few major laboratories. The cathode tube display and photographic record of such an intensity-modulated display present familiar similarity to an x-ray laminogram or planogram of the orbit.

In early 1973, the Bronson-Turner Ophthalmic B-scan instrument became commercially available with the simplistic advantage of contact scanning and no water bath. Grumman Health Systems assisted in developing and engineering this compact unit. The transducer in the hand-held arc scanning head oscillates at 11 scans per second and is contained in a chamber that must be filled with distilled water (never saline!). The chamber face is a thin Mylar film that is moistened with methyl cellulose for coupling with the lid or globe. The scanning head may be sterilized in *cold* ethylene oxide. The display unit and circuitry are self-con-

Fig. 20-1. Bronson-Turner B-scan shown in use with scanning arc positioned horizontally over left upper lid. Display on cathode tube shows anterior segment to left, clear vitreous in midscreen, and posterior bulbar curve to right. Top of screen corresponds to position of knurled screw cap used for filling screening head with water.

Fig. 20-2. Normal B-scan ultrasonogram shown by Polaroid film from screen of Bronson-Turner instrument. Clear vitreous is seen centrally and normal optic nerve is to right.

Fig. 20-3. Normal B-scan ultrasonogram of posterior globe, optic nerve, and retrobulbar fat shown by Polaroid film from screen of Bronson-Turner instrument.

Fig. 20-4. Serous detachment of retina seen in B-scan ultrasonogram taken by Polaroid film from screen of Bronson-Turner instrument. Normal retrobulbar fat to right is to one side of optic nerve and therefore negative outline of the nerve is not seen.

tained in a cabinet the size of a medium screen, home television set that weighs 21 pounds* (Figs. 20-1 to 20-7). With caution this unit may be transported within a building, such as between clinic and operating room.

*Storz Instrument Company, St. Louis, Missouri 63122.

Fig. 20-5. Infrabulbar tumor (plasmocytoma) near orbital floors seen in B-scan ultrasonogram taken by Polaroid film from screen of Bronson-Turner instrument. Scanning head is held vertically in sagittal plane. Orbital floor is seen as curve at bottom of figure. Tumor appears as (black) area with little echo activity from the mass.

A higher resolution, mechanical scanning unit has been developed (1969) by D. Jackson Coleman, M.D., of Columbia Presbyterian Institute of Ophthalmology, with resolution capability of 0.3 mm. in compound scan and 0.1 mm. in linear scan. This couples both A- and B-scanning techniques in real time but requires water immersion of the eye and orbit for coupling with the hand-operated scanner. Frequencies of 2 to 28 million cycles per second are available.* This is a major, fixed instillation that cannot be transported to the operating room.

Available linear or A-scan equipment

Several manufacturers produce ultrasonographic equipment specifically for ocular use. Component parts such as transducers,† generators,‡ amplifiers, and oscilloscopes can be purchased and assembled by acoustical or electronic engineers in most medical centers. Kretztechnik of Zipf, Austria, produces one basic, high-resolution unit for ocular and orbital use: the Kretz 7200 MA (Fig. 20-8) is widely useful and of high quality. It affords coupling for semi-automatic linear and arc

*Sonometrics System, Inc., Bronx, New York 10463.
†Valpey Corp., Holliston, Massachusetts 01746.
‡Hewlett-Packard Corp., Palo Alto, California 94304.

Fig. 20-6. Organized hemorrhage in anterior globe beneath old disorganizing laceration of cornea and iris, seen in B-scan ultrasonogram taken by Polaroid film from screen of Bronson-Turner instrument. Scars and opacities of cornea, iris, and lens preclude light examination.

Fig. 20-7. Recent vitreous hemorrhage extending throughout midvitreous seen in B-scan ultrasonogram taken by Polaroid film from screen of Bronson-Turner instrument.

Fig. 20-8. Kretztechnik A-scan (time-amplitude ultrasound) model 7200 MA for linear biometry and quantitative echography. Oscilloscope screen to right contains linear measuring graticule. This model was introduced in 1970. (Keeney, A. H.: Orbital diagnosis. In NOAO: Symposium on surgery of the orbit and adnexa, St. Louis, 1974, The C. V. Mosby Co.)

scanning with a simplified B display. Siemens Aktiengesellschaft of Erlangen, Germany, and Automation Industries, Inc., of Boulder, Colorado, also manufacture substantial equipment.

Smith-Kline Instrument Co. of Palo Alto, California, has had several years of experience with two models of A-scan ultrasonoscopes applied to ophthalmic use. Their early and pioneering Ekoline 20, is compact enough to roll from examining room to operating room on a light aluminum carriage (Fig. 20-9). The smaller Ekoline 12 has a reduced oscilloscope display. Though portable, this instrument must also be treated with gentle caution and standardized frequently or daily against a Bronson glass plate. This was improved in 1970 with the addition of a built-in attenuator. These units were developed on an average transmission speed of 1,540 m/sec. for all purposes.

Many manufacturers produce specific equipment for continuous-wave Doppler ef-fect examinations,* but all of these call for considerable care in quantitation of energy delivered. Energy levels from continuous wave operations are several log units higher than from pulsed units.

PHYSICAL CHARACTERISTICS

Ultrasound is not heard, seen, or smelled. In the low energies used for ocular diagnosis it cannot be felt as heat or force and gives rise to no known tissue alterations. Thus its patient acceptability is high, and no special preparation or adaptation is required to begin the examination.

Pulsed versus continuous ultrasound. The use of repetitive short bursts of ultrasound allows the same transducer to also act as the echo receiver and reduces the potential for building up damaging levels of energy. Continuous ultrasound is used in Doppler ef-

*Magnaflux Corp., MD Ultrasonic Doppler; Ames Co., Ultradop; Smith-Kline Instrument Co., Doptone.

Fig. 20-9. Smith-Kline Ekoline 20 time-amplitude (A-scan) ultrasonic apparatus with 5-mm. diameter transducer in holder to right of oscilloscope. Polaroid camera is shown opened and turned away from oscilloscope.

fect studies (increasing frequency of sound waves as a moving source approaches the receiver, or decreasing frequency as the source recedes from the receiver) to qualitate blood surge in vessels such as the carotid and ophthalmic arteries. Uncertain, high, and potentially damaging energy levels can be created at various tissue depths with continuous ultrasound. These problems may be intensified by large area or focusing transducer faces.

Frequencies. Five to twenty megacycles per second (megahertz) are commonly needed to obtain soft tissue penetration through the eye and into the orbit. Depth of penetration and indentification of small differences in tissue density are facilitated by higher frequencies. To achieve penetration of high frequencies, however, energy levels must be increased. Low frequencies suffer least absorption or attenuation. Increasing resolution in the deep orbit is achieved with increasing frequencies (up to 15 or 20 MHz) that give relatively narrow beams but are rapidly absorbed by orbital soft tissues. Thus greater energy input is required to obtain deep penetration with higher frequency beams. Unfortunately, normal orbital fat is a very efficient reflector of ultrasound. Echoes generated from these fat lobules obscure all the small vessel and similar anatomic details of retrobular structures.

Energy levels. Energy levels for diagnosis are generally in the range of microwatts per square centimeter per minute. Energies in the range of tenths of a watt per square centimeter per minute are potentially dam-

aging. Higher energy levels have been selectively studied for therapeutic and destructive effects, including the production of corneal edema, cataracts, vitreous liquefaction, chorioretinal scars, and tissue necrosis.

Transducer (crystal) diameter. Every transducer has its individual and particular characteristics that must be matched to the display unit. In ocular and orbital diagnosis narrow beams are more critically localizing, and therefore crystals about 5 mm. in diameter are commonly employed. This affords a light, easily held, and nonfrightening probe similar in size to a cigarette. Alignment of the probe for reception of the reflected and refracted echoes becomes more critical, however, as transducer diameter is reduced. A striking example is that of a spherical steel BB or lead shotgun pellet; this is easily seen on the poorest quality x-ray film, is of markedly different acoustic density in comparison to orbital soft tissues, and affords a gross "acoustic mismatch" at its surface. With a small-diameter transducer, however, the returning echo may easily be reflected beyond or wide of the crystal face if the sonic wave is not coincident or nearly coincident with a radius of the sphere (Fig. 20-10). (In B-scan examination such BB's or bird shot give rise to a series of ringing echoes behind them.)

Coupling. Air is a highly effective insulator to ultrasound, and therefore fluid coupling between the transducer face and bulbar or lid tissue is essential for transmission of the ultrasound. Two to six percent methylcellulose is commonly used as a

Fig. 20-10. Schematic illustration of difficulty in obtaining A-scan ultrasonic echo from a smooth spherical object such as a BB. Illustration at left shows the necessary near coincidence of sonic beam with the diameter of the BB in order for reflected echo to impinge on the 5-mm. transducer face. Higher frequency, larger crystal diameter, and lower energy levels all create narrowing of the beam and make the localization of foreign bodies more difficult.

coupling medium. When the transducer probe is applied to the cornea, a topical anesthetic is instilled first.

FINDINGS

It must be remembered that sonic beams, like light beams, may be absorbed, transmitted, regularly reflected, irregularly reflected, refracted, or scattered by various interfaces and media in their pathway.

A standardized notation of probe placement should be used. Conventionally the five digits 0 through 4 are used indicating the corneal apex as 0, midway between the apex and limbus as 1, the limbus as 2, pars plana roughly as 3, and the most accessible near equator as 4. These locations are further expressed as clock hours of 1 through 12. A third notation should be decibel level. Thus three numbers are recorded for each A-scan echogram: 0-4/1-12/30-80.

Normal results

The normal A-scan ultrasonogram is represented schematically by Fig. 20-11. The base line on the oscilloscope display has linear graduations to aid in measurement. When a sonic beam is undisturbed by variations in acoustic impedance, the display shows no deflection from the base line. When a transducer is fluid-coupled to an eye on its visual axis the first deflection is that of the anterior corneal surface. With equipment that greatly magnifies the length of the globe, it is possible to detect the posterior

Fig. 20-11. Schematic representation of A-scan ultrasonogram made with transducer tip at left in direct fluid coupling to cornea. Opening deflection (opening bang) is shown at corneal surface, A. Reflection from anterior lens capsule is shown at B and posterior lens capsule is shown at C. The clear lens presents no echoes within its depths. Similarly, the clear vitreous presents no echoes. The posterior bulbar wall complex is represented by D and E. The retrobulbar fat at far right shows decreasing irregular spikes.

Fig. 20-12. Normal A-scan ultrasonogram showing posterior bulbar wall and decreasing amplitude of irregular echoes from normal retrobulbar fat; taken by Polaroid film from screen of Kretztechnik A-scan instrument.

corneal surface and also stromal opacities. Normally the aqueous and vitreous are both acoustically homogeneous and therefore give rise to no echoes on the display. The lens, however, shows distinct echo deflections at its anterior and posterior surface; these should be of essentially equal amplitude if the beam is passing axially through the lens center. A large deflection is also created at the posterior bulbar wall or the vitreoretinal interface. Beyond the globe, irregularly decreasing echoes indicate the normal orbital fat pattern. Fig. 20-12 is an actual display of a normal A-scan.

Lens echoes and refractive divergence of the lens on the sonic beam can be avoided in aphakia or by placing the transducer beyond the lens equator (Fig. 20-13, lower tracing).

Altered results

Blood or inflammatory debris in the aqueous or vitreous give irregular, low-amplitude echoes (Fig. 20-14) that disappear at low intensities. Neoplasms, heavy exudates, or old blood clots (Fig. 20-15) give sustained irregular echoes throughout, which persist even at low-intensity examination. The some-

Fig. 20-13. Two ultrasonograms taken through a single eye. Upper tracing (positive deflection) is through the clear lens. Lower tracing (negative deflection) is taken obliquely across the eye. Example shows high myopia. Note 2-mm. scale marking along base line.

Fig. 20-14. Ultrasonogram showing low-amplitude disturbances in vitreous from scattered hemorrhage. Tracing is made peripheral to lens. Note normal retrobulbar fat pattern to right.

times difficult ophthalmoscopic differential of hemangioma vs. malignant melanoma of the choroid is usually assisted by early and bright fluorescence of the hemangioma in intravenous angiography; further, the high sonic absorptiveness of melanomas in either A- or B-scan examination is quite distinct from the high reflectivity (high-amplitude echo spikes) from hemangiomas. Serous detachments of the retina show a sharp isolated spike resembling that of a foreign body; this can be verified from different axes corresponding to the extent and height of elevation. Peculiarly the detached retina gives a far more distinct and higher amplitude echo than does the attached retina in normal position.

Abnormal retrobulbar echoes are generally classifiable into (1) foreign body spikes of high amplitude, (2) dampening or reduction in the normal orbital fat pattern resulting from tumor displacement (Fig. 20-16), (3)

homogeneous or tumor-cyst patterns with very little echo disturbance between distinct interface spikes (Fig. 20-17), and (4) nonhomogeneous tumor-cyst patterns with irregular echoes persisting at low intensities and sometimes delineated by a distinct posterior interface spike (Fig. 20-18). Posterior bulbar wall and deeper echoes are attenuated when the ultrasound beam reaches them through an intraocular mass. The deeper a lesion is in the orbit, the higher the frequency and energy requirements to detect it. Thus masses close to the apex may elude identification or be concealed by reverberation artifacts from the converging bony walls.

Foreign bodies generally afford distinct acoustic mismatch (Fig. 20-19) with identifying high-amplitude echoes. Though both radiopaque and radiolucent foreign bodies yield strong identifying and localizing echograms, the ultrasonic technique is especially indicated and uniquely valuable in the case

Fig. 20-15. Ultrasonogram showing solid tumor extending to midvitreous with sharply localized presenting face and irregular echoes throughout tumor mass to posterior bulbar wall. Echoes do not disappear when intensity is reduced. Histology later confirmed malignant melanoma.

Fig. 20-16. Ultrasonogram of retrobulbar tumor showing dampening or reduction in the usual pattern of echoes from the retrobulbar fat caused by a homogeneous tumor mass.

Fig. 20-17. Retrobulbar pattern of homogeneous or tumor-cyst type showing mass behind the posterior bulbar wall, obliteration of retrobulbar fat echoes, and sharp posterior limit to the lesion.

Fig. 20-18. Ultrasonogram showing solid retrobulbar tumor pattern with sharply localized posterior limit to the tumor mass.

Fig. 20-19. Ultrasonogram showing intraocular foreign body slightly anterior to midvitreous. Sharp, localized echo spike is similar to that from surface of retina in serous detachment. Low amplitude surrounding echoes in the vitreous indicate cellular reaction, especially posterior to the foreign body.

of wood, glass, plastic, and similar materials that are difficult or often impossible to identify, even with the best of soft tissue x-ray techniques. Uniformly spherical foreign bodies such as BB's are more easily and strikingly seen on B-scan than A-scan. One of the most valuable diagnostic findings in the presence of intraocular foreign bodies or detached retina is the state of the vitreous. Echography is essential when a cataract or opaque cornea precludes visualization. Blood or fibrinous changes give low amplitude echoes corresponding to the intensity of vitreous reaction.

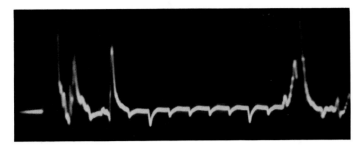

Fig. 20-20. A-scan ultrasonogram through the lens showing increased lens thickness (intumescence). Vitreous depth is indicated to be 18 mm.

Optic nerve. The sudden visual loss of optic neuritis has a serious and treacherous prognosis. The diagnosis, however, until 1972 has been principally one of exclusion. Often a descriptive but embarrassing phrase —"The patient sees nothing and the physician sees nothing"—has been applicable. B-scan ultrasound, however, clearly produces a negative "shadow" or acoustic void that tracks the optic nerve through the irregularly echoing retrobulbar fat. Widening of the optic nerve area with faint to marked reduplication of the nerve outline, is objective evidence of inflammatory swelling, and is known as Coleman's sign (1972).

QUANTITATIVE ULTRASONOGRAPHY

For differential characterization of ultrasound echoes it is essential to perform quantitative studies. Bronson developed a simple attenuator to insert between the transducer and the amplifying system in his Ekoline 12 units. The new Bronson-Turner B-scan (Fig. 20-1) provides finger tip control of attenuation in steps of 10 decibels from 80 to 30. Thus a fresh intravitreal hemorrhage may give high amplitude echoes at 80 or 70 db. but these will disappear at 60 or 50 db. Older fibrin changes in the vitreous may give persistent echoes even at 40 or 30 db. In A-scan quantitative echography, Ossoinig stresses the basic need to establish a maximum echo height at a tissue interface and then trace its drop in amplitude on the oscilloscope. Ossoinig plots an "angle kappa" according to the decreasing amplitude of echoes across the lesion. From this angle he

predicts the vascularity, compactness, and other histologic characteristics of the lesion. A cavernous hemangioma may show excellent sound transmission and little attenuation (small angle kappa) whereas a neurogenic tumor has high acoustic density and poor transmission (large angle kappa).

Oculometric results: A-scan and B-scan

Oculometry, and particularly axial length measurement, is helpful in diagnosing early phthisis (as in hypotony) or early buphthalmos (as in congenital glaucoma), though care must be taken not to press heavily or distort the globe with the probe. Measurement of presumably shrunken lenses and differentiation of normal lens thickness from intumescent lenses can be done with most A-scan equipment (Fig. 20-20) and the Coleman B-scanner. It is also possible to measure normally sized components of the eye that may be present in spite of other congenital anomalies such as microcornea, megalocornea, or posterior microglobus. Staphylomatous distensions of the globe can be localized and measured easily with equipment such as the Bronson B-scan. Refraction of aphakic infants, especially for contact lenses, requires operating room environment and general anesthetic. A-scan measurement of axial length combined with keratometry gives more precise and detailed data than retinoscopy alone. Errors should be under 1 diopter.

In spite of current improvements in resolution of many instruments, it is still generally inaccurate or misleading to interpret echograms as valid in measurements of less than 0.1 mm. Thus the automatic read-out of spectacle prescriptions by ultrasonography requires further refinement in equipment and more accurate knowledge of the speed of sound through individual lenses and individual vitreous bodies.

Preoperative refractive analysis for implantation of artificial lenses following cataract extraction

A careful combination of anterior surface keratometry with A-scan measurement of axial length and anterior chamber depth affords a basis for calculating the desired refractive power of plastic lens inserts. This requires careful use of a water standoff coupling between the transducer and the cornea. The existing lens in situ, always a worrisome source of errors in biometry and other bulbar examinations, must be recognized for its acoustic density being greater than aqueous or vitreous. The speed of ultrasound through the lens is thus greater than through aqueous or vitreous and it creates divergence of the sonic beam.

CURRENT USE STATUS

Ultrasound is now a validated and, valuable diagnostic adjunct, but it presents the limitation of requiring use by the physician or responsible examiner. It cannot be delegated to a technologist unfamiliar with the disease processes that may be affecting the globe or orbit. Wherever several eye physicians practice together, or in any hospital serving a small group of ophthalmologists, there certainly should be facilities for ultrasonic examination. It is essential that at least one physician in the group know the characteristics of the instrument and the technique of standardization, and he should be able to conduct valid and reproducible studies. B-scan equipment at present is commercially available as a handy and rapid, low resolution system (Bronson-Turner), or a complex and expensive immersion scan at high resolution (Coleman-Sonometrics); at least the former should be widely available and understood as to indications and limitations by all practitioners. Differential absorption of ultrasound presents a guide to tissue typing in solid tumors, particularly with the Kretz 7200. Echographic data are steadily approaching the data of tissue characteristics as seen in light microscopy, or offering a noninvasive in vivo approximation of in vitro findings.

REFERENCES

Belkin, M., Ticho, U., Swsal, A., and Livinson, A.: Ultrasonography in refraction of aphakic infants, Br. J. Ophthalmol. 57:845-848, 1973.

Coleman, D. J. and Carroll, F.: Evaluation of optic nerve pathology with B-scan ultrasound, Am. J. Ophthalmol. 74:915-920, 1972.

Gitter, K. A., Keeney, A. H., Sarin, L. K., and Meyer, D.: Ophthalmic ultrasound, St. Louis, 1969, The C. V. Mosby Co.

Introduction to electrophysiologic diagnostic procedures

Several related but somewhat exotic test procedures have reached practicality through development of circuitry and amplification methods to capture or to record electric potentials associated with both sensory and motor ocular function. Much of this has been facilitated by the widespread use of electroencephalography and the polygraphs that record from such brain potentials. Indeed, the electroencephalogram (EEG) itself, when recording potentials from scalp leads over the occipital lobes and augmented by photic driving and visually evoked responses (VER), is a sensitive diagnostic aid to assess integrity of the visual pathways and the "perceptual" responses of the visual cortex.

Chapters 22 through 25 each deal with a specialized field of diagnostic study concerning the visual apparatus. Electroencephalography will be considered later in this chapter. The fields of electroencephalography, electroretinography, electrooculography, and electronystagmography all use similar polygraphs and ink-writing recorders with complete electric shielding and grounding of the room and equipment. These studies can be done in conjunction with existing electroencephalographic laboratories in most hospitals and medical centers. With each new advance, however, necessary equipment becomes more appropriate and less expensive.

The subject of electromyography (Breinin; Jampolsky; Miller; Bjork; Mertens) is less consonant because it requires different amplification and display equipment, involves the somewhat unpleasant problem of inserting needle electrodes into extraocular muscles under no more than topical anesthesia, and is primarily a laboratory and investi-gative, rather than clinical, tool. Similarly the early receptor potential (ERP) of the electroretinogram has not yet reached clinical importance.

The major electrophysiologic diagnostic procedures for the visual apparatus are:

1. Electroencephalography (EEG): the recording of minute electric responses (30 to 100 μv) of the occipital cortex by means of small sets of electrodes inserted into the scalp; the visual evoked response (VER) is actually a refinement of electroencephalography based on detection of electrical responses over the occipital cortex following light stimulation of the eyes

2. Electroretinography (ERG): the recording of light-evoked electric currents originating primarily from the rods, cones, and bipolar cells of the retina (pp. 285-297)

3. Electrooculography (EOG): the recording of changes in resting currents (standing corneoretinal potentials, CRP) that apparently arise in the pigment epithelium of the retina, initiated by excursions of the eye rather than by light (Testing is done in both the light-adapted and the dark-adapted states from skin electrodes affixed to the outer canthi [binocular] or to the inner and outer canthi [monocular].)

4. Electronystagmography (ENG): the recording of fluctuations in resting currents (CRP) occasioned by ocular excursions that may be spontaneous, induced, or modified by opticokinetic or labyrinthian stimuli (pp. 301-306)

5. Electromyography (EMG): the record-

ing of changes in electric potentials of ocular muscles at apparent rest under attempted movement or by stimulation of nerve supply. (Recording is done with needle electrodes inserted into the extraocular muscles; see pp. 307-308.)

Electrophysiologic findings are most meaningful when interpreted in the light of psychophysical tests such as visual acuity, visual fields, dark adaptation, and color discrimination. They are also useful in assessing visual functions in infants and unconscious or nonverbal patients. As largely objective tests, they are helpful in detecting malingerers and hysterics. In detecting some hereditary eye diseases before other signs become evident, these tests strengthen both early diagnosis and family counseling. They can detect retinal function in the presence of opaque media and assess toxic irritation or damage from intraocular metallic foreign bodies.

ELECTROENCEPHALOGRAPHY

Electroencephalography, which dates from the discoveries of Berger in 1929, affords considerable data on the activity of the visual centers, particularly those occupying the large areas in the occipital poles. The normal alpha rhythm of cortical discharges is 8 to 13 c.p.s. Their potential is about 30 to 50 μv* but tends to be less over the primary visual registration area (Brodmann's area 17) of the striate cortex and maximal over the visual association areas 18 and 19. This regular alpha rhythm is easily altered by visual attention or photic stimulation. With an intact visual pathway, the alpha rhythm of the striate cortex can be driven effectively with flashes of light at an intensity of about 80 foot candles; monochromatic light, particularly toward the blue end of the spectrum, appears more effective than white or red light. A maximum acceleration to about 30 to 35 c.p.s. can be achieved in leads from the striate cortex, but rates almost twice this high can be attained in leads from the optic nerve, geniculate body, and optic radia-

*This represents attenuation of as much as 5,000 to 1 between cortex and scalp.

tions. This is sometimes referred to as "flicker following" (Fig. 21-1).

The visual evoked response (VER) is the electrical response to visual stimuli recorded from scalp electrodes over the occipital cortex. The earliest evoked potential recording was done by electroencephalographers who noted changes in the ongoing EEG caused by sensory stimuli. To detect responses to specific stimuli, short time intervals of EEG following visual stimuli were overlaid on film to find similarities within the noise. This was the earliest form of signal averaging.

The waveform of the VER is highly variable from patient to patient, but very stable for the same patient retested under the same conditions (Fig. 21-2). These responses probably reflect signal processing in the underlying cortex, 30 to 300 milliseconds after a stimulus. The variability between patients precludes much analysis beyond the presence or absence of a response. Therefore, tests must rely on the comparison of responses to different stimuli (i.e. pattern sizes) within the same individual. Visual acuity can be calculated by this method. The macular visual field is the most strongly represented area in the VER and therefore this test comes closest to studying the functional integrity of central vision.

Amplitudes of the components of the VER are approximately 1 to 15 μV and are obscured by many extraneous electrical signals such as the ongoing brain waves and muscle potentials in the scalp. Computerized signal averaging must be employed to detect the VER by adding together repetitive responses. The electrical noise in repetitive responses tends to be random and cancels out in the sum, while the VER components are stable and add up with each additional response. Signals as small as one microvolt can be detected by this method. The most effective stimuli are the counterphase type with equal portions of dark and light. The position of the dark and light areas interchange, which causes no change in the total light entering the eye. With this stimulus it is necessary for the visual system to resolve the elements or movement of the elements to produce a VER.

Several other waves of VER can be obtained singularly from the occipital cortex at magnitudes of about 1 μv. Components of this VER wave, known as c^1 and c^2, seem related to photopic and scotopic mechanisms respectively and also to the state of atten-

tion. In the nonattentive state, the c^1 component seems to disappear.

Equipment for recording the VER must include an averaging device. EEG scalp electrodes are placed in a standard outline. For bipolar recording, positions are used that overlie the visual cortex; but larger responses can sometimes be obtained by having one

Fig. 21-1. Sections of normal electroencephalogram showing, at left, response to photic driving at 16 c.p.s. and, at right, response without photic stimulation. Responses appear predominantly in leads over occipital lobes. Designations at right indicate leads according to superimposed lead diagram at left.

electrode higher in the parietal area. A ground electrode is placed on one ear lobe. The VER is usually recorded with the patient sitting, because any movement of the electrodes will cause severe artifacts. The patient faces a screen on which a repetitive stimulus is shown. The patient should concentrate on viewing the stimulus and his continued fixation should be monitored. The complexity of the stimulus has an important effect on the VER. A flashing pattern with multiple borders yields a larger response than a simple flashing light. The most effective stimulus is probably the counterphase checkerboard. This is similar to the bar pattern for the EEG except that it has more borders within the pattern. It can be produced optically or electronically. The examiner should be able to change the size of the elements of the pattern down to the threshold of visual resolution without changing the field size so that objective visual acuity can be estimated. Determining visual acuity with a flashing stimulus is less satisfactory since a pattern

need not be resolved to obtain a response. Amplification for VER is provided by EEG amplifiers that are fed into the averaging device. A gain of 20,000 to 50,000 is usually required. An oscilloscope for constant monitoring of the incoming signal is useful since electrical artifacts caused by muscle discharge or head movement can distort the averaged signal and must be eliminated.

In children with amblyopia, alterations in occipital alpha rhythm are found, and reduced effects of flicker driving may be seen. Where facilities exist for computer averaging* of the VER by an electronic toposcope, the c^1 wave generated from an amblyopic eye seems to be reduced, or the c^2 wave from the nonamblyopic eye is reduced in comparison to that of the amblyopic eye.

Thus electroencephalography with the conventional equipment found in most hospitals, medical centers, or neurologic services affords an objective, though crude, index of functioning in the visual cortex and gross measure of the integrity of the visual pathways from the retina to the occipital lobes (Fig. 21-1). A semiquantitative aspect is also available in demonstration of photic driving or flicker following. These tests give otherwise unobtainable evidence of intact visual pathways in infants, nonresponders, and unconscious patients. The vastly more complex equipment and procedures needed to study VER's (measured at levels of only a few microvolts) hold great promise for objective study of visual fields, form recognition, and even quantitation of visual acuity.

*PDP Lab 8E Digital Electric Corp. Fabritek XXX.

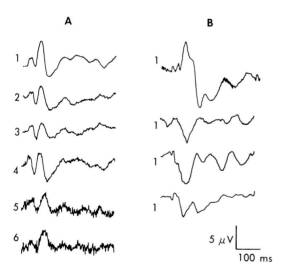

Fig. 21-2. VER recordings from the visual cortex by scalp electrodes. Column A traces were taken from the same individual in several different sessions over several weeks with slightly different size bar pattern stimuli. Column B traces were taken under the same stimulus conditions in several individuals. The lack of similarity among individuals is as striking as the close similarity of responses from the same individual.

REFERENCES

Asselman, P., Chadwick, D. W., and Marsden, C. D.: Visually evoked responses in the diagnosis and management of patients suspected of multiple sclerosis, Brain **98:**261, 1971.

Bourassa, C. M., Singer, M., Mills, L., et al.: Photic evoked cortical potentials in functional amblyopia Can. J. Ophthalmol. **6:**72-78, 1971.

Cohen, J.: Brain waves and blindness: new approaches to evaluation of blind persons, New York, 1970, Am. Foundation for the Blind.

Electroretinography

Theodore Lawwill, M.D.

Electroretinography is the recording through electronic amplification of minute electric potentials in the range of 0.1 to 1 mv. generated by the retina in reponse to changes in light intensity. Stimuli may range from threshold values through increments of approximately 4 logarithmic units. Both light-adapted or photopic patterns of relatively low voltage and dark-adapted or scotopic patterns of higher voltage may be obtained. In addition an objective measurement of the Purkinje shift in maximal color or wavelength sensitivity can be recorded as the retina changes from the dark- to light-adapted state. This accounts for the change in spectral location of the sensation of maximum brightness in scotopic versus photopic vision.

Electroretinography, though subject to modern scientific study since the first of this century, has attained meaningful analysis only in the last few decades (Hartline, 1925; R. Grant, 1933; Riggs, 1941; Karpe, 1945; Henkes, 1949; A. Franceschetti, 1951; François, 1952) and has become a common, useful clinical technique only in the last few years. The United States had only a few electroretinographic laboratories in the 1950s but now almost every major eye department has such facilities. Current visual literature routinely refers to the electroretinogram (ERG) both as a diagnostic modality and more simply in terms of electroretinographic data in relation to case studies or other reports.

ELECTRORETINOGRAPHIC EQUIPMENT

Three components of equipment are required to record an ERG: (1) stimulus light, (2) active and neutral electrodes, and (3) amplifying and recording system. All three components are commercially available. Considerable variability in stimulus light is necessary for the ERG. Jacobson has stressed the wide availability and utility of standard electroencephalographic amplifiers, recorders, and shielded rooms in most general hospitals for adaptation to electroretinographic purposes.

Stimulators. The most usual stimulus is a gas discharge tube (electronic flash or stroboscope), which delivers a high-intensity discharge over a fixed period of milliseconds.* Intensity, wavelength, and frequency can be controlled by filters. A second common stimulus is an incandescent light behind a mechanical or electromagnetic shutter system to control the duration and frequency of stimulations. Ordinary strobe lights for photic driving of the EEG are easily adapted for this purpose. Stimulus duration is commonly controlled at 10 to 100 msec. Background illumination must be controlled.

Electrodes. The active or recording electrode is placed on the eye anteriorly, since posterior or retinal electrodes cannot practically be used in humans. These may be skin leads or may be fitted to contact lenses of either the corneal or scleral type.† Most require the use of contact fluid, such as 1% methylcellulose in saline. The Burian-Allen lens (Fig. 22-1) incorporates a retractor to keep the lids apart.‡ The contact lens

*Photo Stimulator, PS2 Grass Medical Instruments, Quincy, Massachusetts.
†Lo-Vac 1126, Medical Workshop, Groningen, The Netherlands.
‡Manufactured by Hansen Laboratories, Iowa City, Iowa.

Fig. 22-1. Modified Burian-Allen ERG electrode in place supplies an excellent visual opening as well as recording and reference electrodes. Additional earclip grounding electrode is required.

manufactured by Obrig Laboratories* is simpler in design, and small sizes are made for infants and children. Any good contact lens technician can bond a silver wire lead to a narrow scleral flange contact lens for this purpose. An auxiliary filling tube through which additional fluid may be added is convenient. A large neutral or indifferent electrode is usually taped to the skin above the bridge of the nose after cleansing the skin and applying electrolyte jelly. This is not needed if a bipolar contact lens is used. Examining both eyes simultaneously conserves time and gives controlled comparison of the two eyes.

Recorder. The ERG has a time course of about one hundred milliseconds. Amplifying and recording the small electric potentials can be done in many ways. Alternating current amplifiers with a gain of 10,000 to 20,000 times are used to drive recording devices such as pen-writers or storage oscilloscopes (Tectronix XXI). The simplest is the use of a standard electroencephalographic machine or Grass polygraph. The inkwriter gives an

*Sarasota, Florida 33578.

immediate record and is sufficiently detailed for most clinical purposes. Because of the inertia of the inkwriter, however, the wave forms are not recorded as critically as with a cathode ray oscilloscope, which has the disadvantage of requiring a photograph for permanent record. Computer recording and tape storage plus computerized averaging of 60 to 100 responses facilitate the delineation of minute time-related responses that could not be detected on direct records.

ELECTRORETINOGRAPHIC WAVES AND THEIR ORIGIN

The size and shape of electroretinographic waves depend on both conditions of testing and health of the eye. The essential response is biphasic, but four waves may be seen. The first wave is a brief negative deflection called the *a wave;* the following wave is a longer lasting, greater amplitude positive deflection called the *b wave.* A slower, positive *c wave* may also be seen. There may be smaller wavelets superimposed on the b wave; these are oscillatory potentials. Also under high intensity stimuli and with high speed recording, very subtle R_1

(positive) and R_2 (negative) wave deflections may be revealed ahead of the more gross a wave. A long stimulus, as from a shuttered incandescent source may generate an "off response" or d wave as another positive wave. Little clinical significance has been attributed to this wave. For most clinical studies, only the a and b waves are important (Fig. 22-2).

At high intensity both the a and b waves may appear double, and these then are designated a_1 and a_2 or b_1 or b_2. Since they probably represent photopic and scotopic function, they are sometimes called a_p and a_s and b_p and b_s. The b_p wave was originally called the *x wave* or b_x. The most common terms now are those with the photopic or scotopic subscripts.

Precise points of origin of these waves are still somewhat uncertain, but clarification has come from microelectrode studies at various depths in animal retinas, responses in the predominantly rod or cone retinas of certain species, alterations following use of drugs that selectively affect specific retinal areas, and correlating electroretinographic responses with known clinical entities. The a wave probably originates in the outer segments of rods and cones. Bipolar cell activity is probably associated with the b wave, although the inner segments of the rods and cones may also contribute. The high intensity portion of the b wave may come from Mueller cells. The c wave is probably produced by the pigment epithelium. For simplification of understanding it is easiest to associate the a wave with the visual cells and the b wave with the bipolars. The ganglion cells and nerve fibers apparently do not contribute to the ERG. The ERG, however, apparently correlates with the beginning of a chain of electric activity ending in the occipital cortex. Some responses in the optic nerve or even farther back may occur before all of the b wave potential has culminated. The size, shape, and time relationships of the ERG depend on variations in stimulus parameters (intensity, duration, wavelength, frequency), the condition of the eye (state of adaptation, pupil

Fig. 22-2. Normal electroretinograms in 11-year-old female demonstrating **A**, photopic flash responses, **B**, scotopic flash responses, and **C**, scotopic doubled b waves (b), elicited with red filter. Top tracings show stimulus. Middle tracings are from right eye, and bottom tracings are from left eye.

size, pathology), and extraneous nonretinal potentials (lid, bulbar, iris, and ciliary body motion).

The most important ocular variable is the state of adaptation. In the light-adapted state, all components of the normal ERG occur rapidly and are of low voltage. During the early phases of dark adaptation, the amplitude of the a and b waves increases rapidly. At first, this is especially true of a_p and b_p. The a_s and b_s can hardly be distinguished in the light-adapted state. As dark adaptation progresses, a_s and b_s increase and become larger than a_p and b_p. After 20 minutes of dark adaptation, a weak flash will produce a scotopic b wave representing mostly rod-driven elements. When dark adaptation is essentially complete, the a and b waves reach maximum size.

Variations in the stimulus cause greatly different ERG responses. The intensity of the light can change both the amplitude and form of the response. Generally, the amplitude of response increases in proportion to the logarithm of the intensity over a range of about 4 or 5 logarithmic units.

Stimuli of different wavelengths cause different shaped responses. For example, blue light tends to bring out the scotopic waves. A deep red stimulus causes a complex response with a double b wave. This apparently represents the photopic and scotopic b waves rather than a specific red response (Fig. 22-2, C). Absence of one of these specific b_s waves indicates a lack of function of the corresponding system. This may be secondary to loss of the retinal area containing a majority of the related elements (i.e. central vs. peripheral chorioretinitis) or maldevelopment or degeneration of specific elements (i.e. rod achromatopsia).

The phenomenon of flicker fusion is useful in electroretinographic testing. In psychophysiologic tests, the critical flicker fusion frequency is that frequency at which a repetitive stimulus appears to be constant. With the ERG, it is that frequency at which responses are merged and no longer separable. The Grass polygraph can follow 40 to 60 stimuli per second. The cone system is known to be capable of responding separately at a much higher frequency than the rod system. With computer equipment, distinctly separate ERG's can be recorded at rates of over 100 per second. If the electroretinographic responses show fusion of repetitive stimuli at a low rate, this is evidence of cone dysfunction.

LIMITATIONS OF THE ERG

A major limitation of present techniques is in evaluating precise retinal areas and particularly macular function. The usual ERG is a mass response caused by spread of light by the media of the eye and interneuronal connections within the retina. Thus even if a narrow pencil of light is used as a stimulus and directed to the blind spot, the whole retina tends to respond.

Among many efforts to develop "macular ERG," the current "bar pattern ERG" is significantly successful. A patterning of alternating dark and light bars is focused on the retina and position of the bars is alternated. This generates a response only from the area receiving the alternate lightened and darkened pattern. By averaging 60 to 100 signals, reasonable ERG responses can be recorded in a 5° to 10° field using ½° bar width. An essentially normal clinical bar pattern is shown in Fig. 22-3; b wave is the most prominent portion of the response but the a wave is also detectable. This patient has primary pigmentary degeneration of the retina with practically complete extinction of scotopic and photopic flash responses. Absence of the bar pattern ERG in the presence of a normal flash response implies loss of function in the central area. Fig. 22-7 shows absent bar pattern and photopic flash responses with preservation of strong scotopic flash response in a patient with congenital cone dysfunction.

Another limitation of the ERG results from the fact that the rods greatly outnumber the cones. Some estimate that there are 120 million rods compared to 7 million cones in each retina. Though many important clinical disturbances affect the central vision or macular area, the ERG is imprecise in seg-

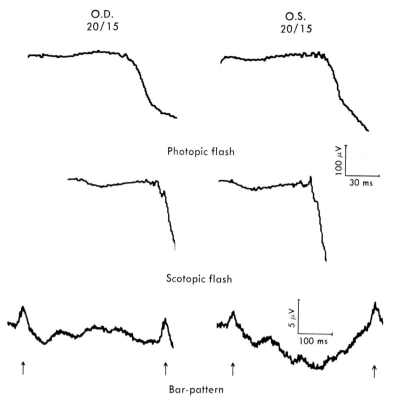

O.D.
20/15

O.S.
20/15

Photopic flash

100 μV

30 ms

Scotopic flash

5 μV

100 ms

Bar-pattern

Fig. 22-3. ERG in primary pigmentary degeneration inherited as a dominant defect. Macular preservation is indicated by essentially normal bar pattern that shows both a and b waves. Both photopic and scotopic flash ERGs are essentially extinct in right and left eye tracings.

regating these functions. In the visual mass response, rod activity overshadows that of the cones. Although the macular area contains almost entirely cones, there may be only about 350,000 cones there out of the total 7 million in the retina. Therefore a discrete macular lesion may entirely destroy these macular cones, but cone ERG responses might appear normal because of the mass response of the overwhelming number of extramacular cones.

However, photopic and scotopic tests, red light, and flicker fusion help separate the rod from the cone waves.

TECHNIQUE OF USE

Where ERG's are to be made in most general hospitals, major clinics, or group practice situations, the usual electrically shielded room for electroencephalography is quite adequate. Shielding may be generally satisfactory with copper wire screen or with thin solid copper plate or foil. The shielding, as well as all equipment, must be grounded through either cold water pipes or a separate ground stake going several feet into the earth. The room should easily accommodate a full-length stretcher with access to the patient. A ceiling lower than 8 ft. or a room length less than 10 ft. is often unpleasant and suggests a torture cell rather than a relaxed diagnostic setting.

Pupils should be fully dilated when possible with drops such as 1% Mydriacyl or 2.5% Neo-Synephrine, after inspection to ensure that the anterior chambers are at least of average depth. If the patient has had narrow-angle glaucoma or has a very shallow chamber, or if gonioscopy in uncertain cases shows a narrow filtration angle, then this aid to electroretinography must be omitted. The desirable use of these topical instillations tends to eliminate iris and ciliary muscle action potential as well as the alterations in stimulus intensity induced by changes in pupillary diameter.

Smoking should be omitted for at least 1 hour before examination. The face should be washed or cleansed of make-up and skin oils in the areas to be used for electrode contact.

The patient should be placed in a comfortable supine position on a padded couch or stretcher as he is given a clear accounting of what will transpire. If contact lens electrodes are used, a topical anesthetic such as proparacaine hydrochloride (Ophthaine) should be instilled. This is omitted if small skin electrodes are substituted for the active poles; they should be taped over a minute amount of electrolyte jelly at a point on the orbital rim below the cornea. The negative or indifferent electrode is taped to the skin above the glabella. The patient is instructed to leave both eyes open, to maintain steady fixation on an overhead point, and not to blink during the tests.

Routines may be quite simplified or complicated by use of many different stimuli and various adaptations. In all cases calibration should be established before and after each examination by recording a linear deflection of the pen equal to a known potential; ordinarily this should be about half of maximum response to be obtained. Preadaptation is achieved with a standard light source such as two 100-watt light bulbs behind a diffusing screen 5 ft. from the eyes for a period of 5 minutes. A light meter may be used to check consistency of this preadaptation light and to avoid unsuspected reduction caused by aging filaments.

Light-adapted responses can be elicited with the stroboscopic flash at maximum intensity. Individual flashes should be separated by at least 3 seconds. Brief bursts of flicker response should also be obtained. When satisfactory light-adapted tracings are recorded, all background and room light is extinguished. Dark adaptation responses are recorded at 1, 3, 5, 9, 15, and 25 minutes or other determined intervals. These brief test flashes even at high intensity do not alter the course of dark adaptation when presented at intervals of greater than 1 second. The patient may close his lids during the period of longer intervals between flashes.

When children are tested it is preferable to have a parent remain in the shielded room beside the child. Infants and very small children will require general or basal anesthesia. Attendants should not touch a patient during examination because this will create electric artifacts.

THE ERG IN PATIENTS WITH OCULAR ABNORMALITIES
Retinal degenerations (involutions)

The large group of retinal degenerations has been one of the most informative areas for use of the ERG. Aid is afforded in diagnosis, recording the functional course of the disease, finding carrier states in unaffected relatives, and providing a better understanding of the disease process. Conversely, correlating electroretinographic changes with the clinical findings has helped in understanding the ERG itself.

Primary pigmentary degeneration of the retina (retinitis pigmentosa). The ERG may be completely absent or of very low amplitude in retinitis pigmentosa. There may be only a small photopic ERG, with almost no scotopic response. This is evidence of widespread rod disease, which precedes the cone involvement with its late reduction of central acuity. This correlates with early impairments of dark adaptation and later night blindness (Fig. 22-3).

In some patients with loss of scotopic vision and early loss of the b wave, there may be no classical findings of bone corpuscle pigmentation. Narrowed vessels and waxy discs, however, help to establish the basic diagnosis of retinitis pigmentosa sine pigmento. In other cases, the pigment shows unusual form or distribution. The ERG may help to differentiate primary from secondary degenerations caused by syphilis, trauma, rubella, vaccinia, or febrile diseases. In the secondary degenerations, the ERG is normal or only slightly reduced in most cases. If the retina is severely affected, however, the ERG may be absent or very low, as in primary disease. If the ERG is near normal, the disease is probably secondary; if it is very abnormal, one cannot be certain.

The ERG is valuable in studying relatives of affected patients. The disease is commonly autosomal dominant, autosomal recessive, or sex-linked recessive, though isolated cases occur. Electroretinography may give early diagnosis in other members of the family, which can help in career planning and genetic counseling. Electroretinography and dark adaptometry are the most sensitive tests in retinitis pigmentosa.

Retinal abiotrophy. In cases of macular degenerations that are really only part of more widespread retinal disorders, as commonly found in children presenting predominantly macular involution, the ERG may show severe changes similar to retinitis pigmentosa. This indicates widespread disease beyond its morphologic manifestations and consequently a poor prognosis. These disturbances are often associated with other systemic or ocular diseases. The finding of an abnormal ERG is evidence of retinal dysfunction that might go unsuspected in myotonic dystrophy, certain cases of Hurler's disease, and high myopia.

Retinitis punctata albescens. Retinitis punctata albescens, a rare form of involution, is characterized by great numbers of small white dot-like areas throughout the retina, with associated narrowing of retinal vessels and pigmentation. The full-blown disease often runs a progressive course with night blindness and contraction of the visual fields. A stationary type also occurs, usually evidenced by night blindness but with no tendency toward progression and therefore a better prognosis. It can be very difficult to distinguish the two types clinically. The ERG may be helpful here, but varying types of response have been recorded. In general, the ERG is severely reduced or absent in the advanced cases and relatively normal in the stationary form. Following the patient with ERG's over a period of years may anticipate progression by revealing depression of the ERG before clinical evidence appears.

Choroideremia

Choroideremia is characterized by progressive atrophy of the choroid and pigment

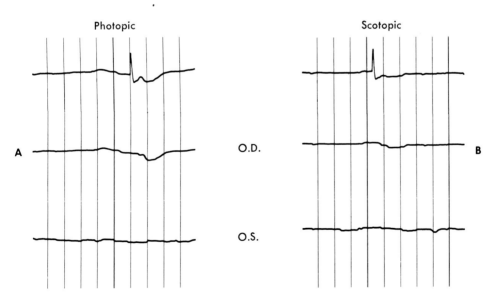

Fig. 22-4. Electroretinographic tracings showing essentially extinguished responses in a 69-year-old male with choroideremia. Top tracings show stimulus flash. Middle tracings are from right eye. Bottom tracings are from left eye. **A**, Photopic examination; **B**, scotopic examination.

epithelium leading to night blindness and gross loss of field. It is a male, sex-linked manifestation, but the carrier females show milder fundus pigment abnormalities with mild or no loss of function. The ERG in choroideremia is usually absent (Fig. 22-4). The ERG is not necessary to establish the diagnosis in characteristic cases but may be helpful in atypical cases.

Circulatory diseases

Central retinal artery occlusion. The ERG usually shows a normal or larger than normal a wave with marked reduction of the b wave, especially b_s. This is the so-called *negative* ERG. Rarely a negative response is seen, with a large a and b_s wave. Electroretinographic findings correlate with the known retinal and choroidal circulation. Thus central retinal artery occlusion affects the inner retinal layers, usually down to the inner nuclear layer, and impairs bipolar cells more than the rods and cones, which derive their supply from the choroidal circulation. This explains retention of the a wave and reduction of the b wave. The amplitude of the b wave may be an indication of the degree of arterial obstruction; that is, a relatively normal b wave indicates only partial obstruction and better prognosis.

Central retinal vein occlusion. Electroretinographic findings are often similar to those of arterial occlusion, but the b wave is retained more often, probably indicating that partial occlusion is more common with the vein than with the artery. Depth of electroretinographic impairment may aid in prognosis, but correlation with the final visual result is not exact.

In branch vein occlusion, the ERG is usually normal or may show a slight reduction of the b wave. Occasionally a greater than normal b wave is seen. Such an ERG is called "supranormal" (Fig. 22-5).

Temporal (cranial) arteritis. A very large a wave, larger than in any other condition, and a slightly reduced b wave may be pathognomonic of temporal arteritis (Burian). The ERG is similar in both eyes, though only one eye is affected clinically. This is usually not seen if steroid therapy has been started.

Carotid artery disease. Ipsilateral diminished b waves are suggestive of carotid insufficiency. In bilateral disease, the ERG may be unequal on the two sides, probably reflecting the status of collateral circulation. Electroretinographic results must be correlated with other studies, such as ophthalmodynamometry and arteriography. The

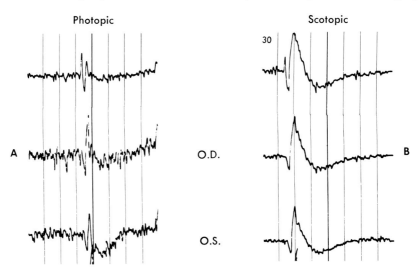

Fig. 22-5. Electroretinograms showing "supranormal" responses in right eye of 65-year-old patient with central retinal vein occlusion. Top tracings show stimulus flash. Middle tracings are from right eye. Bottom tracings are from left eye. **A,** Photopic examination; **B,** scotopic examination.

risks of arteriography should be avoided if other tests can give equally accurate information (pp. 247-251).

Systemic hypertension and arteriosclerosis. Mild degrees of interference with retinal vascular supply may cause an increase in the b wave, while more severe disturbance decreases the b wave. The increased response may result from greater irritability of neurons with mild degrees of anoxia.

Though not completely consistent, the ERG affords some index of the severity of the systemic disease and general prognosis.

Systemic diseases

Diabetes. In general, electroretinographic changes parallel the degree of retinal damage but may not correlate with visual acuity. Wavelets are often missing on rising limb of the b wave. After "glucose loading" by intravenous infusion of 500 ml. of 30% glucose, normal patients show no increase in retinal electric activity; however, long-standing diabetic patients show increased activity even if no retinopathy is visible ophthalmoscopically. Severe diabetic retinopathy is associated with an even greater increase in retinal electric activity. Henkes has coined the term "fundus diabeticus" to indicate the condition of patients with retinal dysfunction in the absence of ophthalmoscopic changes. Similarly fluorescein angiography often shows more widespread retinopathy than is revealed by ophthalmoscopy (Fig. 22-6).

Thyroid disease. Generally the electroretinographic amplitude is found to parallel the thyroid status, being "supranormal" in hyperthyroidism and reduced in hypothyroidism. This returns to normal when either condition is effectually treated.

Myotonic dystrophy. Cataracts and ptosis are commonly found in myotonic dystrophy, and several investigations have found decreased b waves in almost all patients with

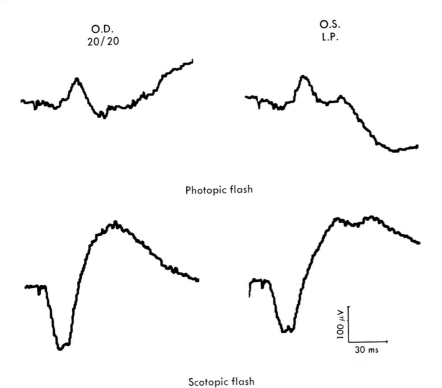

O.D.
20/20

O.S.
L.P.

Photopic flash

100 μV

30 ms

Scotopic flash

Fig. 22-6. ERG from patient with diabetic retinopathy. Wavelets are often missing as in this case on the rising limb of the b wave. Neither amplitude nor latency of the retained ERG responses can be correlated with visual acuity.

myotonic dystrophy, thus adding to understanding of the widespread nature of the disease.

Hurler's disease. Abnormal ERG's are found in many cases of Hurler's disease, which is primarily considered to present corneal opacity as the significant ocular finding.

Liver disease. Both acute or chronic hepatitis and cirrhosis of the liver cause elevated dark-adapted thresholds and reduced b waves. These changes are probably caused by abnormal vitamin A storage or metabolism but are not directly proportional to the degree of liver disease.

Drug toxicity

The ERG can be of value as an objective index both of degree and site of impairment from retinotoxic compounds.

Chloroquine. Chloroquine retinopathy, unlike the reversible corneal impairments caused by crystalline deposits, can cause severe permanent visual loss, and it is difficult to detect in early stages while potentially reversible. Usually the diagnosis is made morphologically or functionally after the characteristic macular pigmentation, or ring scotoma, is noted. In early stages, electroretinography and tests of dark adaptation may be equivocal; electroretinographic impairments are often very subtle until the disease is well established.

Thioridazine hydrochloride (Mellaril). Mellaril, a widely used tranquilizer, can also cause retinal damage after prolonged administration. Depressed ERG's have been found in some cases.

Quinine. Quinine intoxication can cause severe visual loss. In the early and acute stage, the ERG is usually normal despite reduced vision, probably because initial damage is localized to the ganglion cells, which have no appreciable effect on the ERG.

Opaque media

In the presence of dense corneal opacities, pupillary occlusion, or cataract, the ERG gives an objective index of diffuse (mass) retinal function. Other tests of retinal function such as flicker fusion perimetry (pp. 225-226) and auto-ophthalmoscopic perimetry (p. 208), which are applicable when the fundus cannot be visualized, rely on subjective responses. The clinical ERG, however, does not give precise evidence of macular function under these conditions.

Regardless of cataract density, a normal retina will yield a normal ERG. Comparison of ERG's before and after cataract extraction usually shows little or no difference. If the preoperative ERG is normal, there is no widespread retinal disease, but there still can be localized macular or focal disease or optic nerve pathology. If the preoperative ERG is diminished, one must expect some visual limitation after cataract extraction, particularly in the extent of peripheral vision.

Infants and children

The ERG can be objectively helpful in examination of children too young for subjective tests, such as acuity or fields, or when there is suggestion of decreased vision with normal or questionable fundi. In children with abnormal fundi, the ERG may yield information helpful in diagnosis, prognosis, and management. Children age 7 or over can usually be tested with topical anesthesia, as in adults, but younger children may require general or basal anesthesia or strong sedation that may alter their ERG.

Leber's congenital amaurosis. Congenital amaurosis is a defect in which vision is greatly diminished at birth or early in life. Nystagmus, photophobia, and also keratoglobus are common. The fundi may appear normal early in the disease, although pigmentation and vascular narrowing often develop later. The ERG shows greatly reduced or absent photopic and scotopic responses. This proves the presence of widespread retinal dysfunction.

Congenital retinal dysfunction. Congenital retinal dysfunction is a term used by Karpe and Zetterstrom (1958) to describe children with decreased vision, normal fundi, and abnormal ERG's that later improve. This appears to be a developmental delay or retardation at the retinal level.

Congenital cone dysfunction syndromes. Congenital cone dysfunction may occur in complete or partial forms. When complete, the visual acuity is about 20/200 and there is nystagmus, photophobia, and total absence of color discrimination (achromatopsia). Partial forms show visual acuity of 20/40 to 20/100, minimal or no nystagmus and photophobia, and only a partial color vision defect. The fundi are usually normal but may show loss of foveal reflexes and macular abnormalities. This syndrome is frequently misdiagnosed as congenital nystagmus, particularly in children too young to test for color vision or if color vision tests are not done. The ERG is usually diagnostic, showing markedly decreased photopic and bar pattern responses, diminished flicker fusion frequency, and essentially normal scotopic responses (Fig. 22-7).

Albinism. Albinism is distinguished from true retinal degeneration or dysfunction by specific electroretinographic findings. Other ocular functions resemble the cone dysfunction syndrome, with nystagmus, photophobia, and decreased vision caused by macular hypoplasia. The ERG is normal or greater than normal because of increased reflection and scattering of light, in contrast to the various electroretinographic depressions in other types of pathology.

Night blindness. Detecting night blindness in children (as well as in adults) is an area in which the ERG may be very helpful. Progressive patterns, such as in retinitis pigmentosa, choroideremia, or retinitis punctata albescens, can at times be differentiated from stationary defects such as congenital night blindness. If the ERG is greatly decreased or absent, there is severe retinal degeneration, but if there is only modest decrease in scotopic responses, congenital night blindness is likely. Early cases of retinitis pigmentosa, however, may show similar find-

O. D.
20/70

O. S.
20/70

Photopic flash

$100 \mu V$

30 ms

Scotopic flash

$5 \mu V$

100 ms

Bar-pattern

Fig. 22-7. ERG in the presence of cone dysfunction shows total lack of photopic flash response in the presence of well-preserved scotopic flash response. There is no bar pattern response. Tracings are almost identical from right and left eyes.

ings, so that an absolute distinction cannot be made.

Other diseases. In optic nerve lesions, cortical or central blindness, and hysteria or malingering, the ERG is normal and may make unnecessary further and possibly hazardous tests.

In true retinal degenerations, the ERG may make the diagnosis before functional or ophthalmoscopic changes are noted. This will help in genetic counseling and education planning. The ERG may distinguish primary from secondary retinal changes (pp. 290-291).

Neurology

Visually evoked responses. VER's recorded from scalp electrodes over the occiput following photic stimulation of the eyes are elaborations of electroretinographic and electroencephalographic techniques.

Three major aims of response studies are (1) to plot an "objective" visual field by stimulating localized retinal areas, (2) to measure macular function, and (3) to determine the exact location of lesions of the visual pathway anywhere from the retina to the occipital cortex. An objective visual field test would be very helpful in circumstances involving uncooperative or comatose patients and little children. Changes in the VER involve the shape, amplitude, and latency of the waves, which may differentiate the location of lesions causing similar field defects.

The VER in present laboratory conditions offers detection of macular or other localized conditions less identifiable with current ERG's. This is facilitated by the geographically large cortical area of projection associated with the macula. Amblyopia and migraine also seem to present changes in the VER that are becoming clinically useful.

Multiple sclerosis. Multiple sclerosis, a widespread disease of the nervous system with frequent ocular manifestations, has classically been thought to yield a normal ERG because the usual cause of decreased vision is damage to the optic nerve rather than to the retina. However, Gills (1966) has described abnormal ERG's in many multiple sclerosis patients. Some histopathology studies have found decreased cellularity of the inner nuclear layer, raising the possibility of retrograde transsynaptic degeneration.

Other ocular disorders

Glaucoma. Most investigators report a normal ERG in glaucoma except for acute congestive or very advanced stages. Glaucoma damage is primarily to the nerve fibers and ganglion cells, which do not contribute to the ERG. In some advanced cases, however, there is severe impairment of the retinal and choroidal circulation that diminishes or extinguishes the ERG.

In acute glaucoma there may be a temporary increase of the b wave similar to that in hypoxic states, such as hypertension or partial vascular occlusion.

Retinal detachment. In serous detachments, generally the higher the preoperative b wave amplitude, the better the final visual prognosis. The b wave in the "normal" fellow eye should be watched for reductions, which suggest a guarded outlook. Many other variables, however, affect the detached retina and make specific conclusions of limited validity. Nonetheless, patients with retinal detachment should have preoperative electroretinographic tests bilaterally, where these are available.

Siderosis. Early in the course of intraocular ferrous foreign bodies, both a and b waves are increased in amplitude. Later the b wave decreases, and finally the ERG becomes abolished in the late stages. These changes may be present before any subjective or objective manifestations of siderosis. The earliest changes represent a reversible stage, with return toward normal if the foreign body is removed successfully. Later stages are irreversible.

Myopia. The ERG is normal in the mild or usual type of myopia. In severe, progressive, or malignant myopia, however, the b wave is often decreased in proportion to the degree of retinal degeneration. The ERG may even be extinguished, which probably is evidence of other coexisting degeneration.

Harada's disease. Harada's disease is basically a posterior uveitis with exudative retinal detachment, and it is probably a part of the Vogt-Koyanagi syndrome. The ERG is greatly diminished early in the course of the disease because of retinal edema or detachment. The edema may be missed ophthalmoscopically, and the clinician is then faced with the problem of severe loss of vision without obvious cause. Associated neurologic symptoms and signs point to optic nerve or cerebral disease. A diminished ERG is definite evidence of widespread retinal involvement and helps make the correct diagnosis. The scotopic ERG is affected more than the photopic. The abnormal ERG usually returns toward normal as the detachment disappears, paralleling the return of vision.

REFERENCES

Karpe, G., and Zettersttom, B.: Congenital retinal dysfunction, Am. J. Ophthalmol. **45:**249, 1958.

Lawwill, T.: The bar pattern electroretinogram for clinical evaluation of the central retina, Am. J. Ophthalmol. **78:**121-126, 1974.

Electrooculography

Theodore Lawwill, M.D.

Electrooculography is a diagnostic study of the integrity of the pigment epithelium of the retina as determined from changes in the standing corneoretinal potential of the eye. This potential has been known since the 1849 pioneering electrophysiology of DuBois Reymond and subsequently has been found to have a constant or resting value of up to 6 millivolts. The size of this potential varies with the state of light adaptation. Measurement is made indirectly from lightweight electrodes taped to the inner and outer canthal skin (Fig. 23-1). When the eye is rotated horizontally the cornea comes closer to one electrode while the posterior pole comes closer to the other. This alters the voltage across the electrodes in a predictable manner. As the eye moves back and forth through a known angle, the relative amplitude of the potential is found. After calibration, the amplitude and frequency changes may be used, reversely, to record the excursions and rate of involuntary oscillations of the eye (electronystagmography, pp. 302-306).

Changes are elicited by voluntary rotation of the eyes through predetermined arcs in the dark-adapted and subsequently in the light-adapted states. Numerical values are expressed as a ratio or as the arithmetic quotient obtained from dividing the usually higher electric potential of the "light peak" by the usually lower electric potential of the "dark trough."

Primarily investigative studies with the electrooculograph in the last 25 years have shown it to be a clinically sensitive diagnostic device to identify impairments in the retinal pigment epithelium. The ERG is less sensitive than the electrooculogram (EOG) in detecting such deep changes. On the other hand, EOG's in achromatic and nyctalopic patients may be identical to those from normal patients, whereas the ERG in the presence of such pathology will show marked reduction of electric activity. Like most electrophysiologic diagnosis procedures, however, a moderate amount of complex and fragile equipment is required. This is often best protected and operated in a special clinic where such devices are familiar to and cared for by specific technicians. Generally these devices are not expected in the offices of busy practitioners, and probably they should be located in hospitals or medical centers where they may be available to several users.

The EOG is based on a standing current or corneoretinal potential (CRP), which appears to flow through the eye in the direction of the visual axis, thus rendering the globe analogous to a rotatable dipole of positive charge at the cornea and negative charge at the maculopapular area. Because the pickup electrodes (Fig. 23-1) are placed on the canthal skin, remote from the extraocular muscles, the EOG does not reflect action potentials of these muscles, which disturb the ERG. Electric potentials range between 15 and 30 mv. per degree of ocular rotation. The detecting and amplifying system must afford sufficient gain to display these signals on a recorder, such as the Grass polygraphs employed for electroencephalography.

In use, the patient with dilated pupils should be seated comfortably with his occiput resting on a suitably positioned headrest (leaning slightly forward, for a chin and forehead support may be more fatiguing over the 20 or 25 minutes needed for testing). Two conspicuous fixation lights about 30 to 60 degrees apart are located equidistant to each side of the subject's sagittal plane. A screen, diffusing sphere, or other suitable bright illumination source of several hundred ft./lumens is placed between them. The patient is instructed to perform horizontal rotations from one fixation light to the other. Heights of the vertical deflections on the recorder represent the amplitude of the standing potential.

The patient should gain familiarity with

Fig. 23-1. EOG electrodes taped on the inner and outer canthial skin. An electrolyte paste is used between the electrodes and the skin.

Fig. 23-2. Normal EOG tracing. Each vertical excursion corresponds to a rotation of the eye between the two fixation lights. Normally the recorded potentials at least double from the dark adapted state (DT or dark trough) to the light adapted state (LP or light peak; shown here at 7 min.).

the test situation and then be permitted to dark-adapt for 12 minutes while repeating the ocular excursions at intervals of about 1 minute. A "dark trough" of minimal potential is usually reached between 8 and 13 minutes. The eye is then suddenly reilluminated and recording continued at 1-minute intervals for about another 12 minutes. A "light peak" of maximum potential is usually reached in 8 or 9 minutes. In normal patients, the standing potential will at least double between dark and light adaptation (Fig. 23-2).

Because absolute values are difficult to establish and are altered by several factors* in the test situation, more useful information is obtained from the "light peak/dark trough" ratio. Normal ratios are between 3 and 2. Ratios from 2 to 1.75 are borderline, and those between 1.75 and 1.5 are probably subnormal. Those lower than 1.5 are definitely pathologic, and a ratio of 1 shows no light response. (Sometimes these figures are multiplied by 100 and expressed as percentages, which has the unfortunate connotation of suggesting that no light response is "100%.") The EOG is reduced in diffuse

disturbances of the pigment epithelium and vitelliform degeneration. It is also reduced along with the ERG in some retinal degenerations as the retinitis pigmentosa group.

Electrooculography is a functional diagnostic adjunct to verify or interpret morphologic disturbances in the pigment epithelium as seen ophthalmoscopically or with the aid of intravenous fluorescein studies. The EOG, in common with the ERG, tends to provide a diffuse response or to measure a diffuse disturbance, but unlike the ERG it derives primarily from the pigment epithelium and possibly metabolic activity in the outer limbs of the rods. The EOG does not reflect localized disturbances such as those confined to the macula. It does not reflect disturbances of the inner layers of the retina nor of the optic nerve. Thus the EOG is primarily valuable in early detection of abiotrophic processes, particularly those striking the pigment epithelium.

REFERENCES

Arden, G. B., and Kelsey, J. H.: Changes produced by light in the standing potential of the human eye, J. Physiol. **161**:189, 1962.

Marg, E.: Development of electrooculography, Arch. Ophthalmol. **45**:169, 1951.

Reeser, F. W., Weinstein, G. W., Feiock, K. B., and Oser, R. S.: Electrooculography as a test of retinal function, Am. J. Ophthalmol. **70**:505, 1970.

*Preadaptation, light intensity, arc and speed of rotation, amplifying equipment, reduction in skin resistance with time, drowsiness, medications, and so forth.

Nystagmography

NYSTAGMOLOGY

There is no subject within ophthalmic, neurologic, or otologic literature wherein nomenclature is so varied and imprecise as in the field of nystagmology. Nystagmus itself should be defined as involuntary oscillations or tremors of the eyes independent of normal movements. It is usually bilateral but rarely may be unilateral or voluntary. For clarity of description, awareness of mechanism, and diagnostic thinking, the following seven components should be noted:

A. Onset
  1. Congenital and often hereditary: this is usually pendular and horizontal, though it may rarely be vertical or torsional
  2. Acquired
  3. Experimental (induced, opticokinetic)
B. Type or form of movements
  1. Pendular: this is characteristic of ocular nystagmus resulting from visual impairment of 20/100 or worse from birth or very early life
  2. Searching movements of blindisms: these are slow, irregular, inconstant, and not properly considered a true nystagmus
  3. Jerk nystagmus: this may be in any direction but typically has a slow component in one direction (which usually represents the pathologic mechanism) and a fast or recovery component in the opposite direction; it is classically seen in vestibular, central, and induced nystagmus
  4. Latent nystagmus: this is not manifest unless one eye is closed; it is characteristically a jerk nystagmus and is often associated with heterotropia
  5. Disjunctive and seesaw nystagmus: this is a rare manifestation in which the eyes oscillate toward and away from each other, or one ascends while the other descends; it is possibly associated with pineal tumors
  6. Voluntary and fixation nystagmus: these are rare manifestations, usually of fine amplitude and very high frequency (fixation nystagmus is nonvoluntary aside from the fact that usually intent fixation on a nonmoving object is required for its development)

7. Miscellaneous rare forms: these include periodic alternating nystagmus (generally a jerk nystagmus with changes in its laterality); opsoclonus (conjugate but chaotic and apparently random movements in a young child carrying a generally encouraging prognosis); retraction nystagmus (usually a serious midbrain lesion associated with difficulty in vertical gaze and sometimes related to pinealoma in children or vascular lesions in adults); downbeat nystagmus (associated with foramen magnum lesions and especially evoked in extremes of lateral gaze); and ocular flutter and bobbing (series of rapid movements during fixation or at times presenting spontaneously and usually associated with cerebellar lesions)
C. Direction (laterality): mechanistically this should specify the slow component as the pathologically incited phase, though much of the literature has previously named the fast component (recovery) as the direction of the nystagmus
D. Mechanism
  1. Physiologic, end point, or fatigue nystagmus or pseudonystagmus: this appears only in the extremes of ocular versions, particularly horizontal rotation, and is generally normal; it is obliterated by shifting the eyes a few degrees back toward the primary position
  2. Ocular: this is associated with visual impairments and poor fixation ability resulting from (1) congenital defects, such as albinism, cataracts, optic atrophy, or achromatopsia, or (2) acquired disturbances of the visual mechanisms such as head-nodding (spasmus nutans) coming on at the age of 4 to 24 months or miner's nystagmus (allegedly associated with years of labor under poor lighting)
  3. Vestibular or labyrinthine: this is the classical jerk nystagmus with or without conjugate deviation and past pointing; usually acquired; may be experimentally induced by galvanic, caloric, or pressure devices
  4. Central or cerebellar: this is a jerk nystagmus frequently associated with cerebellar disease but which may also accompany disease of medulla, pons, or midbrain; it is accentuated when the eyes are closed or deviated to the side of the lesion; it may be abolished by ocular fixation when the eyes are open, and often this is effected in a particular position of gaze deviation

E. Speed (sometimes called "intensity"): this is expressed in degrees per second as read from the electronystagmographic tracing, or qualitatively described on direct observation as *slow*, *fast*, or *medium* speed.

F. Amplitude (excursion): this is measured in degrees (Electronystagmographs should be adjusted so that a 20-degree eye movement equals a pen deflection of 20 mm. Clinically this is described as "coarse" when the amplitude is over 15 degrees, "fine" when it is less than 5 degrees, and "moderate" when it is between these extremes.)

G. Frequency (rate): this is expressed in oscillations (beats) per second, or qualitatively described on direct observation as *high* (rapid), *moderate*, or *low*

TECHNIQUE OF NYSTAGMOGRAPHY

JOSEPH U. TOGLIA, M.D.

Corneoretinal potential

The electronystagmogram (ENG) is based on recording of the standing corneoretinal potential (CRP). This shows, upon movement of the eyes, the transfer of a positive electric charge from the cornea to the nearest periorbital skin electrode. Its average strength varies up to 400 to 800 mv. and is influenced by physiologic and extraphysiologic factors, among which are light and darkness, alertness and drowsiness, anoxia, acapnia, and medications. Fluctuations as large as 400 mv. occur from day to day, and cannot be correlated with metabolic changes in the human body. Excitement of the patient significantly increases the strength of the CRP, even when the patient has been dark-adapted prior to testing. Some of the tests are performed in absolute darkness to avoid the inhibitory influence of fixation upon vestibular nystagmus. It is recommended that the patient be dark-adapted for 10 to 15 minutes before electronystagmographic examinations are made.

The amplitude of the CRP in dark adaption decreases to a minimum in about 13 minutes and thereafter gradually increases to return in 30 minutes to the original value. In the further course of light adaptation, the amplitude reaches a maximum in about 8 minutes, after which it gradually returns in about 14 minutes to the value observed at the beginning of light adaptation. These factors must be considered when interpreting electronystagmographic records.

Electrodes

Much attention has been devoted to the construction of special electrodes and devices to keep them in firm contact with the skin. Corneal electrodes are not generally recommended. The Beckman biopotential skin electrodes have generally eliminated the problems of stability and are very useful.

The arrangement of the electrodes varies. I use one electrode at the bridge of the nose and one at each lateral canthus for recording horizontal movements of each eye and a pair of vertical electrodes for each eye.

The electrodes are connected to the electroencephalographic amplifiers so that:

1. Upward and downward eye movements are recorded respectively as upward and downward pen deflections on the first two channels. The first channel (left vertical lead) is connected with the left eye, the second (right vertical lead) with the right eye.

2. Right and left horizontal eye movements are recorded correspondingly as upward and downward pen deflections on both the third and fourth channels. The third channel (left horizontal lead) is connected with the left eye and the fourth (right horizontal lead) with the right.

3. Channel five (bitemporal lead) records horizontal gaze movements to the right as upward deflections and to the left as downward deflections, utilizing the bitemporal summation of both corneoretinal potentials.

Recording apparatus

Recording apparatus is selected not only on personal and economic choice but also in regard to specific applications. Otologists interested in labyrinthine function stress the velocities of each phase of nystagmus since they equate speed (degrees per second) of the slow phase to the speed of the endolymphatic flow. Modern apparatus, such as the

LT. VERT. LEAD

RT. VERT. LEAD

LT. HOR. LEAD

RT. HOR. LEAD

BITEMP.

LEAD   SPONT. NYS.   OKN DRUM TO LT.   OKN DRUM TO RT.

Fig. 24-1. Nystagmogram of patient with prosthesis in right orbit following surgical removal of the globe. Vision in the left eye is reduced to poor light projection with resultant pendular nystagmus. No electric activities can be seen on the right. Rotation of opticokinetic drum to left does not change pendular nystagmus. Rotation to the right, however, converts the pendular nystagmus to an irregular nystagmus with slow component to the left and rapid recovery movement to the right.

Beckman Dynograph Type R,* has built-in electronic devices able to derive the speed of each phase. Ophthalmologists, like neurologists, are mainly interested in frequency (rate), amplitude, type, and form of the nystagmus and whether the nystagmus is monocular or binocular.

Some instruments use D.C. and others use A.C. With the D.C. type, the changes in voltage, recorded through the electrodes, are proportional to the angle of ocular deviation, and the position of the eyes is continuously recorded. With the A.C. type, the height of the pen deflection represents the speed and not the amplitude of the eye movements; the higher the spike, the higher the speed of the eye movements (Fig. 24-1).

I use a multichannel electronystagmograph but also use standard electroencephalographic equipment with complete satisfaction. The electroencephalograph is available in almost every hospital. It has suitable filters for eliminating high-frequency potentials, more channels than actually are needed, more than

*Nystagmus Coupler, manufactured by Beckman Instruments, Inc., Bala Cynwyd, Pennsylvania. Electrooculographic equipment can be used for electronystagmography. Two-channel systems with recorders, skin electrodes, and Torok goggles are assembled by Instrumentation and Control Systems, Inc. (ICS), Addison, Illinois 60101.

one paper speed, and more than one time constant. Modifications may be arranged so that a long time constant of 10 seconds is available if desired. The D.C. recording or a long time constant of 10 seconds is advisable for continuously and simultaneously recording the ocular position and the nystagmus. Position information is important because gaze deviation toward the slow phase decreases the nystagmus, whereas deviation toward the fast phase increases the nystagmus (Alexander's law). Convergence and vertical deviation of the eyes also influence the nystagmus to a great extent.

To record eye movements of each eye in both horizontal and vertical planes, at least a four-channel apparatus is needed, and thus the electroencephalograph, available in almost every hospital, remains the first choice. A recording should be obtained using a time constant of 10 seconds (Fig. 24-2).

Photoelectric pickups

Torok's (1951) or Pfaltz's (1956) techniques use a photoelectric cell placed immediately in front of one eye to pick up variations of reflected infrared light focused astride the corneoscleral margin so that it falls partly on the sclera and partly on the iris. During nystagmus, reflections of the infrared beam from the sclera increase and

Fig. 24-2. Electronystagmogram showing marked horizontal jerk type nystagmus predominantly appearing in the abducted eye during extremes of horizontal gaze rotation. Two top tracings show very little vertical activity. Bottom tracing, representing bitemporal leads, shows position of the two eyes first in gaze left and then in gaze right. Patient has multiple sclerosis.

decrease rhythmically. Since the reflection coefficient of light is greater for the white sclera than the darker iris, the total reflected light increases and decreases proportionally with the eye movements. This avoids skin electrodes.

Antonuccio and Galletti (1965) modified the photoelectric technique, eliminating the effect of light and fixation by using a photoresistor. All photoelectric techniques eliminate the problems relative to the variations of CRP, position of electrodes, electric discharges of muscle, cutaneous sweating, and so on. However, the greatest disadvantage of photoelectronystagmography is again that the recording is limited to only one or two channels.

Calibration

Calibration spikes of 10 or 20 mm. are obtained by asking the patient to look alternately at two points marked on the wall or ceiling so as to give a rotational angle of 20 degrees. Two small red lights that alternately flash wtih a preset frequency, varying from 20 to 100 flashes per minute, give calibration by stimulating the patient automatically to move his eyes between the flashing lights. The lights must be at least 3 meters from the patient to avoid convergence unless one eye only is used. Calibration is one of the most important technical aspects if quanti-

tative analysis is desired. Unfortunately the CRP is subject to many influences, some of which are difficult to control, so quantitative analysis remains dubious. Calibrations must be repeated frequently during the examination (Fig. 24-3).

Use

In use, the patient is placed supine on a table with the head elevated 30 degrees. The face is carefully cleaned with alcohol to remove all make-up and facial oils. Small electrodes covered with electrolyte jelly are then taped to the outer canthi and one (ground or indifferent) electrode is taped to the glabella. For vertical tracings, active electrodes are placed immediately below the center of the brow and on the center of the inferior orbital rim. A paper movement speed of 2.5, 5.0, or 10 mm. per second is convenient for calculating frequency and speed in degrees per second. After calibration, the eyes are closed to eliminate visual fixation, which is a very powerful suppressor of vestibular nystagmus. A spontaneous horizontal nystagmus of under 5 or 6 degrees per second may be found in 20% to 25% of the population when the lids are closed. As an aid in observation of fine and evoked nystagmus, internally illuminated Frenzel goggles with +20D lenses fitted over each eye are available from V. Mueller.

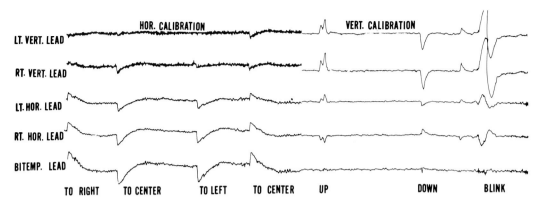

Fig. 24-3. Electronystagmogram in normal subject showing calibration at 10 degrees horizontal and vertical gaze deflections.

Caloric induction of nystagmus

For induced vestibular nystagmus of the horizontal canal alone, it is necessary to elevate the head to 30 degrees before caloric stimulation through either external auditory canal. Two constant-temperature water baths (30° and 44° C.) should be maintained for consistency of cold and hot responses. Irrigating techniques have generally been standardized at 30 seconds for the 30° C. water, with the trace beginning exactly 60 seconds after commencement of irrigation and continuing an additional 30 seconds. A similar routine is then repeated in the opposite ear 5 minutes after the onset of irrigation in the first ear. Subsequently, at 5-minute intervals the two external auditory canals are irrigated with water at 44° C.

From the 30-second tracing, representative 10-second segments of paper are cut and mounted. By measuring the lengths of the fast components in this 10-second segment, adding them, and dividing the sum by 10, the average speed in degrees per second is obtained. When a base line spontaneous nystagmus is present, its amplitude or speed must be subtracted in calculation of the related induced responses.

To diagnose relative impairment of one vestibular mechanism, at least a 20% differential should be quantitated between responses evoked from right and left stimuli before significance can be inferred. In questionable vestibular deficiency, confirmatory irrigation may be done with 30 ml. of ice water.

A competent technician should obtain good nystagmograms and complete induction tests in 30 minutes. The results can be analyzed in a few seconds. Spontaneous nystagmus is often not seen when the eyes are open but is revealed on closing the lids. Normally caloric testing evokes essentially similar nystagmus from either side and by hot or cold stimulus. The normal rhythmic frequency of response varies between 20 and 25 beats per 10-second period. A hyperactive response (increased frequency) with caloric stimulation indicates active end-organ function of the labyrinth, but it may also represent impairment of brainstem inhibition. Nonfunctioning of a vestibular mechanism (incorrectly called "canal paresis") is illustrated by good responses to both cold and hot on one side but no response from irrigations of the opposite canal; this is typical of acoustic neuroma. Directional preponderance from irrigation with cold on one side and hot on the other indicates a disorder somewhere in the vestibular system. Irregular rhythm (dysrhythmia) is commonly associated with brainstem abnormalities. If nystagmus from caloric stimulation with the eyes open and fixed is greater than with the eyes closed, there is failure of fixation suppression and presumptive evidence of central nervous system lesion. Opening the eyes in darkness tends to reduce the speed of spontaneous

Fig. 24-4. Vertically striped drum, which can be rotated slowly to right or left in front of patient for voluntary or involuntary visual fixation and analysis of opticokinetic nystagmus to or away from the side of suspect visual pathway lesions.

nystagmus but not to alter its form or direction.

Simple observation of the character and components of nystagmus in a patient affords immediate information concerning the eyes and local disease as well as the labyrinthian mechanism and the central nervous system. The most revealing items and the ones that must always be recorded are the history and onset (in the patient as well as his family), the type or form of movement, and the direction (when a jerk component is present). These facts, plus the details of ocular examination, usually reveal the mechanism. A test for latent nystagmus is automatically performed whenever one eye is covered, but the observer must note such an event and recall the unfailing impairment of monocular visual performance when it is elicited.

Induced or opticokinetic nystagmus obtained with a drum or tape elicits further diagnostic data regarding the depth or site of lesion. This is well included as a special office examination. The electronic studies of nystagmus, or the reverse studies of electrooculography obtainable with the same equipment, are generally clinical or laboratory procedures requiring considerable equipment and environmental controls. The clinician, however, must be aware of their value and the conditions calling for their use.

REFERENCE

Rubin, W. Nystagmography: terminology, technique, and instrumentation, Arch. Otolaryng. **87:**266, 1968.

CHAPTER 25

Electromyography

Electromyography is the recording of action potentials or integrated voltage discharges of the several related muscle fibers that constitute an individual motor unit. The group of muscle fibers and their motor end plates, which are innervated by a single nerve fiber, discharge synchronously but at various frequencies and amplitudes which depend on the resting or activity state of the muscles and the presence or absence of pathologic alterations. Discharges normally appear as diphasic spikes and are amplified for visual display on a cathode ray oscilloscope or for auditory display through a loudspeaker.

Although human electromyographic studies have been critically made for about two decades (Bjork, 1952; Adler, 1953; Breinin, 1955), the technique is largely a laboratory or research tool and is highly vulnerable to errors and artifacts of instrumentation, techniques, and interpretation. The examiner must be intimately aware of the range of fluctuations and variations within his equipment as well as the alterations generated or imposed by various muscular activities of the patient. Both subtle physiologic movements and overt changes in position of the head, the eyes, and the inserted recording needles can produce gross alterations in the recordings. The examiner must accomplish numerous, repeated observations at any sitting, with critical preparation to discard incompatible recordings and to insist upon more than a few consistent recordings before attempting any interpretations.

Technique with the patient calls for full cooperation, an electrically shielded room, and adequate stretcher space for the patient to recline comfortably. Topical anesthesia is used. General, local block, or infiltration anesthesia grossly impairs or extinguishes electrical activity and hence cannot be used. This precludes testing in most preadolescent patients. Needles are 28- to 30-gauge coaxial type with a separately insulated electrode fixed within the center of the lumen. The outer surface is insulated so that contact is limited to the very tip.

A lid speculum may be used to facilitate placement of the needle electrodes but must be removed during recording. The needles are inserted through the bulbar conjunctiva and into the long axis of the extraocular muscles proximal to their tendinous portions. It is advantageous to have the needles and the recording apparatus connected to auditory signaling during insertion. Thus the examiner's undivided visual attention can be maintained on the insertional path while he attains guidance assistance from changes in the sound of the auditory monitoring.

Just as ocular muscles differ histologically and pharmacologically from skeletal muscles, there is also difference in their electrical activity. The amplitude of discharge is low, measuring 5 to 100 mv. in the resting position and 400 to 600 mv. during rotational or contraction efforts. The duration of the diphasic discharge of a single spike is short, measuring 1 to 5 msec. whether the muscle is "at rest" or in active contracture. The frequency of discharge is high, measuring 100 to 200 per second during rest and increasing by several hundred during activity.

In the so-called position of rest, all extraocular muscles are found to be firing in generally similar patterns. This is in contradistinction to skeletal muscles at rest, which show essentially no electrical activity. Sherrington's law of reciprocal innervation and

Hering's law of equal bilateral innervation are corroborated by increased frequency and amplitude of activity in the agonists and correlated drops in the antagonists. *Complete electrical silence in the absence of disease,* however, is rare except under deep anesthesia, deep sleep, and extremes of opposite gaze.

Areas of electromyographic usefulness beyond strictly research applications are in the identification of lower motor neuron basis for an extraocular muscle paralysis, diagnosis of local muscular dystrophies, establishment of stage or therapeutic responsiveness in myasthenia gravis, identification of inflammatory lesions in the muscles, and possibly the differentiation of central or gaze lesions by their disturbances of agonist-antagonist relationships. The electrodes, however, record only from the motor units with which they are in direct contact, and therefore it is not accurate to generalize widely from such a given point to an entire muscle.

Additional readings

Ocular examination

Berliner, M. L.: Biomicroscopy of the eye, New York, 1966, Hafner Publishing Co.

Blodi, F., Allen, L., and Frazier, O.: Stereoscopic manual of the ocular fundus in local and systemic disease, ed. 2, St. Louis, 1970, The C. V. Mosby Co.

Critchley, M.: The dyslexic child, Springfield, Illinois, 1970, Charles C Thomas, Publisher.

Donaldson, D. D.: Atlas of external diseases of the eye: Cornea and sclera, vol. 3, St. Louis, 1971, The C. V. Mosby Co.

Donaldson, D. D.: Atlas of external diseases of the eye: Anterior chamber, iris, ciliary body, vol. 4, St. Louis, 1974, The C. V. Mosby Co.

Duke-Elder, W. S.: System of ophthalmology, vol. VII, St. Louis, 1962, The C. V. Mosby Co., pp. 231-458.

Eisner, G.: Biomicroscopy of the peripheral fundus, Heidelberg, 1973, Springer-Verlag.

Gass, J. D.: Differential diagnosis of intraocular tumors: A stereoscopic presentation, St. Louis, 1974, The C. V. Mosby Co.

Haining, W. M., editor: Recent advances in technical aspects of fluorescein angiography, Boston, 1974, Little, Brown & Co.

Hanafee, W. N.: Radiology of the orbit, Philadelphia, 1972, W. B. Saunders Co.

Hruby, K.: Slit lamp examination of vitreous and retina, Baltimore, 1967, The Williams & Wilkins Co.

Keeney, A. H., and Keeney, V. T.: Dyslexia: diagnosis and treatment of reading disorders, St. Louis, 1968, The C. V. Mosby Co.

Krill, A. E.: Hereditary retinal and choroidal disease, vol. 1, Evaluation, New York, 1972, Harper and Row.

Norn, M. S.: External eye: Methods of examination, Copenhagen, 1974, Scriptor.

Potts, A. M., editor: The assesssment of visual function, St. Louis, 1972, The C. V. Mosby Co.

Rosen, E. S., and Savir, H.: Basic ophthalmoscopy, New York, 1972, Appleton-Century-Crofts.

Shimizu, K.: Fluorescein microangiography at the ocular fundus, Baltimore, 1973, The Williams & Wilkins Co.

Straub, W.: Ophthalmologic investigational techniques, I, Stuttgart, 1970, Ferdinand Enke Verlag.

Thiel, R.: Atlas of diseases of the eye: typical ocular diseases, differential diagnosis, and histopathology, New York, 1963, Elsevier Publishing Co.

Zismor, J., and Lombardi, G.: Atlas of orbital radiography, Birmingham, 1973, Aesculapius Publishing Co.

Neurologic aspects of examination

Bender, M. B.: The approach to diagnosis in modern neurology, New York, 1967, Grune and Stratton, Inc.

Bickerstaff, E. R.: Neurological examination in clinical practice, ed. 3, Philadelphia, 1973, J. B. Lippincott Co.

Huber, A.: Eye symptoms in brain tumors, translated by F. C. Blodi, ed. 3, St. Louis, 1976, The C. V. Mosby Co.

Kestenbaum, A.: Clinical methods of neuro-ophthalmologic examination, ed. 2, New York, 1961, Grune and Stratton, Inc.

Krayenbuhl, H., and Yesargil, M. G.: Cerebral angiography, ed. 2, Philadelphia, 1968, J. B. Lippincott Co.

Mayo Clinic: Clinical examination in neurology, ed. 3, Philadelphia, 1971, W. B. Saunders Co.

Smith, J. L.: Optokinetic nystagmus: its use in topical neuro-ophthalmologic diagnosis, Springfield, Illinois, 1963, Charles C Thomas, Publisher.

Smith, J. L.: The pupil, Miami, 1974.

Van Allen, M. W.: Pictorial manual of neurologic tests, Chicago, 1969, Year Book Medical Publishers, Inc.

Identification and classification of ocular disturbances

Geeraets, W. J.: Ocular syndromes, ed. 3, Philadelphia, 1976, Lea & Febiger.

Mahlman, H. E.: Handbook of federal visual requirements and information, Chicago, 1971, Professional Press.

Riviere, M.: Rehabilitation codes, classification of impairment of vision function, New York, 1970, National Institute Neurologic Diseases and Blindness.

Roy, F. H.: Ocular differential diagnosis, ed. 2, Philadelphia, 1975, Lea & Febiger.

Scheppart-Kimmijser, J., Colenbrender, J. A., and Franken, S.: Coding systems for disorders of the eye, White Plains, New York, 1968, Phiebig Publishing Co.

Thornton, S. P.: Ophthalmic eponyms and encyclopedia of named signs, syndromes, and diseases, Birmingham, 1967, Aesculapius Publishing Co.

Glaucoma

Becker, S. C.: Clinical gonioscopy, St. Louis, 1972, The C. V. Mosby Co.

Draeger, J.: Tonometry, New York, 1966, Hafner Publishing Co.

Drews, R. C.: Manual of tonography, St. Louis, 1971, The C. V. Mosby Co.

Gloster, J.: Tonometry and tonography, Boston, 1965, Little, Brown & Co.

Kolker, A. E., and Hetherington, J.: Becker-Shaffer's Diagnosis and therapy of the glaucomas, ed. 4, St. Louis, 1976, The C. V. Mosby Co.

Macri, F. J., and Brubaker, R. F.: Methodology of eye pressure measurement, Biorheology **6:**37-45, Apr., 1969.

Perimetry

Harrington, D. O.: The visual fields: A textbook and atlas of clinical perimetry, ed. 3, St. Louis, 1971, The C. V. Mosby Co.

Havener, W. H., and Gloeckner, S. L.: Introductory atlas of perimetry, St. Louis, 1972, The C. V. Mosby Co.

Motility

Burian, H. M., Von Noorden, G. K.: Binocular vision and ocular motility: theory and management of strabismus, St. Louis, 1974, The C. V. Mosby Co.

Gay, A. J., Newman, N. M., Keltner, J. L., et al.: Eye movement disorders, St. Louis, 1974, The C. V. Mosby Co.

Von Noorden, G. K., and Maumenee, A. E.: Atlas of strabismus, ed. 2, St. Louis, 1973, The C. V. Mosby Co.

Electrophysiology

Armington, J. C.: The electroretinogram, New York, 1974, Academic Press.

Fishman, G. F.: The electroretinogram and electro-oculogramin retinal and choroidal disease, Rochester, Am. Acad. Ophthalmol. & Otolaryngol., 1975.

Galloway, N. R.: Ophthalmic electro-diagnosis, Philadelphia, 1975, W. B. Saunders Co.

Color vision

Evans, R. M.: Introduction to color, New York, 1948, John Wiley & Sons, Inc.

Kalmus, H.: Diagnosis and genetics of defective color vision, Elmsford, New York, 1965, Pergamon Press.

Index